Neurologic and Psychiatric Word Book

Helen E. Littrell, CMT

Springhouse
Word Book Series

Springhouse Corporation
Springhouse, Pennsylvania

Printed in the United States of America

Library of Congress Catalog Card Number: 91-5090

ISBN: 0-87434-474-3

SWB 13-010192

Dedication

To my beloved daughter, Sharon, who left us
so suddenly on December 7, 1990.
She dared to follow her dreams.
Success is a measure of what one has over-
come rather than what one has achieved.

How to use this book

All entries in this book are listed alphabetically. When a term may be modified in some way with a variety of other terms, the sub-entries are indented and punctuated as follows:

> meningitis (main entry)
>> occlusive m. (main entry comes after sub-entry)
>> ossificans, m. (main entry comes before sub-entry)

We have also provided extensive cross referencing to help you locate certain terms more easily. You'll find this especially valuable when abbreviations may be used interchangeably with the full entry: for example, TENS (transcutaneous electrical nerve stimulation) - also listed as transcutaneous electrical nerve stimulation (TENS).

As an extra value, plural forms of words which change due to Latin origin are shown following the root word: for example, vertebra (vertebrae). Vertebrae (pl. of vertebra) is also listed alphabetically.

Additionally, you'll discover some medical jargon and slang phrases in this reference. Because they are now an accepted part of everyday medical language, we must recognize them as such.

Acknowledgments

My deepest thanks goes to the staff of Springhouse Corporation, especially to Jean Robinson and Wendy Clarke for their assistance in helping me finalize this manuscript. I consider it an honor to be affiliated with such a fine group of professionals.

I also thank the many friends who encouraged and assisted me in the development of this book. Because you believed in me, you helped me achieve my greatest ambition - to be a writer. I will always be grateful to each of you for the unique part you have played in my success.

Lastly, I must acknowledge a special friend from another time and place, whose brief visit during the completion of this book offered proof that our lives have many dimensions which we are free to accept or deny — the road we follow is up to us.

Helen E. Littrell, CMT

A

A1 segment
Aase syndrome
Abadie's sign
abalienated
abalienatio
   mentis, a.
abalienation
abandoned
abaptiston
abarognosis
abasia
   astasia, a.
   atactica, a.
   choreic a.
   paralytic a.
   paroxysmal trepidant a.
   spastic a.
   trembling a.
   trepidans, a.
abasic
abatic
Abbe neurectomy
Abbott's method
ABC (airway/breathing/circulation) protocol
abdominal reflex
abducens
   nerve (cranial nerve VI), a.
abducent
   nerve, a.
abduct
abduction
abductor
abepithymia
aberrant
   pyramidal tract, a.
aberration
abeyance
ABG (arterial blood gas)
abiatrophy
abient
abionergy
abiosis

abiotic
abiotrophic
abiotrophy
abirritant
abirritation
abirritative
ablate
ablation
ablative
   surgery, a.
ABLB (alternate binaural loudness balance)
ablepsia
abluminal
ablutomania
abnormity
ABR (auditory brain stem response)
abrachiocephalia
abreaction
   motor a.
abscise
abscission
absence
   attack, a.
   seizures, a.
absentia
   epileptica, a.
absolute latency
absorption
abstinence
abstract
abstracting
abstraction
   quotient (AQ)
abulia
   cyclic a.
abulic
abulomania
abuse
   aged a.
   alcohol a.
   child a.
   drug a.

abuse *(continued)*
    psychoactive substance a.
    spousal a.
    substance a.
abused
abusive
academic inhibition
acalculia
acampsia
acantha
acanthesthesia
acanthocytosis
acapnia
acarbia
acarophobia
ACAT (automated computerized axial tomography)
acatalepsia
acatalepsy
acataleptic
acatamathesia
acataphasia
acataposis
acatastasia
acatastatic
acathexis
acathisia
accessiflexor
accessorius nerve
accessory nerve (cranial nerve XI)
accident prone
acclimation
accommodation
    reflex, a.
accommodative
accommodometer
accoucheur's hand
accretion
acculturation
accupoint
acedia
acenesthesia
acephalia
acephalus
acervulus
acetaminophen

acetylcholine (ACh)
    receptor antibody (AChRab), a.
    receptor (AChR), a.
acetylcholinesterase (AChE)
ACh (acetylcholine)
Achard syndrome
Achard-Thiers syndrome
AChE (acetylcholinesterase)
achievement age
Achilles jerk
Achilles reflex
achillodynia
achlorhydria
AChR (acetylcholine receptor)
AChRab (acetylcholine receptor antibody)
achromatopsia
Achucarro's stain
achylia
acidophilic
acidosis
aciduria
acinesia
acinetic
Acland clip
ACLS (advanced cardiac life support)
acoria
Acosta's disease
acouasm
acousma
acousmatagnosis
acousmatamnesia
acoustic
    agraphia, a.
    center, a.
    nerve (cranial nerve VIII), a.
    neurinoma, a.
    neuroma, a.
    neurotomy, a.
acousticophobia
acoustogram
ACPS (acrocephalopolysyndactyly)
acquired immune deficiency syndrome (AIDS)
acquisition time
acragnosis

acral anesthesia
acrania
acranius
acrasia
acratia
acroagnosis
acroanesthesia
acroasphyxia
acroataxia
acrobrachycephaly
acrocephalic
acrocephalopolysyndactyly (ACPS)
acrocephalosyndactyly
acrocephalous
acrocinesis
acrocinetic
acrocontracture
acrocyanosis
acrodynia
acrodysesthesia
acrodysplasia
acroesthesia
acrognosis
acrohypothermy
acrokinesia
acromania
acromegaly
acromial reflex
acromicria
acromyotonia
acromyotonus
acroneuropathy
acroneurosis
acroparalysis
acroparesthesia
acrophobia
acroscleroderma
acrosclerosis
acrotrophodynia
acrotrophoneurosis
ACTH (adrenocorticotropic hormone)
actin
acting out
actinoneuritis
action
    dystonia, a.

action *(continued)*
    potential, a.
    tremor, a.
activated charcoal
activated sleep
active range of motion
activities of daily living (ADL)
activity analysis
activity level
acuity
acupressure
acupuncture
acusection
acusector
acute
    brain syndrome, a.
    confusional state, a.
    disseminated encephalomyelitis
        (ADE), a.
    intermittent porphyria, a.
    mountain sickness, a.
ACUTENS (acupuncture and transcutane-
    ous electrical nerve stimulation)
acystinervia
acystineuria
ad substance
Adair Dighton syndrome
adamantinoma
    pituitary a.
    polycysticum, a.
Adamkiewicz artery
Adamkiewicz demilunes
Adams' disease
Adams-Stokes disease
Adams-Stokes syncope
Adams-Stokes syndrome
adaptation
adapted clothing
adaptive device
adaxial
ADD (attention deficit disorder)
addict
addiction
    polysurgical a.
addictive
addictologist

addictology
Addison's disease
addisonian crisis
addisonism
adducent
adduct
adduction
adductor muscle
adductor reflex
ADE (acute disseminated encephalomy-
    elitis)
adenasthenia
adenocarcinoma
adenochondroma
adenochondrosarcoma
adenocystoma
adenofibroma
adenohypophysectomy
adenohypophysial
adenohypophysis
adenoma
adenoneural
adenovirus
adhesio
    interthalamica, a.
adhesion
adhesive process
adiadochocinesia
adiadochocinesis
adiadochokinesia
adiadochokinesis
adiadokokinesia
adiadokokinesis
adiaphoria
adient
Adie's syndrome
adiposalgia
adiposis
    cerebralis, a.
    dolorosa, a.
    orchalis, a.
    orchica, a.
    tuberosa simplex, a.
adipositas
    cerebralis, a.
adiposity

adiposity *(continued)*
    cerebral a.
    pituitary a.
adipsia
adipsy
aditus
adjunctive
adjustment disorder
adjuvant
Adkins spinal
    fusion
ADL (activities of daily living)
adlerian
Adler's theory
admedial
admedian
admix
admixture
adnerval
adneural
adolescence
adolescent
adrenal
    cortex, a.
    virilism, a.
adrenalectomize
adrenalectomy
Adrenalin
adrenaline
adrenalism
adrenalitis
adrenalopathy
adrenalotropic
adrenarche
adrenergic
    antagonist, a.
adrenoceptive
adrenoceptor
adrenocortical
adrenocorticohyperplasia
adrenocorticomimetic
adrenocorticotrophic
adrenocorticotrophin
adrenocorticotropic
    hormone (ACTH), a.
adrenocorticotropin

adrenogenic
adrenogenital syndrome
adrenogenous
adrenogram
adrenokinetic
adrenoleukodystrophy
adrenolytic
adrenomedullotropic
adrenomegaly
adrenomimetic
adrenomyeloneuropathy
adrenopathy
adrenopause
adrenoprival
adrenoreceptor
adrenostatic
adrenotoxin
adrenotropic
adrenotropin
adromia
Adson brain suction tip
Adson forceps
Adson headrest
Adson maneuver
Adson retractor
Adson saw guide
Adson scalp clip
Adson test
advanced cardiac life support (ACLS)
adynamia
   episodica hereditaria, a.
adynamic
Aeby's muscle
Aeby's plane
AEP (average evoked potential)
aerasthenia
aeremia
aeroasthenia
aerocele
   epidural a.
   intracranial a.
aerodontalgia
aerodromophobia
aeroembolism
aeroemphysema
aerogram

aeroneurosis
aeropathy
aerophagia
aerophobia
Aesculap forceps
affect
   appropriate a.
   blunted a.
   flat a.
affection
affectionless character
affective
   disorder, a.
Affective Disorders Rating Scale
affectivity
affectomotor
affektepilepsie
afferent
A fiber
AFP (alpha-fetoprotein)
African meningitis
African porphyria
afteraction
afterbrain
aftercurrent
afterdischarge
aftereffect
afterhearing
afterhyperpolarization
afterimage
afterimpression
aftermovement
afterperception
afterpotential wave
aftersensation
aftertaste
aftervision
aganglionic
aganglionosis
age
   achievement a.
   anatomical a.
   Binet a.
   chronological a.
   developmental a.
   emotional a.

age *(continued)*
    functional a.
    mental a.
    physical a.
    physiological a.
age regression
agenesia
    corticalis, a.
agenesis
    callosal a.
    gonadal a.
    sacral a.
Agent Orange
agerasia
ageusia
aggression
aggression-turned-inward construct
aggressive
agitated
    depression, a.
agitation
agitographia
agitolalia
agitophasia
agnea
agnosia
    acoustic a.
    auditory a.
    body-image a.
    finger a.
    ideational a.
    tactile a.
    time a.
    visual a.
agnostic
agonadal
agonadism
agonist
agoromania
agorophobia
agrammatica
agrammatism
agrammatologia
agraphia
    absolute a.
    acoustic a.

agraphia *(continued)*
    amnemonica, a.
    atactica, a.
    cerebral a.
    jargon a.
    literal a.
    mental a.
    motor a.
    musical a.
    optic a.
    verbal a.
agromania
agrypnia
agrypnocoma
agrypnode
agrypnotic
agyria
agyrophobia
ahypnia
Aicardi syndrome
aichmophobia
aidoidomania
AIDS (acquired immune deficiency syndrome)
    dementia, A.
ailuromania
ailurophilia
ailurophobia
AIM CPM (continuous passive motion)
air
    conduction, a.
    embolism, a.
    encephalography, a.
    hunger, a.
    swallowing, a.
    ventriculography, a.
air-bone
    conduction, a.
    gap, a.
Air-Dyne bicycle
Airtene
airway
AJ (ankle jerk)
akatamathesia
akatanoesis
akathisia

akinesia
    algera, a.
    amnestica, a.
    reflex a.
akinesis
akinesthesia
akinetic
    mutism, a.
    seizures, a.
aknephascopia
akoria
Akureyri disease
ala (pl. alae)
alabaster skin
alacrima
alae (pl. of ala)
Alajouanine's syndrome
alalia
    cophica, a.
    organica, a.
    physiologica, a.
    prolongata, a.
alalic
alar
alba
Albee spinal fusion
Albers-Schonberg disease
Alberts' Famous Faces Test
albinism
    Forsius-Eriksson type ocular a.
    oculocutaneous a.
    tyrosinase-negative oculocutaneous a.
    X-linked (Nettleship) type ocular a.
albinismus
albinoidism
    oculocutaneous a.
    punctate oculocutaneous a.
albinotic
Albright's syndrome
Albright-McCune-Sternburg syndrome
albuminocytologic dissociation
alcian blue
alcohol
    blood level, a.
    -tobacco amblyopia, a.
    withdrawal, a.

alcohol *(continued)*
    alcoholemia
alcoholic
    amblyopia, a.
    blackout, a.
    brain syndrome, a.
    detoxification, a.
    encephalopathy, a.
    facies, a.
    hallucinosis, a.
    intoxication, a.
    ketoacidosis, a.
    myopathy, a.
    polyneuropathy, a.
alcoholism
alcoholomania
alcoholophilia
aldosterone
aldosteronism
alemmal
alert and oriented x 3 (to person, place, and time)
alert state
alerting response
alertness
alethia
Alexander's deafness
Alexander's disease
Alexander's operation
alexanderism
alexia
    cortical a.
    motor a.
    musical a.
    optical a.
    subcortical a.
Alexian Brothers overhead frame
alexic
alexithymia
Alezzandrini's syndrome
algebraic thinking
algedonic
algesia
algesic
algesichronometer
algesimeter

algesimeter *(continued)*
   Bjornstrom's a.
   Boas' a.
algesimetry
algesiogenic
algesthesia
algetic
algid stage
algiomotor
algiomuscular
algogenesis
algogenic
algolagnia
   active a.
   passive a.
algolagnist
algometer
   pressure, a.
algometry
algophilia
algophily
algophobia
algopsychalia
algorithm
algospasm
aliasing
Alice in Wonderland syndrome
alienate
alienation
alienism
alienist
aligning
aliquot
alkalosis
all-or-none law
all-or-none potential
allachesthesia
   optical a.
Allemann's syndrome
Allen maneuver
allesthesia
   visual a.
alliance
   therapeutic a.
   working a.
alliesthesia

alliteration
allocentric
allochesthesia
allochiria
allocinesia
allocortex
allodynia
alloeroticism
alloerotism
alloesthesia
allokinesis
allokinetic
allolalia
alloplasty
allopsychic
allopsychosis
allotriogeustia
allotriophagy
allotriosmia
allotropic
Allport theory
allude
allusion
alogia
Alper's disease
alpha
   -adrenergic blocking agent, a.
   -adrenergic receptor, a.
   -delta syndrome, a.
   -fetoprotein (AFP), a.
   intrusion, a.
   press, a.
   rigidity, a.
   test, a.
alphalytic
alphamimetic
Alport's syndrome
ALS (amyotrophic lateral sclerosis)
Alstrom's syndrome
alter ego
alter idem
altered level of consciousness
alteregoism
alternate binaural loudness balance
   (ABLB)
alternating

alternating *(continued)*
   hemiplegia, a.
   hypalgesia, a.
   personality, a.
altitude
   anoxia, a.
   sickness, a.
altruism
altruistic suicide
alveus
ALZ-50
Alzheimer baskets
Alzheimer cells
Alzheimer dementia
Alzheimer disease
Alzheimer sclerosis
Alzheimer stain
amantadine
amathophobia
amaurosis
   cat's eye a.
   central a.
   cerebral a.
   congenita of Leber, a.
   congenital a.
   diabetic a.
   fugax, a.
   intoxication a.
   Leber's congenital a.
   partialis fugax, a.
   reflex a.
   saburral a.
   toxic a.
   uremic a.
amaurotic
   familial idiocy, a.
amaxophobia
ambidexterity
ambidextrous
ambient
   cistern, a.
   noise, a.
ambiguospinothalamic paralysis
ambiguous
ambilateral
ambilevosity

ambilevous
ambiopia
ambisexual
ambisinister
ambisinistrous
ambitendency
ambivalence
ambivalent
ambiversion
ambivert
amblyacousia
amblyaphia
amblygeustia
amblyopia
   crossed a.
   ex anopia, a.
   reflex a.
   toxic a.
   uremic a.
Ambu bag
ambulant
ambulation
ambulatory
amenomania
ament
amentia
   agitata, a.
   attonita, a.
   nevoid a,
   occulta, a.
   paranoides, a.
   phenylpyruvic a.
   Stearns' alcoholic a.
amential
American Sign Language
amerisia
ametamorphosis
Amicar
amicula (pl. of amiculum)
amiculum (pl. amicula)
Amigo mechanical wheelchair
amimia
   amnesic a.
   ataxic a.
amino acid
aminoaciduria

Amipaque
Amish albinism
amitriptyline
ammeter
Ammon's horn
amnalgesia
amnemonic
amnesia
   anterograde a.
   auditory a.
   Broca's a.
   circumscribed a.
   concussion a.
   continuous a.
   emotional a.
   episodic a.
   generalized a.
   immunologic a.
   infantile a.
   Korsakoff's a.
   lacunar a.
   localized a.
   olfactory a.
   organic a.
   patchy a.
   postconcussional a.
   posthypnotic a.
   post-traumatic a.
   psychogenic a.
   retroactive a.
   retroanterograde a.
   retrograde a.
   selective a.
   tactile a.
   transient global a.
   traumatic a.
   verbal a.
   visual a.
amnesiac
amnesic
   amimia, a.
   shellfish poisoning, a.
amnestic
   aphasia, a.
   dysnomia, a.
   syndrome, a.

amobarbital interview
amok
amoral
amoralia
amoralis
amorphous
Amoss' sign
amotivational
amphetamine
   psychosis, a.
   sulfate, a.
amphiarkyochrome
amphodiplopia
amphoterodiplopia
amphotony
amplitude modulation
amputation
amputee
amuck
amusia
   instrumental a.
   vocal motor a.
amychophobia
amyelencephalia
amyelencephalus
amyelia
amyelic
amyelineuria
amyelinic
amyelonic
amyelotrophy
amyelus
amygdala
amygdalectomy
amygdaline fissure
amygdalofugal pathway
amyl nitrite
amyloid
amyloidosis
amylopectinosis
amylophagia
amylosis
amyoesthesis
amyoplasia
   congenita, a.
amyostasia

amyostatic
amyosthenia
amyosthenic
amyotaxia
amyotaxy
amyotonia
　　congenita, a.
amyotonic
amyotrophia
　　neuralgic a.
　　spinalis progressiva, a.
amyotrophic
　　lateral sclerosis (ALS), a.
amyotrophy
　　diabetic a.
　　neuralgic a.
amyous
anacamptometer
anacatesthesia
anaclisis
anaclitic
anacousia
anacusia
anacusis
anadrenalism
anadrenia
anagogic
anagogy
anakatesthesia
anakusis
anal
　　erotism, a.
　　personality, a.
　　reflex, a.
　　sex, a.
　　stage, a.
　　wink, a.
analgesia
　　algera, a.
　　audio a.
　　dolorosa, a.
　　epidural a.
　　paretic a.
analgesic
　　neuropathy, a.
　　panaris, a.

analgetic
analgia
analgic
anality
analphalipoproteinemia
analysand
analysis
　　bradycinetic a.
　　character a.
　　ego a.
　　group a.
　　transactional a.
analysor
analyst
analytic
analyzer
anamnesis
anamnestic
ananabasia
ananastasia
anancastic
anandia
anankastic
anaphia
Anafranil
anaphrodisia
anaphrodisiac
anaphrodite
anaphylactic
　　shock, a.
anaphylactogenesis
anaphylactoid
anaphylaxis
anaptic
anarithmia
anarthria
　　literalis, a.
anatomical snuffbox
anatomist's snuffbox
Andernach's ossicles
Anders' disease
Andersch's nerve
Anderson-Green growth prediction
Andes disease
Andre-Thomas sign
androgenic

androgenic *(continued)*
  hyperplasia, a.
androgenicity
androgenization
androgenized
androgyne
androgynism
androgynoid
androgynous
androgyny
android
andromania
andromimetic
andromorphous
androphobia
anelectrotonic state
anelectrotonus
anemophobia
anencephalia
anencephalic
anencephalohemia
anencephalous
anencephalus
anencephaly
anepithymia
anerethisia
anergasia
anergastic reaction
anergia
anergic
anergy
anesthecinesia
anesthekinesia
anesthesia
  bulbar a.
  central a.
  cerebral a.
  compression a.
  crossed a.
  dissociated a.
  dissociation a.
  doll's head a.
  dolorosa, a.
  facial a.
  gauntlet a.
  glove a.

anesthesia *(continued)*
  girdle a.
  gustatory a.
  hypnosis a.
  hysterical a.
  mental a.
  muscular a.
  nausea a.
  olfactory a.
  peripheral a.
  segmental a.
  tactile a.
  thalamic hyperesthetic a.
  thermal a.
  thermic a.
  total a.
  traumatic a.
  unilateral a.
  visceral a.
anesthesimeter
anesthetic
  agent, a.
anesthetization
anesthetize
anesthetospasm
ancuploid
aneuploidy
Aneuroplast
aneurysm
  arterial a.
  arteriovenous a.
  berry a.
  brain a.
  cerebral a.
  Charcot-Bouchard a.
  cirsoid a.
  congenital cerebral a.
  fusiform a.
  innominate a.
  intracranial a.
  miliary a.
  mycotic a.
  PICA a.
  racemose a.
  saccular a.
aneurysm wrapping

aneurysm wrapping *(continued)*
  suprasellar, a.
aneurysmal
aneurysmectomy
aneurysmoplasty
aneurysmorrhaphy
aneurysmotomy
Anexsia
angel dust (PCP)
Angell James hypophysectomy forceps
Angelucci syndrome
anger
angry
Anghelescu's sign
angiasthenia
angiitis
angina
anginal
anginophobia
angioasthenia
angioblastic
  meningioma, a.
angioblastorna
angiocardiogram
angiocardiography
angiochondroma
Angio-Conray
angiocrine
angiocrinosis
angiocyst
angioedema
angioglioma
angiogliomatosis
angiogram
angiographically occult intracranial vascular malformation (AOIVM)
angiography
  carotid a.
  cerebral a.
  digital subtraction a.
angiohemophilia
angioma
  arteriovenous a. of brain
  cavernous a.
  venous a. of brain
angiomatosis

angiomatosis *(continued)*
  cerebroretinal a.
  encephalofacial a.
  encephalotrigeminal a.
  retina, a. of
  retinocerebral a.
angiomatous
angiomyolipoma
angiomyoneuroma
angioneuralgia
angioneurectomy
angioneuropathic
angioneuropathy
angioneurosis
angioneurotic
  edema, a.
angioneurotomy
angioparalysis
angioparesis
angiophakomatosis
angioplastied
angioplasty
angioreticuloendothelioma
angioreticuloma
angiosclerosis
angiosclerotic
angioscotoma
angioscotometry
Angioskop-D
angiospasm
angiospastic
Angiovist
angle of Sylvius
angophrasia
angor
  animi, a.
  ocularis, a.
  pectoris, a.
angst
angular gyrus
anguli (pl. of angulus)
angulus (pl anguli)
anhaphia
anhedonia
anhydrosis
anile

anilinism
anility
anima
animal magnetism
animation
animism
animus
anion gap
anisoaccommodation
anisocoria
ankle clonus
ankle jerk (AJ)
ankyloglossia
ankylophobia
ankylosing spondylitis
ankylosis
annular
annuli (pl. of annulus)
annulospiral endings
annulus (pl. annuli)
   pulposus, a.
anociassociation
anocithesia
anodmia
anodynia
anoesia
anoetic
anoia
anomalad
anomalous
anomaly
anomia
anomic
   aphasia, a.
   suicide, a.
anomie
anophoria
anopsia
anorectic
anorexia
   nervosa, a.
anorexiant
anorexic
anorexigenic
anorgasmia
anorgasmy

anorthography
anosmatic
anosmia
   gustatoria, a.
   preferential, a.
   respiratoria, a.
anosmatic
anosmia
anosmic
anosodiaphoria
anosognosia
anosphrasia
anospinal
anoxemia
anoxia
   altitude a.
   anemic a.
   anoxic a.
   fulminating a.
   histotoxic a.
   myocardial a.
   neonatorum, a.
   stagnant a.
anoxiate
anoxic
   anoxia, a.
   encephalopathy, a.
   insult, a.
ANS (autonomic nervous system)
ansa (pl. ansae)
   cervicalis, a.
   hypoglossi, a.
   lenticularis, a.
   lenticular nucleus, a. of
   subclavia, a.
   Vieussens, a. of
ansae (pl. of ansa)
   nervorum spinalium, a.
ansate
ansiform
ansotomy
antagonism
antagonist
antagonistic
   reflexes, a.
antalgesic

antalgic
    gait, a.
antaphrodisiac
antapoplectic
antarthritic
antasthenic
antatrophic
antebrachium
antecollis
antecubital
    fossa, a.
    space, a.
antecurvature
anteflect
anteflexed
anteflexion
antegrade
antephialtic
antergia
antergic
anterior
    communicating artery, a.
    horn cell, a.
anterocollis
anterograde amnesia
anterolisthesis
anterotic
anteversion
antexed
antexion
anthophobia
anthrax
anthropomorphism
anthropophobia
anthypnotic
anthysteric
antiacetylcholine receptor antibodies
antiadrenergic
antianxiety
antiapoplectic
antiarrhythmic
anticachectic
anticarcinogenic
anticathexis
anticephalalgic
anticheirotonus

anticholinergic
anticholinesterinase
anticoagulant
anticoagulation
anticonvulsant
anticonvulsive
anticurare
anticus
antidepressant
    tricyclic a.
antidinic
antidromic
    volley, a.
antiembolic
antiemetic
antiepileptic
antifibrinolytic
antigonadotropic
antihallucinatory
antihistamine
antihypertensive
antihypnotic
antihypotensive
antihysteric
anti-La antibody
antimongolism
antimongoloid
antimyasthenic
antinarcotic
antinauseant
antineuralgic
antineuritic
antineurotoxin
antinion
antiparalytic
antiparasympathomimetic
antiparkinsonian
antiphlogistic
antipsychomotor
antipsychotic
anti-Ro antibody
antisocial
antisocialism
antispasmodic
antispastic
antisympathetic

antitetanic
antithenar
antitonic
antitrismus
Antivert
antivertiginous
Anton's syndrome
anuli (pl. of anulus)
anuloplasty
anulus (pl. anuli)
anxietas
   presenilis, a.
   tibiarum, a.
anxiety
   castration a.
   free-floating a.
   separation a.
anxiety attack
anxiety component
anxiety disorder
anxiety equivalent
anxiety hysteria
anxiety neurosis
anxiety overlay
anxiety state
anxiety tension state (ATS)
anxiety tremor
anxiolytic
anxious facies
AOA/CHICK halo system
AOIVM (angiographically occult intracranial vascular malformation)
aortic arch
   syndrome, a.
aosmic
APACHE (acute physiology and chronic
   health evaluation)
APACHE II score
apallesthesia
apandria
apanthropia
apanthropy
aparalytic
apareunia
apastia
apastic

apathetic
apathic
apathism
apathy
A-pattern strabismus
ape hand
apertura (pl. aperturae)
aperturae (pl. of apertura)
aperture
Apert's disease
Apert's syndrome
Apert-Crouzon disease
apex (pl. apices)
APGAR (Family APGAR Questionnaire)
Apgar score
aphagia
   algera, a.
aphagopraxia
aphasia
   acoustic a.
   ageusic a.
   amnemonic a.
   amnesic a.
   amnestic a.
   anomic a.
   anosmic a.
   associative a.
   ataxic a.
   auditory a.
   Broca's a.
   combined a.
   commissural a.
   complete a.
   conduction a.
   cortical a.
   expressive a.
   expressive-receptive a.
   fluent a.
   frontocortical a.
   frontolenticular a.
   functional a.
   gibberish a.
   global a.
   graphomotor a.
   Grashey's a.
   impressive a.

aphasia *(continued)*
   intellectual a.
   jargon a.
   Kussmaul's a.
   lenticular a.
   lethica, a.
   Lichtheim's a.
   mixed a.
   motor a.
   nominal a.
   nonfluent a.
   optic a.
   parieto-occipital a.
   pathematic a.
   pictorial a.
   psychosensory a.
   receptive a.
   semantic a.
   sensory a.
   subcortical a.
   syntactical a.
   tactile a.
   temporoparietal a.
   total a.
   transcortical a.
   true a.
   verbal a.
   visual a.
   Wernicke's a.
aphasiac
aphasic
aphasiology
aphemesthesia
aphemia
aphemic
aphephobia
apheter
aphonia
   clericorum, a.
   hysteric a.
   paralytica, a.
   paranoica, a.
   spastic a.
aphonic
aphonogelia
aphose

aphrasia
aphrodisia
aphrodisiac
aphrodisiomania
aphthongia
apicotomy
apinealism
apiphobia
apituitarism
aplasia
   axialis extracorticalis congenita, a.
Apley sign
apnea
   sleep a.
apnea alarm mattress
apneic
   oxygenation, a.
   spell, a.
apneusis
apneustic
   breathing, a.
apocarteresis
apokamnosis
aponeurectomy
aponeurosis
apophyseal
apophysis
   cerebral a.
   cerebri, a.
   genial a.
apoplectic
apoplexia
apoplexy
   adrenal a.
   asthenic a.
   Broadbent's a.
   bulbar a.
   capillary a.
   cerebellar a.
   cerebral a.
   delayed a.
   embolic a.
   fulminating a.
   heart a.
   ingravescent a.
   meningeal a.

apoplexy *(continued)*
    neonatal a.
    pituitary a.
    pontile a.
    pontine a.
    Raymond's a.
    spinal a.
    thrombotic a.
    traumatic late a.
apparatus
    Perroncito, a. of
    Timofeew, a. of
appendicular
    ataxia, a.
    test, a.
apperception
apperceptionism
apperceptive
appersonation
appersonification
appestat
appetition
appetitive behavior
apposed
apposition
apprehension
apprehensive
apractic
apractognosia
apraxia
    akinetic a.
    algera, a.
    amnestic a.
    Bruns' a. of gait
    classic a.
    constructional a.
    cortical a.
    developmental a.
    dressing a.
    gait a.
    ideational a.
    ideokinetic a.
    ideomotor a.
    innervation a.
    limb-kinetic a.
    Lipmann's a.

apraxia *(continued)*
    motor a.
    oculomotor a.
    sensory a.
    transcortical
apraxic
aprophoria
aprosexia
aprosody
apselaphesia
apsithyria
apsychia
apsychosis
AQ (abstraction or achievement quotient)
aquaphobia
aqueduct
    cerebral a.
    midbrain, a. of
    Sylvius, a. of
aqueductal syndrome
aqueductus
    cerebri, a.
AR (achievement radio)
arachnitis
arachnoid
    cyst, a.
    trabeculae, a.
    villi, a.
arachnoidal
arachnoidea
    encephali, a.
    spinalis, a.
arachnoiditis
arachnophobia
arachnopia
Aran's law
Aran-Duchenne disease
Aran-Duchenne muscular atrophy
Arantius
    ventricle of A.
araphia
ARAS (ascending reticular activating system)
arbitrary inference
arbor
    medullaris vermis, a.

arbor *(continued)*
    vitae cerebelli, a.
arborization
arbovirus
arc
    motion, a. of
archaeocerebellum
archaeocortex
archencephalon
archeocerebellum
archeocortex
archeokinetic
archetype
archicerebellum
archicortex
archineuron
archipallial
archipallium
architectonic
Arctic hysteria
ardanesthesia
area
    association a.
    Betz cell a.
    Broca's motor speech a.
    Broca's parolfactory a.
    Brodmann's a.
    excitable a.
    excitomotor a.
    facial nerve, a. of
    Flechsig's a.
    glove a.
    hypothalamic a.
    language a.
    motor a.
    Obersteiner-Redlich a.
    olfactory a.
    parolfactory a. of Broca
    postcentral a.
    postpterygoidea, a.
    postrema, a.
    postrolandic a.
    precentral a.
    prefrontal a.
    premotor a.
    primary a.

area *(continued)*
    primary receptive a.
    projection a.
    psychomotor a.
    pterygoidea, a.
    receptive a.
    rolandic a.
    sensorimotor a.
    sensory a.
    silent a.
    somatosensory a.
    somesthetic a.
    subcallosal a.
    supplementary a.
    suppressor a.
    trigger a.
    vagus a.
    visual a.
    visuopsychic a.
    visuosensory a.
    Wernicke's a.
areflexia
areflexic
arenavirus
Arenberg-Denver inner-ear valve
argininosuccinic aciduria
argumentative
Argyll Robertson pupil
Argyll Robertson sign
arhigosis
arhinencephalia
Arica movement
arithmomania
arm
    bird a.
    Saturday-night a.
arm board
arm swings
Armstrong's disease
Arndt's law
Arndt-Schulz law
Arnold lumbar brace
Arnold's canal
Arnold's nerve
Arnold's nerve reflex cough syndrome
Arnold-Chiari malformation

AROM (active range of motion)
Aron Alpha adhesive
arousal
   level, a.
arouse
arrhaphia
arrhythmokinesis
Artane
arterial
   beading, a.
   blood gas (ABG), a.
   hypertension, a.
arteriogram
arteriography
arteriosclerosis
arteriosclerotic
arteriovenous (AV)
   malformation (AVM), a.
arteritis
   cranial a.
   temporal a.
artery of Adamkiewicz
arthralgia
arthresthesia
arthritic
arthritides (pl. of arthritis)
arthritis (pl. arthritides)
arthrochalasis
arthrodynia
arthrodysplasia
arthroereisis
arthrogryposis
arthrolysis
arthroneuralgia
arthropathy
articular
   capsule, a.
   facet, a.
articulare
articulate
articulating
   facet, a.
   surface, a.
articulatio (pl. articulationes)
articulation
articulationes (pl. of articulatio)

articulator
artifact
artifactitious
artifactual
artificial palate
artisan's cramp
arylcyclohexylamine
asaphia
ascending reticular activating system
   (ARAS)
asceticism
Aschner's sign
asemasia
asemia
   graphica, a.
   mimica, a.
   verbalis, a.
Asendin
asexuality
ash leaf spot
Asherson's syndrome
asonia
aspartane
aspartylglucosaminuria
aspergillosis
asphyctic
asphyxia
asphyxiation
aspirate
aspiration pneumonitis
assault
   sexual a.
assaultive
assertive
assertiveness training
ASSI (Accurate Surgical and Scientific
   Instruments Corporation)
ASSI bipolar coagulating forceps
ASSI craniotomy blade
ASSI wire pass drill
assimilation
assisted ventilation
associated movements
association
   clang a.
   dream a.

association *(continued)*
   free a.
association areas
association center
association neurosis
association test
association time
associationism
associative
astasia
   -abasia, a.
astatic
astereocognosy
astereognosis
astereopsis
asterion
asterixis
asthenia
   myalgic a.
   neurocirculatory a.
   periodic a.
   tropical anhidrotic a.
asthenic
asthemometer
asthenope
asthenophobia
asthenopia
   hysterical a.
   muscular a.
   nervous a.
   neurasthenic a.
astral body
astral projection
astraphobia
astroblast
astroblastoma
astrocyte
   fibrous a.
   gemistocytic a.
   plasmatofibrous a.
   protoplasmic a.
astrocytoma
   anaplastic a.
   fibrillare, a.
   gemistocytic a.
   pilocytic a.

astrocytoma *(continued)*
   protoplasmaticum, a.
astrocytosis
astroglia
astrogliosis
astroid
astrophobia
asyllabia
asylum
asymbolia
asymboly
asymmetrical
asymmetry
asynchronism
asyndesis
asynergia
asynergy
   appendicular a.
   axial a.
   axioappendicular a.
   truncal a.
asyntaxia dorsalis
atactic
ataractic
Atarax
ataraxia
ataraxic
ataxaphasia
ataxia
   acute a.
   acute cerebellar a.
   adult onset a.
   alcoholic a.
   autonomic a.
   Briquet's a.
   Broca's a.
   central a.
   cerebellar a.
   cerebral a.
   family a.
   Fergusson and Critchley's a.
   Friedreich's a.
   frontal a.
   Greenfield classification of
      spinocerebellar a.
   hereditary a.

ataxia *(continued)*
  hysterical a.
  intermittent a.
  intrapsychic a.
  kinetic a.
  labyrinthic a.
  Leyden's a.
  locomotor a.
  Marie's a.
  motor a.
  nondirectional a.
  noothymopsychic a.
  ocular a.
  optic a.
  periodic a.
  progressive a.
  proprioceptive a.
  Sanger Brown a.
  sensory a.
  spastic a.
  spinal a.
  spinocerebellar a.
  static a.
  telangectiasia, a.
  thermal a.
  truncal a.
  vasomotor a.
  vestibular a.
ataxiadynamia
ataxiagram
ataxiagraph
ataxiameter
ataxiamnesia
ataxiamnesic
ataxiaphasia
ataxic
  atelophobia, a.
  breathing, a.
  gait, a.
  lymphopathy, a.
ataxiophemia
ataxiophobia
ataxoadynamia
ataxophemia
ataxophobia
ataxy

ateleiosis
atelencephalia
atelia
atelocephaly
atelomyelia
athalposis
atheist
athetoid
athetosis
athetotic
  idiocy, a.
athiaminosis
Ativan
ATL real-time NeurosectOR scanner
atlantad
atlantal
atlantoaxial
  articulation, a.
atlanto-occipital
atlas
atloaxoid
atloido-occipital
ATLS (advanced trauma life support)
atonia
  choreatic a.
atonic
  bladder, a.
  seizure, a.
atonicity
atony
atopognosia
atraumatic needle
atremia
atresia
atretic
atrophia
atrophied
atrophy
  alcoholic cerebral a.
  Aran-Duchenne muscular a.
  Charcot-Marie a.
  Charcot-Marie-Tooth a.
  cerebral a.
  circumscribed a. of brain
  convolutional a.
  corticostriatospinal a.

atrophy *(continued)*
   Cruveilheir's a.
   Dejerine-Sottas type a.
   Dejerine-Thomas a.
   denervated muscle a.
   disuse a.
   Duchenne-Aran muscular a.
   Eichhorst's a.
   Erb's a.
   facial a.
   facioscapulohumeral muscular a.
   Fazio-Londe a.
   gray a.
   hemifacial a.
   hemilingual a.
   Hoffman's a.
   Hunt's a.
   idiopathic muscular a.
   ischemic muscular a.
   Landouzy-Dejerine a.
   leaping a.
   Leber's optic a.
   lobar a.
   multisystem a.
   muscular a.
   myelopathic muscular a.
   myopathic a.
   neural a.
   neuritic muscular a.
   neuropathic a.
   neurotic a.
   neurotrophic a.
   olivopontocerebellar a.
   pallidal a.
   Parrot's a. of the newborn
   peroneal a.
   Pick's convolutional a.
   progressive neuromuscular a.
   progressive neuropathic muscular a.
   progressive spinal muscular a.
   progressive unilateral facial a.
   pseudohypertrophic muscular a.
   spinal muscular a.
   spinoneural a.
   Sudeck's a.
   Tooth's a.

atrophy *(continued)*
   trophoneurotic a.
   Vulpian's a.
   Werdnig-Hoffmann spinal muscular a.
   white a.
   Zimmerlin's a.
atropine
   coma, a.
   psychosis, a.
attack
   anxiety a.
   drop a.
   panic a.
   vagal a.
   vasovagal a.
ATS (anxiety tension state)
attention deficit disorder (ADD)
attenuate
attenuation
attitude
attitudinal reaction
atypia
atypical
   absence seizures, a.
   psychosis, a.
atypism
Aubert's phenomenon
audible thought
audile
audioanalgesia
audiogram
audiometry
AudioScope
audiovisual
audition
   chromatic a.
   gustatory a.
   mental a.
auditive
auditognosis
audito-oculogyric reflex
auditory
   agnosia, a.
   amnesia, a.
   brainstem response (ABR), a.
   discrimination, a.

auditory *(continued)*
    evoked potential, a.
    evoked response, a.
    hallucinations, a.
    reflex, a.
aula
aulatela
aulic
auliplexus
aura
    auditory a.
    epileptic a.
    hysterica a.
    intellectual a.
    kinesthetic a.
    motor a.
    procursiva, a.
    reminiscent a.
aural
Australian X disease
authoritarian
authority figure
autism
    akinetic a.
    early infantile a.
    infantile a.
autistic
autoamputation
autoanalysis
autocastration
autocatharsis
autocerebrospinal
autochthonous idea
autoecholalia
autoenucleation
autoerotic
autoeroticism
autoerotism
Autoflex II CPM unit
autogenous bone graft
autognosis
autognostic
autohypnosis
autohypnotic
autokinesis
autokinetic

autokinetic *(continued)*
    visible light phenomenon, a.
autolesion
autologous fat graft
automania
automatic
    behavior, a.
    memory, a.
    reflex bladder, a.
    writing, a.
automatism
    ambulatory a.
    command a.
automatograph
automysophobia
autonomic
    ataxia, a.
    dysfunction, a.
    dysreflexia, a.
    function, a.
    ganglia, a.
    manifestation, a.
    nervous system (ANS), a.
    plexus, a.
    reflex, a.
    response, a.
autonomotropic
autonomous bladder
autonomy
autophagia
autophilia
autophobia
autophonomania
autophonometry
autoplastic change
autoplasty
autopsychic
autopsychorhythmia
autopsychosis
autopsychotherapy
autopunition
autoscopic hallucinations
autosmia
autosomal
    -dominant, a.
    -recessive, a.

autosomatognosis
autosomatognostic
autosuggestibility
autosuggestion
autosynnoia
autotopagnosia
autotrepanation
auxiliomotor
AV (arteriovenous)
   crossing changes, AV
   fistula, AV
   nicking, AV
   shunt, AV
avalanche law
avalanche theory
avascular
   plane, a.
   space, a.
Avellis' paralysis
Avellis' syndrome
Aventyl
average evoked potential (AEP)
averaged electroencephalic
audiometry
aversion
   therapy, a.
aversive
   conditioning, a.
aviator's disease
avitaminosis
Avitene
AVM (arteriovenous malformation)
avoidance
avoidant
awake-alert state
awareness
Axenfeld-Krukenberg spindle
axes (pl. of axis)
axial loading of spine

axifugal
axilemma
axilla (pl. axillae)
   nerve root, a. of
axillae (pl. of axilla)
axillocephalic suspension
axion
axipetal
axis (pl. axes)
   cylinder, a.
axoaxonal
axoaxonic
axodendritic
axofugal
axoid
axoidean
axolemma
axolysis
axon
   hillock, a.
   reaction, a.
axonal
axonapraxia
axonopathy
axonotmesis
axopetal
axophage
axoplasm
axoplasmic transport
axosomatic
axospongium
Axsaine
Ayala's quotient
Ayer's test
Ayer-Tobey test
Azima battery
Aztec idiocy
Aztec type

Additional entries

B

Baastrup's disease
Baastrup's syndrome
Babcock needle
Babcock-Levy test
Babe's tubercles
Babinski reflex
Babinski sign
Babinski toe sign
Babinski's downgoing
Babinski's law
Babinski's phenomenon
Babinski's platysma sign
Babinski's pronation sign
Babinski's syndrome
Babinski's test
Babinski-Frohlich syndrome
Babinski-Nageotte syndrome
Babinski-Vaquez syndrome
Babinski-Weil test
Babkin reflex
bacciform
bacillophobia
bacitracin
back
   board, b.
   brace, b.
   manipulation, b.
   precautions, b.
backache
backalgia
backbone
background
   activity, b.
   rhythm, b.
backpack palsy
backward progression
baclofen
Bacon forceps
bacteremia
bacterial antigen screen
bad trip
BADS syndrome

BAEP (brain stem auditory evoked potential)
BAER (brain stem auditory evoked response)
bagged
Bailey conductor
Bailey leukotome
Bailey-Badgley cervical spine fusion
Baillarger's lines
Baillarger's sign
Baillarger's stripes
Bailint syndrome
Balint theory
Balkan frame
Balkan splint
ball-bearing feeder
Ballenger swivel knife
Baller-Gerold syndrome
Ballet's disease
Ballet's sign
ballism
ballismus
ballistic
ballooning
Balo's disease
Bamberger's disease
Bamberger's sign
bamboo spine
bandlike
Bane forceps
Barany's syndrome
Bannwarth's syndrome
bar-reading test
Barany's pointing test
Barany's sign
Barany's symptom
barber chair position
barbituism
barbiturate
Bard's sign
Bard-Parker scalpel
Bardet-Biedl syndrome
baresthesia

Barker's point
Barlow's maneuver
Barlow's sign
baroagnosis
baroelectroesthesiometer
barognosis
baroreceptor
baroreflexes
barotrauma
Barr body
Barre's pyramidal sign
Barre's sign
Barre-Guillain syndrome
Barre-Lieou syndrome
Barret test
Barrett-Adson retractor
barrier
    blood-brain b.
    blood-cerebral b.
    blood-cerebrospinal fluid b.
    hematoencephalic b.
barrier-free design
Barron pump
Barton tongs
Barton-Cone tongs
Bartschi-Rochain syndrome
Bartter's syndrome
baryesthesia
baryglossia
barylalia
baryphonia
basal
    cell nevus syndrome, b.
    ganglia, b.
    metabolism, b.
    nucleus of Meynert, b.
    skull fracture, b.
Basedow's disease
baseline
basement membrane
bases (pl. of basis)
basial
basialis
basiarachnitis
basiarachnoiditis
basibregmatic

basic life support (BLS)
basicranial axis
basifacial axis
basilad
basilar
    invagination, b.
basilaris
    cranii, b.
basilateral
basinasial
basioccipital
basion
basirhinal
basis (pl. bases)
    pontis, b.
basisphenoid
basisylvian
basitemporal
basivertebral
basket
    Alzheimer's b.
basket of veins
basograph
basolateral
basophilic
basophobia
Bassen-Kornzweig syndrome
Bassett electrical stimulation device
Bastian's law
Bastian-Bruns law
Bastian-Bruns sign
bathmotropic
bathmotropism
bathophobia
bathrocephaly
bathyanesthesia
bathyesthesia
bathyhyperesthesia
bathyhypesthesia
Batten disease
Batten-Mayou disease
battered-child syndrome
battered-spouse syndrome
battered-woman syndrome
battery
Battle's sign

Bayle's disease
Bayley Scale of Infant Development
bayonet thumb forceps
B-D (Becton-Dickinson) spinal needle
beach chair position
Beal's syndrome
BEAM (brain electrical activity map)
beam splitter
beans (street drug)
Beard's disease
beaten silver appearance
Bebax shoe
BEC (blood ethanol concentration)
Bech-Rafaelsen Mania Scale
Bech-Rafaelsen Melancholia Scale
Bechterev's reflex
Beck Depression Inventory
Beck's syndrome
Becker's dystrophy
Becker's phenomenon
Becker's sign
Beckman retractor
Beckman-Adson retractor
Beckman-Eaton retractor
bed phase
bed-wetting
bedbound
bedewing of cornea
bedlamism
bedridden
bedsore
Beevor's sign
behavior
    automatic b.
    invariable b.
    operant b.
    respondent b.
    variable b.
behavior modification
Behavior Problem Checklist
behavior therapy
behavioral science
behaviorism
behaviorist
Behcet's syndrome
Behler-Hardy sign

Behr complicated optic atrophy
Bekesy audiometry
Bekhterev's disease
Bekhterev's reaction
Bekhterev's sign
Bekhterev's spondylitis
Bekhterev's test
Bekhterev's tract
Bekhterev-Mendel reflex
Bell's mania
Bell's nerve
Bell's palsy
Bell's paralysis
Bell's phenomenon
Bell's sign
Bell's spasm
Bell-Dally cervical dislocation
Bell-Magendie law
belladonna
belle indifference
belonephobia
Bence Jones protein
Benda's stain
Bender Gestalt test
Bender Visual Motor Gestalt test
bends
Benedikt's syndrome
benign
    epileptiform transients (BET), b.
    essential tremor, b.
    intracranial hypertension (BIH), b.
    mesenchymoma, b.
    positional vertigo (BPV), b.
Benjamin proverbs
Benton Visual Retention Test
benzodiazepine
berdache
bereavement
Berens 3-character test
Berger rhythm
Berger's paresthesia
Berger's sign
Bergeron's chorea
Bergeron's disease
beriberi
    atrophic b.

beriberi *(continued)*
   cerebral b.
   dry b.
   paralytic b.
Berkow formula
Berlin's disease
Bernard's puncture
Bernard's syndrome
Bernard-Horner syndrome
Bernard-Soulier syndrome
Berne theory
Bernhardt's disease
Bernhardt's disturbance of sensation
Bernhardt's paresthesia
Bernhardt-Roth disease
Bernhardt-Roth syndrome
Bernreuter Personality Inventory Test
berry aneurysm
berserk
Bertolotti's syndrome
bestiality
BET (benign epileptiform transients)
beta
   -adrenergic, b.
   buzz, b.
   -endorphin, b.
   press, b.
   rhythm, b.
   test, b.
   waves, b.
Bethe's method
betweenbrain
Betz's cell area
Betz's cells
Bevan Lewis cells
bevel
bevelled
bhang
Bianchi's syndrome
bibliomania
bibliotherapy
bicap cautery
Biceps bipolar coagulator
biceps jerk
bicipital
Biegel Manic State Scale

Bielschowsky head-tilting test
Bielschowsky silver stain
Bielschowsky-Jansky disease
Biemond's syndrome
Biernacki's sign
bifid
bifida
bifidus
biforate
bifrontal
   craniotomy, b.
   headache, b.
bifurcate
bifurcation
bigeminal
BIH (benign intracranial hypertension)
Bilderbeck's disease
bilirubin encephalopathy
Billroth's disease
bilobate
bind web
Binda's sign
Binet age
Binet test
Binet-Simon test
Bing test
binge
   -drinker, b.
   -eater, b.
bingeing
Binswanger's dementia
Binswanger's disease
Binswanger's encephalitis
Binswanger's encephalopathy
Biobrane
bioccipital
Biocclusive dressing
biochemical
   marker, b.
Biocoral
biodynamics
bioelectricity
bioenergetics
biofeedback
   alpha b.
biogenic amine hypothesis

Biograft
biologic depression
biologic sex
biological clock
biological rhythm
biomechanics
biopsy bed
biopsychic
biopsychology
biopsychosocial
biorhythm
biosocial theory
biothesiometer
Biot's breathing
biparietal
biparietal craniotomy
bipolar
    affective disorder, b.
    cautery, b.
    coagulation, b.
    forceps, b.
    neuron, b.
bipotentiality
bird's head type
bird-arm
bird-headed dwarf
bird-leg
Birkitt-type non-Hodgkin's lymphoma
Birtcher cautery
birth palsy
Bischoff myelotomy
bisexual
bisexuality
bistoury
bisynchronous
bitemporal
biventer cervicis
bizarre
Bjerrum's scotoma
Bjerrum's sign
Bjornstad's syndrome
Bjornstrom's algesimeter
black locks
black magic
Black Mass
Black and Decker battery-operated drill

blackout
bladder Crede
bladder spasm
Blair saw guide
blank spell
blanket roll
Blaskovics operation
bleed
bleeding points
Blenoxane
bleomycin
blepharoclonus
blepharoplasty
blepharoplegia
blepharoptosis
blepharospasm
    essential b.
    symptomatic b.
blepharosphincterectomy
Bleuler's theory
Bleulerian schema
blind sight
blind spot
blindism
blindness
    amnesic color b.
    blue b.
    blue-yellow b.
    Bright's b.
    color b.
    concussion b.
    cortical b.
    cortical psychic b.
    day b.
    eclipse b.
    electric-light b.
    epidemic b.
    flight b.
    functional b.
    green b.
    hysterical b.
    legal b.
    letter b.
    mind b.
    moon b.
    night b.

blindness *(continued)*
 note b.
 object b.
 psychic b.
 red b.
 red-green b.
 river b.
 snow b.
 soul b.
 syllabic b.
 taste b.
 text b.
 total b.
 twilight b.
 word b.
 yellow b.
blink reflex of Descartes
block
 caudal b.
 dynamic b.
 epidural b.
 field b.
 intercostal nerve b.
 intraspinal b.
 mental b.
 methadone b.
 nerve b.
 paraneural b.
 parasacral b.
 paravertebral b.
 perineural b.
 presacral b.
 pudendal b.
 sacral b.
 saddle b.
 spinal b.
 spinal subarachnoid b.
 splanchnic b.
 stellate b.
 subarachnoid b.
 sympathetic b.
 transsacral b.
 vagal b.
 vagus nerve b.
 ventricular b.
blockade

blockade *(continued)*
 adrenergic b.
 adrenergic neuron b.
 alpha adrenergic b.
 alpha b.
 beta adrenergic b.
 beta b.
 cholinergic b.
 narcotic b.
 neuromuscular b.
blocking
 adrenergic b.
 thought b.
Blocq's disease
blood
 alcohol level, b.
 -brain barrier, b.
 -cerebral barrier, b.
 dyscrasia, b.
 ethanol concentration (BEC), b.
 patch, b.
bloodless field
bloody tap
Bloom syndrome
Blount brace
Blount-Schmidt Milwaukee brace
blow-by oxygen
blow-in fracture
blow-out fracture
blown pupil
BLS (basic life support)
Blumberg's sign
blunted affect
blunting
blurred disk
blurring of vision
BNMSE (Brief Neuropsychological Mental Status Examination)
Boas' algesimeter
Bock's ganglion
Bock's nerve
Bodal's test
body
 buffer zone, b.
 dysmorphic disorder, b.
 habitus, b.

body *(continued)*
-image agnosia, b.
language, b.
mechanics, b.
Luys, b. of
packer syndrome, b.
rocking, b.
schema, b.
Bohlman cervical vertebrectomy
bolster
Bolton point
Bolton triangle
bondage
bonding
bone
age according to Greulich and Pyle, b.
bank, b.
bleeding, b.
cement, b.
chip, b.
conduction, b.
debris, b.
dowel, b.
dust, b.
edge margin, b.
flap, b.
fragment, b.
graft, b.
island, b.
pain, b.
plug, b.
punch, b.
rongeur, b.
scan, b.
sensibility, b.
slurry, b.
spur, b.
wax, b.
Bonhoeffer's syndrome
Bonnet's sign
Bonnet's syndrome
Bonnier's syndrome
bony
architecture, b.
bridging, b.
landmarks, b.

bony *(continued)*
overhang, b.
ridge, b.
spicule, b.
spur, b.
boopia
Boplant surgibone
border fibrils
borderline
features, b.
personality, b.
Bordier-Frankel sign
Borjeson's syndrome
Borjeson-Forssman-Lehmann syndrome
bosselated
bosselation
Boston Arm
Boston Diagnostic Aphasia Battery
Boston Naming Test
Boston thoracic brace
Boston's sign
Bosworth spinal fusion
Botterell classification
botulism
bouche de tapir
boulimia
bouquet
Bourneville's disease
Bovie electrocautery
bovied
Bowditch's law
boxer's encephalopathy
Boyes brachioradialis transfer
BPV (benign positional vertigo)
brace
Arnold lumbar b.
Blount b.
Blount-Schmidt Milwaukee b.
Boston thoracic b.
chairback b.
Cook walking b.
Dennyson cervical b.
Fisher b.
Florida cervical b.
four-point cervical b.
four-poster cervical b.

brace *(continued)*
   Guilford cervical b.
   Jewett b.
   King cervical b.
   Knight back b.
   MacCausland lumbar b.
   McKee b.
   Milwaukee b.
   Philadephia Plastizote cervical b.
   TLSO (thoracolumbosacral orthosis) b.
bracelet test
brachial
   plexus, b.
   plexus neuritis, b.
   syndrome, b.
brachialgia
   statica paresthetica, b.
brachiocephalic
brachiocrural
brachiocubital
brachiocyllosis
brachiocyrtosis
brachiofaciolingual
brachium
Brachmann-de Lange syndrome
brachybasia
brachycephalic
brachycephaly
brachycranic
brachystasis
brachytherapy
bracing
Bradford frame
bradyacusia
bradyarthria
bradycardia
bradycinesia
bradyecoia
bradyesthesia
bradyglossia
bradykinesia
bradykinetic
bradykinin
bradylalia
bradylexia

bradylogia
bradyphagia
bradyphasia
bradyphemia
bradyphrasia
bradyphrenia
bradypnea
bradypragia
bradypsychia
bradytachycardia
bradyteleocinesia
bradyteleokinesis
Bragard's sign
Bragg peak
braidism
Brailey stretching of supratrochlear nerve
braille
brailler
Brain's reflex
brain
   new b.
   old b.
   olfactory b.
   smell b.
   respirator b.
   'tween b.
   wet b.
brain activity
brain biopsy
brain biopsy needle
brain cannula
brain clip
brain concussion
brain contusion
brain damage
brain dead
brain death
brain edema
brain electrical activity map (BEAM)
brain engorgement
brain-exploring cannula
brain-exploring trocar
brain forceps
brain-heart infusion
brain hook
brain irradiation

brain knife
brain laceration
brain mantle
brain metastasis
brain retractor
brain sand
brain scan
brain scissors
brain spatula
brain speculum
brain spoon
brain stem
    auditory evoked potential (BAEP), b.
    auditory evoked response (BAER), b.
    lesion, b.
brain suction tip
brain test
brain tumor
brain wave
brainstorm
brainwashing
brake phenomenon
brancher deficiency
brancher glycogen storage disease
branchial neuritis
Brauch-Romberg symptom
Braun's canal
Braun-Yasargil right-angle clip
Bravais-Jacksonian epilepsy
Brazelton Behavior Scale
Brazelton Neonatal Assessment Scale
breakdown
break-off phenomenon
Breathalyzer
breathing
    apneustic b.
    ataxic b.
    Biot's b.
    cluster b.
    frog b.
    glossopharyngeal b.
    intermittent positive pressure
      (IPPB) b.
    periodic b.
bredouillement
bregma

bregmatic
bregmatodynia
Bremmer halo
Breschet's canals
Brescio-Cimino AV fistula
breviflexor
breviradiate
Brickner's sign
bridge
    Varolius, b. of
bridging
    osteophytes, b.
    veins, b.
Brief Neuropsychological Mental Status
    Examination (BNMSE)
brief short-action potential (BSAP)
Bright's blindness
Brighton electrical stimulation system
Briquet's ataxia
Briquet's hysteria
Briquet's syndrome
brisement
    force, b.
Brissaud's dwarf
Brissaud's infantilism
Brissaud's reflex
Brissaud's scoliosis
Brissaud-Marie syndrome
Brissaud-Sicard syndrome
Bristowe's syndrome
brittle bone syndrome
broach
broaching
Broadbent registration point
Broadbent's apoplexy
Broadbent's test
Broca's amnesia
Broca's aphasia
Broca's center
Broca's convolution
Broca's fissure
Broca's gyrus
Broca's motor speech area
Broca's parolfactory area
Brodie's disease
Brodie's pain

Brodmann's area
Brodmann's classification system
bromides
brominism
bromism
bromocriptine
bromomania
Brompton cocktail
Brompton solution
bronchoplegia
brontophobia
bronzed disease
Brooks-Jenkins atlantoaxial fusion technique
   nique
Broviac catheter
brow
   pang, b.
Brown forceps
Brown Personality Inventory
Brown's vertical retraction syndrome
Brown-Roberts-Wells (BRW) CT stereotaxic guide
   taxic guide
Brown-Sequard disease
Brown-Sequard lesion
Brown-Sequard paralysis
Brown-Sequard syndrome
Brown-Symmers disease
Bruce's tract
Bruch's membrane
Bruck's disease
Brucke's lines
Brudzinski's sign
bruissement
bruit
Brun bone curette
Bruns' apraxia of gait
Bruns' syndrome
brushes of Ruffini
Brushfield spots
Brushfield-Wyatt syndrome
brux
bruxism
bruxomania
BRW (Brown-Robert-Wells) CT stereotaxic guide
   taxic guide
B-scan ultrasonography

BSAP (brief short-action potential)
bubble ventriculography
buccal smear test
buccolingual dyskinesia
buccolinguomasticatory movement
Buck's traction
Bucy knife
Bucy retractor
Bucy-Frazier cannula
Budd-Chiari syndrome
Budge's center
buffalo hump
buffalo type
bulb
bulbar
   palsy, b.
   syndrome, b.
bulbi (pl. of bulbus)
bulbiform
bulbonuclear
bulbopontine
bulbs of Krause
bulbus (pl. bulbi)
bulesis
bulging disk
bulimia
   nervosa, b.
bulimic
bulimorexia
bulldog reflex
Bumke's pupil
bundle
Bungner's bands
Bunina bodies
buphthalmos
bur
   drill, b.
   hole, b.
   hole cap, b.
   hole incision, b.
Burdach's tract
Buretrol
burned out
burning feet syndrome
burning tongue
burnout

burred
burring
bursa (pl. bursae)
bursae (pl. of bursa)
burst
   suppression, b.
Buspar

buspirone
butterfly glioma
butterfly needle
butterfly rash
button
by-the-numbers phenomenon

Additional entries

_____

_____

_____

_____

_____

_____

_____

_____

_____

_____

_____

_____

_____

_____

_____

_____

_____

_____

_____

_____

_____

_____

C

CA (chronological age)
cabala
cabalism
cacesthenic
cachectic
cachergasia
cachesthenic
cacesthesia
cachexia
cachinnation
cacodemonomania
cacogeusia
cacosmia
cadaver graft
cadaver plug
cadaveric
reaction
CADD-PLUS intravenous infusion pump
cafard
cafe au lait spot
Cafergot
caffeinc
caffeinism
Caffey's disease
CAGE (cut-down, annoyed, guilty, eye-
opener) test for alcoholism
cainotophobia
Cairn clamp
Cairns forceps
caisson disease
Cajal's double method
calamus scriptorius
calcar
calcarine fissure
Calcitite
calcium channel blocker
calculation
calculi (pl. of calculus)
calculus (pl. calculi)
Caldwell view
calibration
California encephalitis
California Personality Inventory

caliper
Callahan extension of cervical injury
Callahan fusion technique
callomania
callosal
callosomarginal
callosum
callus
calmative
caloric testing
Calvare's disease
calvaria
calvarial
calvarium
calyculi (pl. of calyculus)
calyculus (pl. calyculi)
Campbell's elevator
Camino intracranial pressure monitor
camisole
cAMP (cyclic adenosine monophosphate)
campimeter
campimetry
campospasm
campotomy
camptocormia
camptodactylism
camptodactyly
camptomelia
camptomelic
dwarfism, c.
camptospasm
Camurati-Engelmann disease
Canadian crutch
canal
canales (pl. of canalis)
canalis (pl. canales)
canalization
Canavan's disease
Canavan-van Bogaert-Bertrand disease
cancerphobia
candidiasis
cane
English c.

cane *(continued)*
 quadripod c.
 tripod c.
cane-walking
cannabinoids
cannabis
cannabism
cannibalism
cannibalistic compulsion taxon
Cannon's law of denervation
cannula
cannulate
cannulation
cannulization
Cantelli's sign
Capener rhachotomy
Capgras' syndrome
capita (pl. of caput)
Capps' sign
capsaican
capsula (pl. capsulae)
capsulae (pl. of capsula)
capsulation
capsule
capsulitis
 adhesive c.
capsulothalamic syndrome
caput (pl. capita)
carbamazepine
carbide bur
carbodopa
carbon dioxide (CO2)
carbon monoxide
carcinoma
carcinomata
carcinomatophobia
carcinophobia
cardiac
 arrest, c.
cardiasthenia
cardinal direction
cardiogenic shock
cardiomalacia
cardiomyopathy
cardioneural
cardioneurosis

cardiophobia
cardiospasm
C-arm fluoroscopy
C-arm image intensifier
carnal
carnophobia
Carnett's sign
carnosinemia
Carolina rocker
Caroll Rating Scale for Depression
carotid
 amytal speech test, c.
 angiogram, c.
 arteriogram, c.
 artery, c.
 artery stenosis, c.
 bifurcation, c.
 bruit, c.
 bulb, c.
 canal, c.
 -cavernous fistula, c.
 Doppler, c.
 endarterectomy (CEA), c.
 ischemia, c.
 massage, c.
 nerve, c.
 phonoangiography, c.
 pulse tracing, c.
 sheath, c.
 sinus nerve, c.
 sinus pressure, c.
 sinus syncope, c.
 siphon, c.
 triangle, c.
 ultrasound, c.
carotidynia
carpal
carpal tunnel
 decompression, c.
 release, c.
 syndrome, c.
Carpenter's syndrome
carphologic movement
carphology
carpopedal spasm
carpoptosis

car sickness
cartilage
cartilaginous
CASH brace
Caspar alligator forceps
Casser's fontanelle
casserian
Castellani-Low symptom
castration
    anxiety, c.
    complex, c.
CAT (computerized axial tomography)
CAT scan
cat's cry syndrome
cat's eye amaurosis
cat's eye pupil
cat's eye reflex
cat's eye syndrome
catalepsy
cataleptic
cataleptiform
cataleptoid
catalogia
cataphasia
cataphora
cataphoria
cataphrenia
cataplectic
cataplexie
    dui reveil, c.
cataplexis
cataplexy
catapophysis
catathymic
catatonia
catatonic
    excitement, c.
    negativism, c.
    rigidity, c.
    schizophrenia, c.
    stupor, c.
catatony
catch-give sensation
catecholamines
catelectrotonic state
catharsis

catharsisovert
cathartic
cathectic
Cathelin's method
cathexis
cathisophobia
cat-scratch fever
Cattell Infant Intelligence Scale
Cattell theory
cauda (pl. caudae)
    equina, c.
    nuclei caudati, c.
caudad
caudae (pl. of cauda)
caudal
    area, c.
    myotome, c.
caudalward
caudocephalad
caumesthesia
causal lesion
causalgia
causative
caustic euphoria
cauterization
cauterizer loop
cautery
cautionary
cavalry bone
cavernous sinus
cavitary
cavitas (pl. cavitates)
cavitates (pl. of cavitas)
cavitation
Cavitron ultrasonic aspirator (CUSA)
cavity
cavum
Cawthorne-Cooksey vestibular exercises
CBS (chronic brain syndrome)
CCT (computerized cranial tomography)
CEA (carotid endarterectomy)
cecocentral scotoma
ceftazidime
cell
    button, c.
    count, c.

cella (pl. cellae)
    lateralis ventriculi lateralis, c.
    media ventriculi lateralis, c.
cellae (pl. of cella)
celliform
Cellolite
cellular
    edema, c.
cellulose gauze
celluloneuritis
    acute anterior c.
Celontin
Celsus' quadrilateral
cenesthesia
cenesthopathy
cenopsychic
cenotophobia
censor
    freudian c.
    psychic c.
censorship
center
    acoustic c.
    apneustic c.
    auditopsychic c.
    auditory c.
    auditory word c.
    autonomic c.
    brain c.
    Broca's c.
    Budge's c.
    cardioaccelerator c.
    cardioinhibitory c.
    cheirokinesthetic c.
    ciliospinal c.
    coordination c.
    correlation c.
    cortical c.
    deglutition c.
    eupraxic c.
    facial c.
    feeding c.
    ganglionic c.
    glossokinesthetic c.
    gustatory c.
    heat-regulating c.

center *(continued)*
    higher c.
    inhibitory c.
    lower c.
    Lumsden's c.
    medullary c. of cerebellum
    micturition c.
    motor c.
    nerve c.
    optic c.
    panting c.
    phrenic c.
    pneumotaxic c.
    polypneic c.
    psychocortical c.
    reflex c.
    respiratory c.
    satiety c.
    Sechenow's c.
    sensory c.
    sex-behavior c.
    speech c.
    swallowing c.
    taste c.
    temperature c.
    thermoregulatory c.
    trophic c.
    vasoconstriction c.
    vasodilator c.
    vasomotor c.
    visual word c.
    Wernicke's c.
    word c.
centigray (cGy)
central
    canal of spinal cord, c.
    core disease, c.
    effector neuron, c.
    European encephalitis, c.
    excitatory state (CES), c.
    lesion, c.
    line, c.
    nervous system (CNS), c.
    nervous system depression, c.
    nervous system dysfunction, c.
    pontine myelinolysis, c.

central *(continued)*
   summation, c.
centration
centrencephalic
centriciput
centrifugation
centrocecal scotoma
centrokinesia
centrokinetic
centrostaltic
centrotherapy
centrum
   semiovale, c.
   vertebrae, c.
cephalad
cephalalgia
   histaminic c.
   pharyngotympanic c.
   postcoital c.
   quadrantal c.
cephaledema
cephalematocele
cephalematoma
cephalgia
cephalhematocele
   Stromeyer's c.
cephalhematoma
   deformans, c.
cephalhydrocele
   traumatica, c.
cephalic
   index, c.
   suspension, c.
   triangle, c.
cephalitis
cephalization
cephalocaudad
cephalocaudal
   pattern of development, c.
cephalocele
   orbital c.
cephalocentesis
cephalochord
cephalodactyly
   Vogt's c.
cephalodynia

cephalogram
cephalogyric
cephalohematocele
cephalohematoma
cephalohemometer
cephaloma
cephalomeningitis
cephalometer
cephalometry
cephalomotor
cephalone
cephalonia
cephalopathy
cephaloplegia
cephalorachidian
cephalostat
cephalostyle
cephalotetanus
cephalotropic
cephalotrypesis
ceptor
   chemical c.
   contact c.
   distance c.
   nerve c.
cerea flexibilitas
cerebellar
   angioblastoma, c.
   ataxia, c.
   biventral lobule, c.
   ciliary body, c.
   cortex, c.
   declive, c.
   dentate nucleus, c.
   dyssynergia, c.
   emboliform nucleus, c.
   fasciculus uncinatus, c.
   fastigial nucleus, c.
   fimbriate nucleus, c.
   fissure, c.
   fit, c.
   folium, c.
   gait, c.
   globose nucleus, c.
   gracile lobule, c.
   lenticular nucleus, c.

cerebellar *(continued)*
    lobe, c.
    motor tectal nucleus, c.
    outflow tremor, c.
    peduncle, c.
    pontine angle (CPA), c.
    posterior inferior ansiform lobule, c.
    posterior lobe, c.
    pressure cone, c.
    pyramis, c.
    region, c.
    roof nucleus, c.
    signs, c.
    stalk, c.
    tonsil, c.
    tuber, c.
    vein, c.
    vermis, c.
    white matter, c.
cerebellifugal
cerebellipetal
cerebellitis
cerebellofugal
cerebellomedullary cistern
cerebello-olivary
cerebellopontile
cerebellopontine
    angle (CPA), c.
    angle tumor, c.
cerebellorubral
cerebellorubrospinal
cerebellospinal
cerebellum
    agenesis, c.
cerebra
cerebral
    angiography, c.
    anoxia, c.
    arcuate fibers, c.
    arteriography, c.
    arteriosclerosis, c.
    artery, c.
    artery thrombosis, c.
    atherosclerosis, c.
    atrophy, c.
    blood flow, c.

cerebral *(continued)*
    cortex, c.
    cortex electrode, c.
    dorsum, c.
    edema, c.
    elastance, c.
    embolism, c.
    epidural space, c.
    fissure, c.
    fossa, c.
    gigantism, c.
    gray matter, c.
    hemisphere, c.
    hemorrhage, c.
    herniation, c.
    infarct, c.
    insufficiency, c.
    lacunae, c.
    medial surface, c.
    metabolic rate, c.
    nerves, c.
    palsy (CP), c.
    peduncle, c.
    perfusion, c.
    porosis, c.
    rheumatism, c.
    salt wasting, c.
    sarcoma, c.
    sphingolipidosis, c.
    superolateral surface, c.
    thrombosis, c.
    vascular accident, c.
    vein, c.
    vein thrombosis, c.
    ventricle, c.
    white matter, c.
cerebrasthenia
cerebration
    unconscious c.
cerebriform
cerebrifugal
cerebripetal
cerebritis
    saturnine c.
cerebroatrophic hyperammonemia
cerebrocardiac

cerebrocerebellar
cerebrogalactose
cerebrohepatorenal syndrome
cerebrohyphoid
cerebroid
cerebrol
cerebrolein
cerebrology
cerebroma
cerebromacular
cerebromalacia
cerebromedullary
cerebromeningeal
cerebromeningitis
cerebrometer
cerebro-ocular
cerebron
cerebropathia
   psychica toxemica, c.
cerebropathy
cerebrophysiology
cerebropontile
cerebropsychosis
cerebrorachidian
cerebroscintigraphy
cerebrosclerosis
cerebroscope
cerebroscopy
cerebrose
cerebroside
cerebrosidosis
cerebrosis
cerebrospinal
   axis, c.
   fever, c.
   fluid (CSF), c.
   fluid assay, c.
   fluid culture, c.
   fluid electrophoresis, c.
   fluid pressure, c.
   ganglia, c.
   meningitis, c.
   nerves, c.
   puncture, c.
   rhinorrhea, c.
cerebrospinant

cerebrospinase
cerebrostimulin
cerebrostomy
cerebrotendinous
   xanthomatosis, c.
cerebrotomy
cerebrotonia
cerebrovascular
   accident (CVA), c.
   insufficiency, c.
   obstructive disease, c.
   resistance, c.
cerebrum
certifiable
certification
ceruloplasmin
Cerva Crane halter
cervical
   collar, c.
   cordotomy, c.
   disk, c.
   disk excision, c.
   disk syndrome, c.
   diskectomy, c.
   ganglion, c.
   lamina propria, c.
   myotome, c.
   nerves, c.
   orthosis, c.
   plexus, c.
   radiculopathy, c.
   rib, c.
   somatosensory evoked potential, c.
   spinal cord, c.
   spine (C-spine), c.
   spondylolisthesis, c.
   spondylolysis, c.
   spondylosis, c.
   traction, c.
   vertebrae
cervicobrachial
cervicobrachialgia
cervicodorsal
cervicodynia
cervicofacial
cervico-occipital

cervicoscapular
cervicothoracic
cervicothoracolumbosacral orthosis
cervix of axon
CES (central excitatory state)
Cestan's syndrome
Cestan-Chenais syndrome
Cestan-Raymond syndrome
C-fiber
CFIDS (chronic fatigue and immune dys-
    function syndrome)
cGMP (cyclic guanosine monophosphate)
cGy (centigray)
Chaddock's reflex
Chaddock's toe sign
Chaddock's wrist sign
Chagas' disease
Chagas-Cruz disease
chagasic
chaining
chairback brace
Chamberlain's line
Chance vertebral fracture
Chandler felt
collar splint
Chandler forceps
channeling
chaos
chaotic
character
    acquired c.
    anal c.
character armor
Charcot's disease
Charcot's gait
Charcot's joint
Charcot's sign
Charcot's syndrome
Charcot's triad
Charcot-Bouchard aneurysm
Charcot-Marie atrophy
Charcot-Marie type
Charcot-Marie-Tooth atrophy
Charcot-Marie-Tooth disease
Charcot-Marie-Tooth type
Charcot-Weiss-Baker syndrome

Charest head frame
charleyhorse
Charnley pillow
Chassaignac's tubercle
Chastek paralysis
Chatfield-Girdleston splint
Chaussier's line
Chaves-Rapp paralysis
checking
cheek phenomenon
cheirobrachialgia paresthetica
cheirocinesthesia
cheirognostic
cheirokinesthesia
cheirokinesthetic
cheirology
cheiropodalgia
cheirospasm
chelation
chemanesia
chemical dependence
chemical warfare
chemonucleolysis
chemopallidectomy
chemopallidothalamectomy
chemopsychiatry
chemoreception
chemoreceptor
chemoreflex
chemothalamectomy
chemotherapeutic
chemotherapy
Cherchevski's disease
cheromania
cherophobia
Cherry osteotome
Cherry tongs
Cherry-Kerrison forceps
chest roll
Chestnut Lodge Prognostic Scale
Chevreul pendulum
Cheyne-Stokes psychosis
Cheyne-Stokes respiration
CHH cervical brace
Chiari's syndrome
Chiari-Arnold syndrome

chiasma
   syndrome, c.
chiasmal arachnoiditis
chiasmatic
Chievitz's layer
child abuse
child molestation
child molester
child within
Children's Apperception Test
Children's Hospital clip
Chimani-Moss test
chin jerk
chin-occiput piece
chin reflex
chin-retraction sign
chin-up bar
Chinese reds (heroin)
Chinese restaurant syndrome
chionablepsia
chiralgia
chirismus
chirobrachialgia
chirognostic
chirokinesthesia
chiropodalgia
chiropractic
chiropractor
chirospasm
chisel
chloral hydrate
chloroformism
chlorpromazine
chocked reflex
choked disk
chokes
choke-saver
cholecystokinin
choleromania
cholerophobia
cholesteatoma
cholesterol emboli
cholesterol ester storage disease
choline
   acetylase, c.
   acetyltranferase, c.

cholinergic
cholinesterase
cholinoceptive
cholinoceptor
cholinolytic
cholinomimetic
chondral
chondralgia
chondralloplasia
chondritis
   costal c.
   intervertebralis calcanea, c.
chondrodynia
chondrodysplasia
   hereditary deforming c.
   punctata, c.
chondrodystrophia
   calcificans congenita, c.
   congenita punctata, c.
   fetalis calcificans, c.
chondrodystrophy
   familial c.
   hereditary deforming c.
   hyperplastic c.
   hypoplastic c.
   hypoplastic fetal c.
   malacia, c.
chondromalacia
chondromatosis
chorda (pl. chordae)
   saliva, c.
chordae (pl. of chorda)
chordoma
chorea
   acute c.
   automatic c.
   Bergeron's c.
   button-maker's c.
   chronic progressive hereditary c.
   chronic progressive nonhereditary c.
   cordis, c.
   dancing c.
   degenerative c.
   diaphragmatic c.
   dimidiata, c.
   Dubini's c.

chorea *(continued)*
electric c.
epidemic c.
festinans, c.
fibrillary c.
gravidarum, c.
habit c.
hemilateral c.
Henoch's c.
hereditary c.
Huntington's c.
hyoscine c.
hysterical c.
imitative c.
insaniens, c.
juvenile c.
laryngeal c.
limp c.
local c.
major, c.
malleatory c.
maniacal c.
methodic c.
mimetic c.
minor c.
mollis, c.
Morvan's
nocturna, c.
nutans, c.
one-sided c.
paralytic c.
posthemiplegic c.
prehemiplegic c.
procursive c.
rhythmic c.
rotary c.
saltatory c.
school-made c.
Schrotter's c.
scriptorum, c.
senile c.
simple c.
Sydenham's c.
tetanoid c.
tic c.
choreic

choreic *(continued)*
athetoid movements, c.
choreiform
movements, c.
choreoacanthocytosis
choreoathetoid
choreoathetosis
choreoid
choreomania
choreophrasia
choriocarcinoma
choriomeningitis
choroid
plexotomy, c.
plexus, c.
plexus papilloma, c.
choroidectomy
choroideremia
Chotzen's syndrome
Christoferson's disk implant
chromaffin
chromaffinoma
medullary c.
chromaffinopathy
chromaphil
chromatolysis
chromatopsia
chromatotropism
chromesthesia
chromophil tumor
chromophobe
tumor, c.
chromopsia
chromosomal aneuploidy
chronaxie
chronic
anxiety state, c.
back pain, c.
brain syndrome (CBS), c.
factitious disorder, c.
fatigue and immune dysfunction syndrome (CFIDS), c.
fatigue syndrome, c.
motor tic disorder, c.
pain syndrome, c.
subdural hematoma, c.

chronobiology
chronognosis
chronological age
chronophobia
chronotaraxis
chthonophagia
chunking
Churg-Strauss vasculitis
Chvostek's sign
Chvostek-Weiss sign
Chymodiactin
chymonucleolysis
cicatricial
cicatrix
ciguatera
ciliary
   body, c.
   nerve, c.
   reflex, c.
ciliospinal
   center, c.
   reflex, c.
ciliotomy
cillo
cillosis
cimbia
cimetidine psychosis
Cimino arteriovenous fistula
Cimino catheter
cinchonism
cinclisis
cincture sensation
cinerea
cinereal
cinesalgia
cingula (pl. of cingulum)
cingulate
   fasciculus, c.
   gyrus, c.
   sulcus, c.
cingule
cingulectomy
cingulotomy
cingulum (pl. cingula)
   hemispherii, c.
cingulumotomy

cinology
cinometer
circadian
   rhythm, c.
   sleep-wake cycle, c.
circinate
circle
   Willis, c. of
CircOlectric bed
circuit
circuli (pl. of circulus)
circulus (pl. circuli)
circumcallosal
circumduct
circumduction
   gait, c.
circumlocution
circumstantiality
circumvolute
circumvolutio
   cristata, c.
circus movement
cistern
   basal c.
   cerebellomedullary c.
   chiasmatic c.
   fossa of Sylvius, c. of
   great c.
   interpeduncular c.
   lateral fossa, c. of
   Pecquet, c. of
   posterior c.
   subarachnoidal c.
   Sylvius, c. of
cisterna (pl. cisternae)
   ambiens, c.
   basalis, c.
   cerebellomedullaris, c.
   chiasmatica, c.
   chiasmatis, c.
   corpus callosum, c.
   fossae lateralis cerebri, c.
   fossae Sylvii, c.
   intercruralis profunda, c.
   interpeduncularis, c.
   magna, c.

cisterna (pl. cisternae) *(continued)*
  subarachnoideales, c.
  sulci lateralis, c.
  Sylvii, c.
  venae magnae cerebri, c.
cisternae (pl. of cisterna)
cisternal
  puncture, c.
cisternography
  metrizamide c.
cisvestitism
Citelli's syndrome
citrullinemia
citta
CJD (Creutzfeldt-Jakob disease)
CK (creatine kinase)
cladosporiosis
clairaudience
clairsentience
clairvoyance
clairvoyant
clamping habit
clang association
clanging
clapping
clarification
Clarke's column
clasp-knife reflex
clasp-knife rigidity
clasp-knife spasticity
Claude's hyperkinesis sign
Claude's syndrome
Claude-Bernard-Horner syndrome
claudicant
claudication
claudicatory
claustra (pl. of claustrum)
claustral
claustrophilia
claustrophobia
claustrum (pl. claustra)
clausura
clawfoot
clawhand
claw toe
clear sensorium

clearing of sensorium
cleft cheek
cleft lip
cleft palate
cleft tongue
clefting
cleidocranial
  dysostosis, c.
cleisiophobia
cleithrophobia
clenching
Clerambault's syndrome
clicking
client-centered psychotherapy
climacteric
climacterium
climbing-up on body
Clinitron bed
clip-shave
clipped speech
clipping of aneurysm
clipping of cerebral artery
clithrophobia
clitoris crises
clival
clivography
clivus
  Blumenbachii, c.
clock-drawing
clomipramine
clonal selection
clonazepam
clonic
  convulsion, c.
  seizure, c.
  spasm, c.
clonic-tonic
clonicity
clonicotonic
clonism
clonismus
clonograph
clonospasm
clonotonic
clonus
Cloquet's ganglion

closed-angle glaucoma
closed chest cardiac massage
closed head injury
closed skull fracture
Clos-O-Mat
Clostridium tetani
clothespin spinal fusion graft
clouded consciousness
clouded sensorium
clouding of consciousness
clouding of sensorium
clouding of sinus
cloven spine
Cloward anterior spinal fusion
Cloward cervical disk approach
Cloward chisel
Cloward drill
Cloward fusion diskectomy
Cloward hammer
Cloward puka procedure
Cloward punch
Cloward technique
Cloward vertebral spreader
Cloward-Hoen retractor
clownism
clozapine
Clozaril
clubfoot
clubhand
cluster breathing
cluster headaches
cluttering
CMV (cytomegalovirus)
cnemoscoliosis
CNS (central nervous system)
CO2 (carbon dioxide)
coagulation cautery
coarctation of aorta
coast erysipelas
COATS (Comprehensive Occupational
    Assessment and Training System)
coaxial needle
Cobb osteotome
Cobb periosteal elevator
Cobb scoliosis measuring technique
Cobb syndrome

cocaine
    baby, c.
    metabolite assay, c.
cocainism
coccidioidomycosis
coccygeal
coccygodynia
coccyodynia
coccyx
cochlear
    implant, c.
    nerve, c.
    prosthesis, c.
cochleo-orbicular reflex
cochleopalpebral reflex
cochleovestibular
Cockayne's syndrome
coconscious
coconsciousness
cocontraction
codependence
codependency
codependent
Codman exercise
Codman's sign
COEPS (cortically originating ex-
    trapyramidal system)
coffin formation
Cogan's syndrome
Cogentin
cognate
cognition
cognitive
    ability, c.
    capacity screening examination, c.
    disorder, c.
    dissonance, c.
    dysfunction, c.
    function, c.
cognizant
cogwheel
    gait, c.
    phenomenon, c.
    rigidity, c.
    sign, c.
cogwheeling

Cohen syndrome
coherence
coherent
Cohn's test
Cohnheim's areas
coin counting
coin test
coitophobia
coitus
Colclough laminectomy rongeur
cold
    calorics, c.
    cautery, c.
    intolerance, c.
    pressor test, c.
    water calorics, c.
colicoplegia
collar brace
collateral
    flow, c.
    sprouting, c.
collective unconscious
Collet's syndrome
Collet-Sicard syndrome
colliculi (pl. of colliculus)
colliculus (pl. colliculi)
Collier's sign
collimation
collimator
Colliver's syndrome
collodion
colloid
    cyst, c.
    oncotic pressure (COP), c.
coloboma (pl. colobomata)
colobomata (pl. of coloboma)
Coloplast wafer
color
    agnosia, c.
    blindness, c.
    deficient, c.
    -flow Doppler, c.
    gustation, c.
    hearing, c.
    sense, c.
    taste, c.

Colorado tick fever
colostomy
Columbia Mental Maturity Scale
column
    anterior c. of spinal canal
    anterolateral c.
    autonomic c. of spinal cord
    Burdach, c. of
    dorsal c.
    dorsal gray c.
    dorsal c. of spinal cord
    Goll, c. of
    Gowers' c.
    gray c. of spinal cord
    interomediolateral c. of spinal cord
    Kolliker, c. of
    lateral c. of spinal cord
    Lissauer, c. of
    muscle c.
    posterior c. of spinal cord
    posteroexternal c.
    posteromedian c. of medulla oblongata
    posteromedian c. of spinal cord
    spinal c.
    Spitzka-Lissauer, c. of
    striomotor c.
    Turck's c.
    ventral c. of spinal cord
    vertebral c.
columna (pl. columnae)
columnae (pl. of columna)
coma
    agrypnodal c.
    alcoholic c.
    alpha c.
    apoplectic c.
    depasse, c.
    diabetic c.
    hepatic c.
    hyperosmolar nonketotic c.
    irreversible c.
    Kussmaul's c.
    metabolic c.
    prehepatic c.
    scale, c.
    somnolentium, c.

coma *(continued)*
   uremic c.
   vigil, c.
comatose
   state, c.
combat fatigue
combat neurosis
combat stress
combative
Combid
combination therapy
combined system disease
comedown
comma tract of Schultze
command automatism
command hallucinations
comminuted
comminution
commissura (pl. commissurae)
commissurae (pl. of commissura)
commissural
commissure
common
   carotid artery, c.
   dural sac, c.
   peroneal nerve, c.
commotio
   cerebri, c.
   retinae, c.
   spinalis, c.
commune
communicans
communicating hydrocephalus
communication board
communication deviance
comparison film
compartmental syndrome
compass turns
compatibility
compatible
compensation
   neurosis, c.
competence
competent
completed stroke
complex

complex *(continued)*
   castration c.
   Electra c.
   inferiority c.
   Oedipus c.
complex partial seizures
compos mentis
compound skull fracture
Comprehensive Occupational Assessment and Training System (COATS)
compressed spectral array (CSA)
compression
   fracture, c.
   hook, c.
   rod, c.
compulsion
   repetition c.
compulsion neurosis
compulsive
compulsive ideas
compulsive personality
compulsive speech
compulsive tic
compulsory
computed tomographic mapping of EEG
   (CTM/EEG)
computed tomography (CT)
computerized cranial tomography (CCT)
Comrey Personality Scale
conamen
conarium
conation
conative
concave
concavity
concavoconcave
concavoconvex
concealed straight leg raising
concentration camp neurosis
concentric
   sclerosis, c.
concept
Concept bipolar coagulator
Concept hand-held cautery
conception
conceptual quotient (CQ)

conceptualize
conceptus
concha of cranium
concrete
   thought process, c.
concreteness
concretism
concussion
concussive
condensation
conditioned
   insomnia, c.
   orientation reflex audiometry, c.
   reflex, c.
   response, c.
   stimulus, c.
conditioning
   aversive c.
   classical c.
   instrumental c.
   operant c.
   respondent c.
conduct disorder
conduction
   aphasia, c.
   deafness, c.
   studies, c.
   velocity, c.
conductive hearing loss
conductor
Cone cannula
Cone needle
Cone wire twister
confabulate
confabulation
confidentiality
configurationism
conflict
   approach-approach c.
   approach-avoidance c.
   avoidance-avoidance c.
   extrapsychic c.
   intrapersonal c.
   intrapsychic c.
confluence
confluens

confluens *(continued)*
   sinuum, c.
confluent
conformer
confrontation
   therapy, c.
confrontational
confusion
confusional
   state, c.
congenital
   anomaly, c.
   facial diplegia, c.
coning
conjoint therapy
conjugal paranoia
conjugate
   eye movements, c.
   gaze, c.
conjure
Conn's syndrome
connatal
connectedness
connective tissue
Conners Hyperactivity Rating Scale
Connoly system
Conradi's disease
conscience
conscious
consciousness
   disturbance, c.
   raising, c.
consensual
   light index, c.
   light reflex, c.
   reflex, c.
   response, c.
consenting adult
constant touch perception
constellation
constitution
   ideo-obsessional c.
   psychopathic c.
constitutional psychopathic inferiority
constricted affect
constructional apraxia

content
   latent c.
   manifest c.
contiguous gene syndrome
continence
continent
continuous passive motion (CPM)
Contour retractor
contractile
contractility
   idiomuscular c.
   neuromuscular c.
contraction
contracture
   Dupuytren's c.
   ischemic c.
   organic c.
   postpoliomyelitic c.
   veratrin c.
   Volkmann's c.
contralateral
   reflexes, c.
   sign, c.
contraparetic
contrast
   CT scan, c.
   enhancement, c.
   -enhancing lesion, c.
   material, c.
   medium, c.
contrastimulant
contrastimulism
contrastimulus
contraversion
contravolitional
contrecoup
   injury, c.
control
   associative automatic c.
   aversive c.
   idiodynamic c.
   reflex c.
   stimulus c.
   synergic c.
   tonic c.
   vestibuloequilibratory c.

control *(continued)*
   volitional c.
   voluntary c.
controlled substance
contusion
conus
   medullaris, c.
convergence-retraction nystagmus
conversion
   disorder, c.
   reaction, c.
   symptom, c.
convex
convexity
convexobasia
convexoconcave
convexoconvex
convoluted
convolution
   Broca's c.
   cerebrum, c's of
   Heschl's c.
   occipitotemporal c.
   Zuckerkandl's c.
convolutional
convolutionary
convolutions of Gratiolet
convulsant
convulsion
   central c.
   choreic c.
   clonic c.
   coordinate c.
   epileptiform c.
   essential c.
   febrile c.
   hysterical c.
   hysteroid c.
   local c.
   mimetic c.
   mimic c.
   myoclonic c.
   puerperal c.
   salaam c.
   spontaneous c.
   static c.

convulsion *(continued)*
   tetanic c.
   tonic-clonic c.
   uremic c.
convulsive
   disorder, c.
   reflex, c.
   seizure, c.
   shock therapy, c.
   syncope, c.
   tic, c.
Cook shingle
Cook TPN catheter
Cook walking brace
cooling blanket
Cooper cannula
Cooper's irritable breast
Coopernail sign
coordinated
coordination
COP (colloid oncotic pressure)
cope
coping
   skills, c.
   technique, c.
copodyskinesia
copper-wire effect
copper-wiring
coprolagnia
coprolalia
coprolalomania
coprophagia
coprophagy
coprophilia
coprophobia
coprophrasia
copropraxia
coprostasophobia
cord
   compression, c.
   decompression, c.
   sign, c.
cordectomy
cordotomy
core
   conductor theory, c.

core *(continued)*
   gender identity, c.
Cori cycle
corneal reflex
corneals
Cornelia de Lange syndrome
corneomandibular reflex
Corning puncture
cornu (pl. cornua)
cornua (pl. of cornu)
cornucommissural
cornucopia
cornuradicular zone
corona (pl. coronae)
   radiata, c.
coronad
coronae (pl. of corona)
coronal
   cut, c.
   plane, c.
   sulcus, c.
   suture, c.
coronale
coronalis
coronary personality
corpora (pl. of corpus)
corpus (corpora)
corpuscula
corpusculum (corpuscula)
correlation
corset
cortex (pl. cortices)
   cerebral c.
   limbic c.
   precentral c.
   premotor c.
cortical
   atrophy, c.
   blindness, c.
   deafness, c.
   dementia, c.
   evoked response, c.
   function, c.
   hyperplasia, c.
   mapping, c.
   modality, c.

cortical *(continued)*
   neuron, c.
   sensory loss, c.
   thumb, c.
corticectomy
cortices (pl. of cortex)
corticifugal
corticipetal
corticoadrenal
corticoafferent
corticoautonomic
corticobulbar
corticocerebral
corticodiencephalic
corticoefferent
corticofugal
corticoid
corticomesencephalic
corticopeduncular
corticopetal
corticopontine
corticospinal
corticosteroid
corticothalamic
corticotroph
corticotrophic
corticotrophin
corticotropic
corticotropin
Cortrosyn
coruscation
corybantism
Cosman ICP Tele-Sensor
Cosman Tele-Monitor System
cosmesis
cosmetic effect
cosmetic prosthesis
cosmic consciousness
costal
costalgia
Costen's syndrome
costicervical
costispinal
costocentral
costocervical
costocervicalis

costoclavicular
costotransverse
costotransversectomy
costovertebral
   angle (CVA), c.
   articulation, c.
   joint, c.
cot death
Cotard's syndrome
co-therapy
Cotrel scoliosis
Cotrel scoliosis cast
Cotrel traction
Cotrel-Dubousset spinal system
Cotte operation
Cotte presacral neurectomy
cotton-ball lesion
cotton-wool lesion
cotton-wool spot
cottonoid patty
Cotugno's disease
cough syncope
counseling
counselor
count fingers vision
countercathexis
counterconditioning
counterculture
counterdependence
counterimmunoelectrophoresis
counterincision
counterinvestment
counterphobia
Counter Rotation System (CRS)
countersuggestion
countersunk
countertraction
countertransference
coup
   de fouet, c.
   de sabre, c.
   de sang, c.
   de soleil, c.
   sur coup, c.
courbature
coursing

couvade syndrome
Cover-Roll adhesive
cover-uncover test
covert
cowboy story
Cowen's sign
COWS (cold to the opposite, warm to the
    same) caloric testing
coxalgia
coxitic scoliosis
coxodynia
coxsackievirus
CP (cerebral palsy)
CPA (cerebellar pontine or cerebellopont-
    ine angle)
CPK (creatine phosphokinase)
CPM (continuous passive motion)
    device, C.
CQ (conceptual quotient)
crack (street drug)
    baby, c.
    cocaine, c.
cracked-pot sound
Crafts' test
Craig head rest
Craig scissors
Crane mallet
cramp
    accessory c.
    heat c.
    recumbency c.
    stoker's c.
    writer's c.
crania (pl. of cranium)
craniad
cranial
    arteritis, c.
    bone, c.
    bur, c.
    cavity, c.
    drill, c.
    duplication, c.
    dura mater, c.
    epidural space, c.
    fossa, c.
    insufflation, c.

cranial (continued)
    nerve palsy, c.
    nerve paralysis, c.
    nerves I through XII (see below), c.
    pia mater, c.
    reflex, c.
    retractor, c.
    rongeur, c.
    subarachnoid space, c.
    subdural space, c.
    trephine, c.
cranial nerves
    I   olfactory
    II   optic
    III oculomotor
    IV   trochlear
    V   trigeminal
    VI   abducens
    VII facial
    VIII vestibulocochlear (acoustic)
    IX   glossopharyngeal
    X   vagal
    XI   accessory
    XII hypoglossal
cranialis
craniamphitomy
craniectomy
cranioacromial
cranioaural
craniobuccal
    cyst, c.
    pouch, c.
craniocaudal
    craniocaudal projection
craniocele
craniocerebral
craniocervical
craniocleidodysostosis
craniofacial
    appliance, c.
    dysostosis, c.
    suspension wiring, c.
craniofenestria
craniography
craniolacunia
craniomalacia

craniomeningocele
craniometer
craniometric
    point, c.
craniometry
craniopathy
    metabolic c.
craniopharyngeal
    duct cyst, c.
craniopharyngioma
craniophore
cranioplastic powder
cranioplasty
craniopuncture
craniorachischisis
craniosacral
cranioschisis
craniosclerosis
cranioscopy
craniospinal
    space, c.
craniostenosis
craniostosis
craniosynostosis
craniotabes
craniotome
craniotomy
    flap, c.
craniotonoscopy
craniotopography
craniotrypesis
craniotympanic
craniovertebral
cranitis
cranium (pl. crania)
    bifidum, c.
    bifidum occultum, c.
    cerebral c.
    cerebrale, c.
    visceral c.
    viscerale, c.
crank (street drug)
crateriform
craterization
Crawford head frame
crazy bone

creatine kinase (CK)
creatine phosphate
creatine phosphokinase (CPK)
Crede maneuver
Creed dissector
cremasteric reflex
cremasterics
cremnomania
cremnophobia
crenated
crepuscular
crescentic
crescent-shaped disk
cresomania
crest
CREST syndrome
cresta (pl. crestae)
crestae (pl. of cresta)
cretin
cretinism
cretinistic
cretinoid
Creutzfeldt-Jakob dementia
Creutzfeldt-Jakob disease (CJD)
crib death
cribriform plate
Crichton-Browne's sign
crick (spasm)
cricket thigh
cri du chat syndrome
Crigler-Najjar disease
Crigler-Najjar syndrome
Crile forceps
Crile head traction
Crile knife
criminaloid
criminosis
cripple
crippling
crises (pl. of crisis)
crisis (pl. crises)
    addisonian c.
    adrenal c.
    anaphylactoid c.
    catathymic c.
    cholinergic c.

crisis (pl. crises) *(continued)*
    identity c.
    Ludvall's blood c.
    myasthenic c.
    ocular c.
    oculogyric c.
    parkinsonian c.
    Pel's c.
    pharyngeal c.
    tabetic c.
    thoracic c.
    thyroid c.
    thyrotoxic c.
crisis intervention
crispation
cristai
critical flicker fusion test
critical fusion frequency
crocidismus
crocodile tears
Crocq's disease
Cronholm-Ottosson Scale
Cross syndrome
cross-bridges
cross-dependency
cross-dressing
cross-gender wish
cross-table x-ray
cross-tolerance
crossclamp
crossed laterality
crossed-leg progression
crossed reflexes
crossed straight leg raising
crossing changes
Cross-McCusick-Breen syndrome
crotaphion
Crouzon's craniofacial dysostosis
Crouzon's disease
crown
    drill, c.
    saw, c.
CRS (Counter Rotation System)
CRST syndrome
crura (pl. of crus)
crural palsies

crus (pl. crura)
crush syndrome
crutch
    paralysis, c.
    -walking, c.
Crutchfield tongs
Crutchfield drill
Crutchfield-Raney tongs
Cruveilhier's atrophy
Cruveilhier's disease
Cruveilhier's joint
Cruz-Chagas disease
cryalgesia
cryanesthesia
cryesthesia
crymodynia
cryoablation
cryoanalgesia
cryobank
cryocautery
cryodestruction
cryofibrinogenemia
cryogenic
cryohypophysectomy
cryonics
cryopreservation
cryoprobe
cryoprotectants
cryosurgery
cryothalamectomy
cryothalamotomy
cryotherapy
cryptamnesia
cryptesthesia
cryptic
cryptococcal meningitis
cryptococcosis
cryptogenic drop attack
cryptomeroarachischisis
cryptomnesia
cryptoneurous
cryptophthalmos syndrome
cryptopsychic
cryptopsychism
cry reflex
CSA (compressed spectral array)

CSF (cerebrospinal fluid)
   cytology, CSF
   manometrics, CSF.
   otorrhea, CSF.
   protein, CSF.
   rhinorrhea, CSF.
   shunting, CSF.
   sugar, CSF.
C-spine (cervical spine)
   precautions, C.
CT (computerized tomography)
   scan, CT.
CTAT (computerized transaxial tomography)
   scan, C.
CTM/EEG (computed tomographic mapping of EEG)
cubebism
cubital
   fossa, c.
   tunnel, c.
cuboidodigital reflex
cue
cued speech
cuffed tracheostomy tube
Cuignet's test
culmen (pl. culmina)
   monticuli, c.
culmina (pl. of culmen)
cult
cultism
culture-bound syndrome
culture shock
culture-specific
cunei (pl. of cuneus)
cuneiform
cuneus (pl. cunei)
cunnilingus
Cuprimine
cupulolithiasis
cupulometry
curare
curaremimetic
curarization
curse
cursive epilepsy

curvature
curve
CUSA (Cavitron ultrasonic aspirator)
Cushing's disease
Cushing's law
Cushing's medulloblastoma
Cushing's phenomenon
Cushing's response
Cushing's spatula
Cushing's spoon
Cushing's syndrome
cushingoid
   facies, c.
cutaneous nerve
cutdown
   catheter, c.
cutting bur
cutting current
cutting loop electrode
CVA (cerebrovascular accident OR costovertebral angle)
cyanose
cyanosed
cyanosis
cyanotic
   crisis, c.
cybernetics
cyberphilia
cyberphobia
Cybex test
cycle
cyclencephalus
cyclic
   abulia, c.
   adenosine monophosphate (cAMP), c.
   guanosine monophosphate (cGMP), c.
cyclodamia
cyclophoria
cycloplegia
cycloplegic
cyclospasm
cyclothyme
cyclothymia
cyclothymiac
cyclothymic
cyclothymosis

cyclotropia
cycrimine hydrochloride
Cylert
cylindrodendrite
cymbocephaly
cynanthropy
cynic spasm
cynomania
cynophobia
Cyon's experiment
cypridophobia
cypriphobia
Cyriax's syndrome
cyrtosis
cystencephalus
cysticercosis

cystometrogram
cystometry
cystoneuralgia
cystoplegia
cystosarcoma
cystospasm
cytheromania
cytoarchitectonics
cytoarchitecture
cytodistal
cytogenetic
cytomegalovirus (CMV)
cyton
cytoskeletal
cytotoxic
cytotoxicity

Additional entries

D

Daae's disease
DaCosta's syndrome
dacnomania
dactylocampsodynia
dactylography
dactylogryposis
dactylology
dactylospasm
daily living skills
Dalgan
Dalmane
Dalrymple's sign
daltonism
Dana posterior rhizotomy
dance
dancing chorea
dancing disease
dancing mania
Dandy nerve hook
Dandy scalp hemostat
Dandy scissors
Dandy ventriculostomy
Dandy-Cairns brain needle
Dandy-Cairns ventricular needle
Dandy-Walker syndrome
Danlos' syndrome
Darco shoe
Darco splint
dark adaptation
Darkschevich's nucleus
Darkschewitsch's fibers
Darkschewitsch's nucleus
Darlodel
dartos muscle reflex
darwinian theory
darwinism
date rape
David's disease
Davidoff retractor
Davidsohn's sign
Davidson retractor
Davis conductor
Davis retractor

Davis spatula
Davis system
Dawson's encephalitis
Daxolin
day blindness
day terrors
daydream
dazzle reflex
DBI (development-at-birth index)
DCS (dorsal column stimulation OR stimulator)
de Andrade-MacNab occipitocervical arthrodesis
de Lange's syndrome
de Morsier's syndrome
de Musset's sign
de Quervain's disease
De Sanctis-Cacchione syndrome
deaf
  -mute, d.
  -mutism, d.
  point, d.
deafferentation
deafness
  acoustic trauma d.
  Alexander's d.
  apoplectiform d.
  aviator's d.
  bass d.
  boilermaker's d.
  central d.
  cerebral d.
  ceruminous d.
  conduction d.
  cortical d.
  functional d.
  high frequency d,
  hysterical d.
  labyrinthine d.
  Michel's d.
  midbrain d.
  Mondini's d.
  music d.

deafness *(continued)*
nerve d.
neural d.
occupational d.
organic d.
ototoxic d.
pagetoid d.
paradoxic d.
perceptive d.
postlingual d.
prelingual d.
psychic d.
Scheibe's d.
sensorineural d.
tone d.
toxic d.
vascular d.
word d.
dealcoholization
death
death with dignity
debilitating
debility
debrancher glycogen storage disease
Debre-Semelaigne syndrome
debris
debulk
debulking
deburring
Decadron
decerebellation
decerebrate
posturing, d.
rigidity, d.
decerebration
decerebrize
decibel
decidophobia
decision-making
deck plate
Decker pituitary rongeur
deckplatte
declinator
decline
declive
monticuli cerebelli, d.

declivis
decompensation
sickness, d.
decomposition of movement
decompress
decompression
cerebral d.
nerve d.
spinal cord, d. of
suboccipital d.
subtemporal d.
decompression laminectomy
decompression sickness
decompressive laminectomy
deconditioning
decorticate posturing
decortication
decrement
decremental
decrementing response
decubitus
position, d.
decursus
fibrarum cerebralium, d.
decussate
decussatio (pl. decussationes)
decussation
Forel's d.
fountain d. of Meynert
decussationes (pl. of decussatio)
decussorium
dedolation
de-efferented state
DEEG (depth electroencephalogram)
deep
middle cerebral vein, d.
pain, d.
palpation, d.
peroneal nerve d.
sleep d.
temporal nerve d.
tendon reflexes (DTRs) d.
defatigation
defecalgesiophobia
defecation syncope
defect

defective
  insight, d.
  judgment, d.
  recent memory, d.
  remote memory, d.
defeminization
defense
  mechanism, d.
  psychoneurosis, d.
  reflex, d.
deferred limitation
deferred shock
deficiency
deficit
deflect
deflection
deformation
deforming
deformity
degeneracy
degenerate
degenerated intervertebral disk
degeneration
  alcoholic cerebellar d.
  axonal d.
  Holmes' d.
  spongiform d.
  striatonigral d.
  wallerian d.
degenerative
  changes, d.
  disease, d.
  disk disease, d.
  tic, d.
degenere
degenitalize
degustation
dehumanization
dehypnotize
Deiters' tract
deja entendu
deja eprouve
deja fait
deja degenere
deja pense
deja raconte

deja vecu
deja voulu
deja vu
dejected
dejection
dejecture
Dejerine's disease
Dejerine's sign
Dejerine's syndrome
Dejerine's type
Dejerine-Klumpke paralysis
Dejerine-Klumpke syndrome
Dejerine-Landouzy dystrophy
Dejerine-Landouzy type
Dejerine-Lichtheim phenomenon
Dejerine-Roussy syndrome
Dejerine-Sottas atrophy
Dejerine-Sottas disease
Dejerine-Sottas syndrome
Deklene
de la Camp's sign
delayed sleep phase syndrome
delimitation
delinquency
delinquent
deliquium
  animi, d.
delire
  de toucher, d.
deliria (pl. of delirium)
deliriant
delirifacient
delirious
delirium (pl. deliria)
  acute d.
  alcoholic d.
  alcoholicum, d.
  alcohol withdrawal d.
  chronic d.
  constantium, d.
  epilepticum, d.
  exhaustion d.
  febrile d.
  lingual d.
  low d.
  mussitans, d.

delirium (pl. deliria) *(continued)*
    negation, d. of
    persecution, d. of
    partial d.
    senile d.
    schozophrenoides, d.
    sine delirio, d.
    toxic d.
    traumatic d.
    tremens, (DT), d.
delta activity
    intermittent rhythmic d.
    polymorphic d.
delta rhythm
delta sleep
delta wave
delusion
    being controlled, d. of.
    bizarre d.
    control, d. of
    depressive d.
    encapsulated d.
    expansive d.
    fixed d.
    fleeting d.
    fragmentary d.
    grandeur, d. of
    grandiose d.
    mood-congruent d.
    mood-incongruent d.
    negation, d. of
    nihilistic d.
    paranoid d.
    persecution, d. of
    persecutory d.
    poverty, d. of
    reference, d. of
    somatic d.
    systematized d.
    unsystematized d.
de lunatico inquirendo
delusional
    state, d.
demarcation
DeMartel scissors
demasculinization

dematerialize
dement
demented
dementia
    alcoholic d.
    apoplectic d.
    Alzheimer's d.
    atherosclerotic d.
    axial d.
    Binswanger's d.
    cortical d.
    Creutzfeldt-Jakob d.
    dialysis d.
    epileptic d.
    Huntington d.
    hydrocephalic d.
    multi-infarct d.
    myoclonica, d.
    paralytic d.
    paralytica, d.
    paranoides, d.
    paretic d.
    Parkinson's d.
    Pick's d.
    postfebrile d.
    postpump d.
    praecox, d.
    praesenilis, d.
    presenile d.
    primary degenerative d.
    progressive d.
    pugilistica, d.
    semantic d.
    senile d.
    static d.
    syphilitic d.
    terminal d.
    toxic d.
    Wernicke's d.
dementing process
Demianoff's sign
demoniac
demoniacal
demonic
demonism
demonology

demonomania
demonophobia
demorphinization
Demser
demutization
demyelinate
demyelinating disease
demyelination
demyelinization
denarcotize
dendraxon
dendric
dendriceptor
dendrite
dendritic lesion
dendrodendritic
dendron
dendrophagocytosis
denervate
denervation
denial
denial and isolation
Denis Browne clubfoot splint
Denis Browne talipes hobble splint
Dennie-Marfan syndrome
Dennyson cervical brace
Dens view
dense
    hemiparesis, d.
    hemiplegia, d.
    paralysis, d.
    paresis, d.
density
dental dissector
dental roll
dentaphone
dentate ligament
Denver Development Screening Test
Denver hydrocephalus shunt
Denver peritoneal venous shunt
deossification
deoxyribonucleic acid (DNA)
Depakene
Depakote
dependence
    alcohol d.

dependence *(continued)*
    psychoactive substance d.
    substance d.
dependency
dependent
depersonalization
depersonalize
depolarization
depolarize
depolarizer
depravation
depraved
deprenyl
depressant
depressed
    fracture, d.
    fragment, d.
    mood, d.
depression
    agitated d.
    anaclitic d.
    bipolar d.
    endogenous d.
    involutional d.
    major d.
    neurotic d.
    pacchionian d.
    postdormital d.
    postpartum d.
    psychoneurotic d.
    psychotic d.
    reactive d.
    retarded d.
    situational d.
    unipolar d.
depressive
    equivalent, d.
    neurosis, d.
    psychosis, d.
    reaction, d.
depressomotor
depressor nerve
depressor reflex
deprivation
    emotional d.
    maternal d.

deprivation *(continued)*
    sensory d.
    thought d.
deprive
deprogramming
depth electrode
depth electroencephalogram (DEEG)
depth electrography
depth psychology
DePuy head halter
derailment
deranencephalia
deranged
derangement
Dercum's disease
derealization
dereism
dereistic
dereistic
    thinking, d.
derencephalocele
derencephalus
derivation
dermatalgia
dermatodynia
dermatoglyphics
dermatomal rule
dermatome
dermatomic area
dermatomyositis
dermatoneurology
dermatophobia
dermatopolyneuritis
dermoid
dermoneurotropic
D'Errico bur
D'Errico chisel
D'Errico perforator drill
D'Errico retractor
D'Errico skull trephine
D'Errico spatula
D'Errico-Adson retractor
DeSanctis-Cacchione syndrome
Descemet's membrane
desecration
desensitization

desensitization *(continued)*
    systematic d.
desensitize
desexualize
desiccant
desiccate
desiccation
desipramine
desmalgia
Desmarres' law
desmocranium
desmodynia
desmoid
    tumor, d.
desmoma
Desoxyn
d'Espine's sign
D-spine (dorsal spine)
destructive
desynapsis
desynchronization
desynchronized sleep
detached
    mood, d.
detachment
detain
detention
determinism
    psychic d.
detox (detoxification)
detoxed (detoxified)
detoxification
detoxify
detrusor instability
detrusor muscle
devasation
development
    arrested d.
    cognitive d.
    psychosexual d.
    psychosocial d.
development-at-birth index (DBI)
developmental
    age, d.
    anomaly, d.
    arrest, d.

developmental *(continued)*
   defect, d.
   disorder, d.
   milestones, d.
   stage, d.
Devereaux Rating Scale
deviant
   sexual d.
deviant behavior
deviated
deviation
Devic's disease
Devic's syndrome
DeVilbiss cranial rongeur
DeVilbiss cranial trephine
devious
devitalization
devitalize
DeWald spinal appliance
Dewar-Harris paralysis
dexamethasone
   suppression test, d.
Dexedrine
dexterity
dextrad
dextral
dextrality
dextraural
dextrocerebral
dextrocular
dextrocularity
dextromanual
dextropedal
dextrophobia
dextroposition
dextrorotoscoliosis
dextroscoliosis
dextrosinistral
Dextrostix
dezocine
DHE 45 (dihydroergotamine)
diabetes
diabetic
   acidosis, d.
   coma, d.
   myelopathy, d.

diabetic *(continued)*
   neuritis, d.
   neuropathy, d.
   paraplegia, d.
   puncture, d.
   retinopathy, d.
   tabes, d.
diabolic
diabolism
diacele
diadochocinesia
diadochocinetic
diadochokinesia
diadochokinesis
diadochokinetic
diagonal band of Broca
diagraph
dialysis
   dementia, d.
   dysequilibrium syndrome, d.
dialytic
dialyze
diameter
diametrical
diametrically opposite
diamond bur
Diamox
Diana complex
dianoetic
diaphemetric
diaphragma
   sellae, d.
diapophysis
diaschisis
diastaltic
diastatic skull fracture
diastematocrania
diastematomyelia
diastomyelia
diastrophic
diataxia
   cerebral d.
   cerebralis infantilis, d.
diathermal
diathermy
   microwave d.

diathermy *(continued)*
    shortwave d.
    ultra-shortwave d.
diathesis
diathetic
diaxon
diazepam
DIC (disseminated intravascular coagulation)
dichromacy
dichromatopsia
dichotomy
Dickson paralysis
Didronel
diencephalic
    syndrome, d.
diencephalohypophysial
diencephalon
differentiation
diffuse idiopathic skeletal hyperostosis (DISH)
diffuse meningiomatosis
DiGeorge syndrome
Dighton-Adair syndrome
digit retention
digital reflex
digital subtraction angiography (DSA)
Digitron
diglossia
DiGuglielmo disease
dihydroergotamine (DHE 45)
Dilantin
dilantinization
dilantinize
dilated pupils
dildo
DILE (drug-induced lupus erythematosus)
dilemma
dimenhydrate
diminished
    capacity, d.
    reflexes, d.
Dimitri's disease
DIMOAD (diabetes insipidus, diabetes mellitus, optic atrophy, deafness)
dineuric

dinomania
diocoele
Diogenes syndrome
diogenism
diopsimeter
diparesis
diphasic meningoencephalitis virus
diphenhydramine
diphonia
diphtheroid
diphthongia
diplacusia
diplacusis
    binaural d.
    disharmonic d.
    echo d.
    monaural d.
diplegia
    atonic-astatic d.
    facial d.
    infantile d.
    mastication d.
    spastic d.
diploe
diploetic
diploic
diplomyelia
diploneural
diplophonia
diplopia
diplopiaphobia
dipsomania
dipsopathy
dipsophobia
dipsosis
dipstick test
direct
    consensual light reflex, d. and light reflex, d.
    reflex, d.
    response, d.
directionality
director
dirigomotor
disability
disabled

disabling
Discase
discharge
disci (pl. of discus)
discogenic
discoid
discography
discoidectomy
disconjugate
   gaze, d.
disconjugation
disconnected
disconnection
   syndromes, d.
discopathy
   traumatic d.
discrete
   lesion, d.
discrimination
   one-point d.
   tonal d.
   two-point d.
discus (pl. disci)
disdiaclast
disdiadochokinesia
disease
   Acosta's d.
   Adams' d.
   Adams-Stokes d.
   Addison's d.
   Akureyri d.
   Albers-Schonberg d.
   Alexander's d.
   Alper's d.
   Alzheimer's d.
   Andes d.
   Apert's d.
   Apert-Crouzon d.
   Aran-Duchenne d.
   Armstrong's d.
   Australian X d.
   aviator's d.
   Azorean d.
   Baastrup's d.
   Ballet's d.
   Balo's d.

disease *(continued)*
   Bamberger's d.
   Basedow's d.
   Batten d.
   Batten-Mayou d.
   Bayle's d.
   Beard's d.
   Bekhterev's d.
   Bergeron's d.
   Berlin's d.
   Bernhardt's d.
   Bernhardt-Roth d.
   Bilderbeck's d.
   Billroth's d.
   Binswanger's d.
   Blocq's d.
   Bourneville's d.
   brancher glycogen storage d.
   bronzed d.
   Brown-Symmers d.
   Bruck's d.
   Brushfield-Wyatt d.
   Caffey's d.
   Calvare's d.
   Camurati-Engelmann d.
   Canavan's d.
   Canavan-van Bogaert-Bertrand d.
   central core d. of muscle
   Chagas' d.
   Chagas-Cruz d.
   Charcot's d.
   Charcot-Marie-Tooth d.
   Cherchevski's d.
   Cotugno's d.
   Creutzfeldt-Jakob d.
   Crigler-Najjar d.
   Crocq's d.
   Crouzon's d.
   Cruveilhier's d.
   Cruz-Chagas d.
   Cushing's d.
   cytomegalic inclusion d.
   Daae's d.
   David's d.
   debrancher glycogen storage d.
   Dejerine's d.

disease *(continued)*
    Dejerine-Sottas d.
    demyelinating d.
    de Quervain's d.
    Dercum's d.
    Devic's d.
    Di Guglielmo d.
    Dimitri's d.
    Down's d.
    Dubini's d.
    Dubois' d.
    Duchenne's d.
    Duchenne-Aran d.
    Duchenne-Griesinger d.
    Dupre's d.
    Durante's d.
    Economo's d.
    Edsall's d.
    Erb's d.
    Erb-Charcot d.
    Erb-Goldflam d.
    Erb-Landouzy d.
    Eulenburg's d.
    extensor process d.
    extrapyramidal d.
    Fabry's d.
    Farber d.
    Feer's d.
    Flajani's d.
    Flatau-Schilder d.
    Forestier d.
    Fothergill's d.
    Frankl Hochwart's d.
    Friedreich's d.
    Furstner's d.
    Gamstorp's d.
    Gaucher d.
    Gerhardt's d.
    Gerlier's d.
    Gilles de la Tourette's d.
    Glanzmann's d.
    glycogen storage d.
    Goldflam's d.
    Goldflam-Erb d.
    Graves' d.
    Greenfield's d.

disease *(continued)*
    Guinon's d.
    Gull's d.
    H d.
    Hammond's d.
    Hartnup d.
    Hashimoto's d.
    Heine-Medin d.
    heredodegenerative d.
    Hodgkin's d.
    Horton's d.
    Hunt's d.
    Huntington's d.
    Hutchinson-Gilford d.
    hydrocephaloid d.
    Iceland d.
    Jaffe-Lichtenstein d.
    Jakob's d.
    Jakob-Creutzfeldt d.
    Janet's d.
    Jansky-Bielschowsky d.
    Joseph d.
    jumping d.
    Kalischer's d.
    Kashin-Beck d.
    Kienbock's d.
    Klippel's d.
    Koshevnikoff's d.
    Krabbe's d.
    Krishaber's d.
    Kufs' d.
    Kugelberg-Welander d.
    Kummell's d.
    Kummell-Verneuil d.
    Lafora's d.
    Landry's d.
    Lasegue's d.
    Leber's d.
    Legal's d.
    Leigh's d.
    Lichtheim's d.
    Little's d.
    Lobstein's d.
    Lorain's d.
    Lowe's d.
    Lyme d.

disease *(continued)*
   Machado-Joseph d.
   maple syrup urine d.
   March's d.
   Marchiafava-Bignami d.
   Marie-Strumpell d.
   Marie-Tooth d.
   Marsh's d.
   Meniere's d.
   Menkes' d.
   mental d.
   Merzbacher-Pelizaeus d.
   Mills' d.
   Minamata d.
   Minor's d.
   Mitchell's d.
   mixed connective tissue d.
   Mobius' d.
   Monge's d.
   Morel-Kraepelin d.
   Morvan's d.
   Moschcowitz's d.
   motor neuron d.
   mountain d.
   moyamoya d.
   Mozer's d.
   multicore d.
   Munchmeyer's d.
   Murray Valley d.
   Niemann d.
   Niemann-Pick d.
   Norrie's d.
   Oguchi's d.
   Oppenheim's d.
   Paas' d.
   Parkinson's d.
   Parrot's d.
   Pel-Ebstein d.
   Pelizaeus-Merzbacher d.
   Pick's d.
   Pott's d.
   pulseless d.
   Raynaud's d.
   Recklinghausen's d.
   Reed-Hodgkin d.
   Refsum d.

disease *(continued)*
   Rendu-Osler-Weber d.
   Romberg's d.
   Rot's d.
   Rot-Bernhardt d.
   Roth's d.
   Roth-Bernhardt d.
   Rust's d.
   Sachs' d.
   Schilder's d.
   Schmorl's d.
   Scholz's d.
   Schuller's d.
   Schuller-Christian d.
   Seitelberger's d.
   Selter's d.
   shuttlemaker's d.
   sickle cell d.
   Simmonds' d.
   Spielmeyer-Sjogren d.
   Spielmeyer-Vogt d.
   Steiner's d.
   Steinert's d.
   Sternberg's d.
   Strumpell's d.
   Sturge's d.
   Sturge-Weber-Dimitri d.
   swineherd's d.
   Takayasu's d.
   Talma's d.
   Tay-Sachs d.
   thalassemia-sickle cell d.
   Thomsen's d.
   Tooth's d.
   Tourette's d.
   Unverricht's d.
   Verse's d.
   vibration d.
   Vogt's d.
   Vogt-Spielmeyer d.
   Voltolini's d.
   von Economo's d.
   von Hippel d.
   von Hippel-Landau d.
   von Recklinhausen's d.
   Vrolik's d.

disease *(continued)*
   Wartenberg's d.
   wasting d.
   Weber's d.
   Werdnig-Hoffman d.
   Wernicke's d.
   Whytt's d.
   white matter d.
   Wilson's d.
   Winckel's d.
   Winkelman's d.
   Ziehen-Oppenheim d.
disease-modifying antirheumatic drugs
   (DMARDs)
disengagement
disequilibration
disequilibrium
DISH (diffuse idiopathic skeletal hyperostosis)
   syndrome, D.
disharmony
DISHEVEL (dependent, immature, seduc-
   tive, histrionic, egocentric, vain,
   emotionally labile)
disimpaction
disinhibit
disinhibition
disintegration
disjunction
disjunctive nystagmus
disk
   bulging d.
   cervical d.
   crescent-shaped d.
   herniated d.
   intervertebral d.
   protruding d.
   ruptured d.
   slipped d.
disk excision
disk extrusion
disk fragment
disk grabber
disk herniation
disk material
disk protrusion

disk rupture
disk space
disk space narrowing
Diskard head halter
diskectomy
   cervical d.
   Cloward fusion d.
   lumbar d.
   microlumbar d.
   Williams d.
diskiform
diskitis
diskogenic
diskogram
diskography
   cervical d.
   lumbar d.
dislocation
disorder
   adjustment d.
   affective d.
   amnestic d.
   anxiety d.
   attention-deficit d.
   autistic d.
   avoidant d.
   behavior d.
   bipolar d.
   body dysmorphic d.
   character d.
   conduct d.
   conversion d.
   cyclothymic d.
   delusional d.
   depersonalization d.
   dissociative d.
   dysthymic d.
   emotional d.
   expressive d.
   factitious d.
   functional d.
   generalized anxiety d.
   identity d.
   induced psychotic d.
   intermittent explosive d.
   isolated explosive d.

disorder *(continued)*
   major mood d.
   manic-depressive d.
   mental d.
   mood d.
   multifactorial d.
   multiple personality d.
   obsessive-compulsive d.
   organic mental d.
   overanxious d.
   panic d.
   paranoid d.
   personality d.
   pervasive developmental d.
   post-traumatic stress d.
   psychoactive substance-induced organic mental d.
   psychoactive substance use d.
   psychogenic pain d.
   psychosexual d.
   psychosomatic d.
   receptive d.
   schizoaffective d.
   schizophrenic d.
   schizophreniform d.
   seasonal affective d.
   seasonal mood d.
   separation anxiety d.
   shared paranoid d.
   sleep terror d.
   sleepwalking d.
   somatization d.
   somatoform d.
   somatoform pain d.
   substance use d.
   Tourette's d.
   unipolar d.
disordered
   action of heart, d.
   sleep, d.
   thought process, d.
disorganization
disorganized
   schizophrenia, d.
disorientation
   spatial d.

disoriented
dispersonalization
displacement
disruption
disruptive
disseminated intravascular coagulation (DIC)
disseminated sclerosis
dissociated vertical divergence (DVD)
dissociation
   reaction, d.
dissociative
   disorder, d.
dissolution
dissonance
   cognitive d.
distal tingling on percussion (DTP)
distalward
distaxia
distorted
distortion
   parataxic d.
distortor
distractibility
distractible
distraction
   hook, d.
   rod, d.
distraught
distress
disturbance
   emotional d.
   sexual orientation d.
   transient situational d.
disturbed
disuse atrophy
disvolution
disvagation
Diulo
diurnal
divagation
diver's palsy
divergence
divergent
diving reflex
divisio (pl. divisiones)

divisiones (pl. of divisio)
divot
Dix-Hallpike test for nystagmus
Dixon-Mann sign
dizziness
dizzy spell
DMARDs (disease-modifying antirheumatic drugs)
DNA (deoxyribonucleic acid)
DNA-ploidy
dog-ear
dol
doll the eye
doll's eye movements
doll's eye sign
doll's head anesthesia
doll's head maneuver
doll's head phenomenon
dolor (pl. dolores)
    capitis, d.
    coxae, d.
    vagus, d.
dolores (pl. of dolor)
dolorific
dolorimeter
dolorimetry
domatophobia
dominance
dominant
    background activity, d.
    laterality, d.
dominate
domineering
domoic acid
Don Juanism
Donders' law
Donohue's syndrome
dopamine
dopaminergic
Dopar
Doppler
Doppler carotid ultrasound
Doppler color-flow
Doppler effect
Doppler ultrasonic angiogram
Doppler ultrasound

Dorello's canal
Doriden
dormifacient
dorophobia
dorsa (pl. of dorsum)
dorsad
dorsal
    column stimulation (DCS), d.
    column stimulator (DCS), d.
    fasciculus of Schutz, d.
    gray column, d.
    inertia posture, d.
    kyphosis, d.
    kyphotic curvature, d.
    motor nucleus, d.
    phthisis, d.
    raphe nucleus, d.
    reflex, d.
    root, d.
    root entry zone (DREZ), d.
    root ganglion, d.
    spinal nerve root, d.
    spine (D-spine), d.
    spinocerebellar tract, d.
    spinothalamic tract, d.
    vertebra, d.
    zone of His, d.
dorsalgia
dorsalis
dorsalward
dorsiduct
dorsiflex
dorsiflexion
dorsiflexors
dorsispinal
dorsocephalad
dorsocuboidal reflex
dorsodynia
dorsointercostal
dorsolateral
dorsolumbar
dorsomedian
dorsomesial
dorsonuchal
dorsum (pl. dorsa)
dotage

double
    bind, d.
    bubble flushing reservoir, d.
    -crush syndrome, d.
    depression, d.
    disharmonic hearing, d.
    floor, d.
    -lumen catheter, d.
    personality, d.
    simultaneous stimulation, d.
    -step gait, d.
    vision, d.
doubting insanity
doughnut headrest
dowager's hump
dowel
    cutter, d.
    dissector, d.
    spinal fusion, d.
doweling spondylolisthesis
Down's disease
Down's syndrome
downbeat jerk nystagmus
downbeat nystagmus
down-biting rongeur
Downey hemilaminectomy retractor
downgoing lumbar curette
downgoing toes
doxepin
Doyere's eminence
drag
drag-to gait
Drake clip
Dramamine
dramatism
dramatization
drapetomania
Draw-a-Bicycle test
Draw-a-Person test
drawn ankle clonus
dream
    analysis, d.
    anxiety attack, d.
    clairvoyant d.
    interpretation, d.
    sleep, d.

dream *(continued)*
    symbolism, d.
    veridical d.
    work, d.
dressing
    apraxia, d.
    stick, d.
DREZ (dorsal root entry zone)
DREZ lesion
drift
drill
    bit, d.
    guide, d.
    -out laminotomy, d.
drive
    aggressive d.
    sexual d.
    controls, d.
driver's thigh
driving response
dromedary hump
dromomania
dromophobia
dromotropic
dromotropism
droop
drooping
drop
    attack, d.
    foot d.
    hand d.
    phalangette, d.
    spell, d.
    wrist d.
dropsy of brain
drowsiness
drowsy state
drug
    abuse, d.
    addict, d.
    addiction, d.
    dependence, d.
    desensitization, d.
    holiday, d.
    -induced lupus erythematosus
        (DILE), d.

drug *(continued)*
  -induced paresis of accommodation, d.
  level, d.
  overdose, d.
  screen, d.
  -seeking behavior, d.
  toxicity, d.
  trafficking, d.
  use, d.
  withdrawal, d.
  -withdrawal insomnia, d.
drunkenness
DSA (digital subtraction angiography)
DSM (Diagnostic and Statistical Manual
  of Mental Disorders)
D-state sleep
DT (delirium tremens)
DTP (distal tingling on percussion)
DTRs (deep tendon reflexes)
dual diagnosis
dual personality
dualism
dualistic
Duane's retraction syndrome
Duane's syndrome
Dubini's chorea
Dubois' abscess
Dubois' method
DuBois-Reymond's law
Dubowitz criteria
Dubowitz scale
Duchenne's disease
Duchenne's muscular dystrophy
Duchenne's syndrome
Duchenne's type
Duchenne-Aran disease
Duchenne-Aran muscular atrophy
Duchenne-Aran type
Duchenne-Erb paralysis
Duchenne-Erb syndrome
Duchenne-Griesinger disease
Duchenne-Landouzy dystrophy
Duchenne-Landouzy type
duck waddle
Duckworth's phenomenon
Duckworth's sign

duct
DUI (driving under the influence)
dullness
dumb
  rabies, d.
dumbbell tumor
dumbness
Dumont jeweler's forceps
Duncan's ventricle
Dunn anterior spinal system
duoparental
duplex scan
duplication
Dupre's disease
Dupre's syndrome
Dupuytren's contracture
dura
  mater, d.
dural
  cul-de-sac, d.
  flap, d.
  membrane, d.
  plate, d.
  sac, d.
  space, d.
  tear, d.
duramatral
Duramorph
Durante's disease
duraplasty
Durck's nodes
Duret hemorrhage
Duret lesion
Durham's decision
duroarachnitis
durosarcoma
durotomy
duskiness
dusky
Duval's nucleus
DVD (dissociated vertical divergence)
Dwyer scoliosis cable
Dwyer screws
Dwyer spinal instrumentation
Dwyer-Wickham electrical stimulation
  system

dyad
dyadic
Dyke-Davidoff syndrome
dynamic
   splint, d.
dynamism
dynamogenesis
dynamogenic
dynamograph
dynamometer
   squeeze d.
dynamoneure
dynamopathic
dynamoscopy
dyne
dysacousia
dysacousis
dysacousma
dysacusis
dysadrenalism
dysanagnosia
dysantigraphia
dysaphia
dysarthria
   literalis, d.
   syllabaris spasmodica, d.
dysarthria-clumsy hand syndrome
dysarthric
dysarthrosis
dysautonomia
dysbasia
   angiosclerotica, d.
   angiospastica, d.
   lordotica progressiva, d.
   neurasthenica intermittens, d.
dysbulia
dysbulic
dyscalculia
dyscephaly
   mandibulo-oculofacial d.
dyschiasia
dyschiria
dyschondroplasia
dyschondrosteosis
dyschronism
dyscinesia

dyscoimesis
dyscontrol
dyscorticism
dysdiadochocinesia
dysdiadochocinetic
dysdiadochokinesia
dysdiadochokinetic
dysecoia
dysencephalia splanchnocystica
dysequilibrium
dyserethesia
dyserethism
dysergasia
dysergastric reaction
dysergia
dysesthesia
   auditory d.
   pedis, d.
dysesthetic
dysfunction
   minimal brain d.
   myofascial pain d.
dysgenesis
dysgenetic
dysgerminoma
dysgeusia
dysgnathia
dysgnosia
dysgrammatism
dysgraphia
dyskinesia
   algera, d.
   biliary d.
   intermittens, d.
   tardive d.
   uterine d.
dyskinetic
dyskoimesis
dyslalia
dyslexia
dyslexic
dyslogia
dysmegalopsia
dysmetria
dysmetropsia
dysmimia

dysmnesia
dysmnesic
dysmorphia
dysmorphic
    features, d.
dysmorphism
dysmorphophobia
dysmorphopsia
dysmorphosis
dysmyotonia
dysnomia
dysomnias
dysopia
    algera, d.
dysopsia
dysorexia
dysosmia
dysosteogenesis
dysostosis
    cleidocranial d.
    craniofacial d.
    mandibulofacial d.
    metaphyseal d.
    multiplex, d.
    Nager's acrofacial d.
    orodigitofacial d.
dyspareunia
dysphagia
dysphasia
dysphasic
dysphemia
dysphonia
    clericorum, d.
    spasmodic d.
dysphonic
dysphoretic
dysphoria
dysphoriant
dysphoric
dysphrasia
dysphylaxia
dysplastic
dysponesis
dyspragia
dyspraxia
    ideational d.

dyspraxia *(continued)*
    ideomotor d.
    innervatory d.
    limb-kinetic d.
dyspraxic
    reflex, d.
dysprosody
dysraphia
dysreflexia
    autonomic d.
    cerebral d.
    dysrhythmia d.
    electroencephalographic d.
dysrhythmic
dyssocial
dyssomnia
dysstasia
dysstatic
dyssymbolia
dyssymboly
dyssynergia
    cerebellaris myoclonica, d.
    cerebellaris progressiva, d.
dystasia
    hereditary ataxic d.
    Roussy-Levy hereditary ataxic d.
dystaxia
    agitans, d.
dystectia
dysthymia
dysthymic
    disorder, d.
dysthyreosis
dysthyroid
dysthyroidism
dystonia
    cranial d.
    deformans progressiva, d.
    lenticularis, d.
    musculorum deformans, d.
    tardive d.
    torsion d.
dystonic
dystrophia
    myotonica, d.
dystrophic

dystrophoneurosis
dystrophy
    adiposogenital d.
    autosomal-dominant distal d.
    Becker's d.
    Becker's muscular d.
    craniocarpotarsal d.
    Dejerine-Landouzy d.
    distal muscular d.
    Duchenne type muscular d.
    Duchenne-Landouzy d.
    Erb's d.
    facioscapulohumeral muscular d.
    Gowers type muscular d.
    infantile neuroaxonal d.
    Landouzy d.

dystrophy *(continued)*
    Landouzy-Dejerine d.
    Leyden-Mobius d.
    limb-girdle muscular d.
    muscular d.
    myotonic d.
    oculocerebrorenal d.
    oculopharyngeal d.
    progressive muscular d.
    pseudohypertrophic muscular d.
    reflex sympathetic d.
    scapulohumeral d.
    scapuloperoneal d.
    Simmerlin's d.
    tapetochoroidal d.
    thyroneural d

Additional entries

E

EAE (experimental allergic encephalomy-
    elitis)
EAN (experimental allergic neuritis)
ear-minded
ear oximeter
earlobe crease
early morning arousal
eastern equine encephalitis (EEE)
easy fatigability
Eaton-Lambert syndrome
Ebbinghaus' test
Eberle contracture release technique
ebonation
eburnated
eburnation
eccentric
eccentricity
eccentrochondroplasia
eccentro-osteochondrodysplasia
ecchordosis physaliphora
ecdemomania
ecdysiasm
ECG (electrocardiogram)
echo
    sign, e.
    -free space, e.
    -ranging, e.
ECHO (enteric cytopathogenic human or-
    phan) virus
echoacousia
echocardiography
echodense
echoencephalogram
echoencephalography
echogenic
echogenicity
echogram
echographia
echography
echokinesis
echolalia
echolalus
echolocation

Echols retractor
echolucent
echomatism
echomimia
echomotism
echopathy
echophotony
echophrasia
echopraxia
echopraxis
echovirus
ECI (electrocerebral inactivity)
EC-IC (extracranial-intracranial) bypass
Ecker's fissure
eclampsia
eclamptic
eclamptogenic
eclysis
ecmnesia
ecomania
Economo's disease
Economo's encephalitis
ecophobia
ecphoria
ecphorize
ecphory
ECS (electroconvulsive shock OR elec-
    trocerebral silence)
ecstasy
ecstatic
ECT (electroconvulsive therapy)
ectocinerea
ectocinereal
ectopic ACTH syndrome
edeomania
Edepryl
Edinger's law
Edinger-Westphal nucleus
edipism
edrophonium chloride
Edsall's disease
educable
educative

Edwards Personal Preference Schedule
Edwards' syndrome
EEA (electroencephalic audiometry)
EEA stapler
EEC syndrome
EEE (eastern equine encephalitis)
EEG (electroencephalogram)
effector field
effeminate
effemination
efferent
   nerve, e.
   neuron, e.
effort
   syndrome, e.
   training, e.
effortful processing
egersimeter
egersis
eggcrate mattress
ego
   -alien, e.
   -dystonic, e.
   -dystonic homosexuality, e.
   -id conflict, e.
   ideal, e.
   identity, e.
   instinct, e.
   -libido, e.
   strength, e.
   -syntonic, e.
   trip, e.
egocentric
egocentrism
egodystonic
egoism
egoistic suicide
egomania
egosyntonic
egotism
egotistical
egotropic
Ehlers-Danlos syndrome
Ehrenritter's ganglion
Eichhorst's atrophy
Eichhorst's type

eicosanoids
eidetic
   image, e.
eight-ball
eighth cranial nerve
EIWA (Escala Inteligencia Wechsler Para
   Adultes)
ejaculation
Ekbom syndrome
EKG (electrocardiogram)
ekiri
ekphorize
elaboration
elasticity
elation
Elavil
elbow jerk
elbow reflex
Eldepryl
Electra complex
electric
   light baker, e.
   shock, e.
   shock therapy (EST), e.
electrical stimulation
electroacupuncture
electroanalgesia
electrocardiogram (ECG or EKG)
electrocardiography
electrocautery
electrocerebral
   inactivity (ECI), e.
   silence (ECS), e.
electrocoagulation
electrocochleogram
electrocochleography
electrocontractility
electroconvulsive
   shock (ECS), e.
   therapy (ECT), e.
electrocorticogram
electrocorticography
electrocution
electrode
electrodiagnosis
electroejaculation

electroencephalic
  audiometry (EEA), e.
  response, e.
electroencephalogram (EEG)
  flat e.
  isoelectric e.
  normal waking e.
electroencephalograph
electroencephalography
electroencephaloscope
electroexcision
electrofocusing
electrogoniometer
electrogram
electrographic
  seizure, e.
electrography
electrogustometry
electrohemostasis
electrokinetic
electrolepsy
electrolyte
  balance, e.
  imbalance, e.
electromanometer
electromyogram (EMG)
electromyography
electron microscopy
electronarcosis
electroneurography
electroneurolysis
electroneuromyography
electronic voice
electronystagmogram
electronystagmography (ENG)
electro-oculogram (EOG)
electro-oculography
electro-olfactogram (EOG)
electrophysiologic
electrophysiology
electroplexy
electroretinogram (ERG)
electroscission
electrosection
electroshock
  therapy (EST), e.

electrosleep
electrospectrogram
electrospectrography
electrospinogram
electrostimulation
electrostriatogram
electrosurgery
electrothanasia
electrotherapeutic
electrotherapy
electrotomy
electrotonic
electrotonus
electrovagogram
electroversion
elephantiasis neuromatosa
eleuthromania
elevator
eleventh cranial nerve
elfin facies syndrome
ELISA (enzyme-linked immunosorbent
  assay)
Elliott's sign
ellipsis
Ellis-van Creveld syndrome
elopement
  precautions, e.
Elsberg cannula
Ely's sign
Ely's test
emasculate
emasculation
embolalia
embolectomy
emboli (pl. of embolus)
embolic
emboliform
embolism
embolization
embololalia
embolophrasia
embolus (pl. emboli)
embrace reflex
embryogenesis
Emery-Dreifuss dystrophy
EMG (electromyogram)

EMI (Electric and Musical Industries)
  brain scanner, E.
  scan, E.
eminence
eminentia (pl. eminentiae)
eminentiae (pl. of eminentia)
emissary vein
emission
  tomography (ET), e.
emotiomotor
emotiomuscular
emotion
emotional
  anesthesia, e.
  headache, e.
  instability, e.
  insulation, e.
  lability, e.
  need, e.
  overlay, e.
  response, e.
  stability, e.
emotionalism
emotive
  imagery, e.
emotivity
empathic
empathize
empathy
empirical
emprosthotonos
empty delta sign
empty nest syndrome
empty sella syndrome
empyema
empyematic scoliosis
EMS (eosinophilia-myalgia syndrome)
EMV (eyes, motor, voice) grading of
  Glasgow Coma Scale
en bloc
en cuirasse
en face
en mass
en plaque
enabler
encapsulated

encephalalgia
encephalatrophy
encephalauxe
encephalemia
encephalic
  trunk, e.
encephalitic
encephalitides (pl. of encephalitis)
encephalitis (pl. encephalitides)
  A, e.
  acute demyelinating e.
  acute disseminated e.
  acute necrotizing e.
  Australian X e.
  B, e.
  benign myalgic e.
  Binswanger's e.
  C, e.
  California e.
  Central European e.
  chronic subcortical e.
  cortical e.
  Dawson's e.
  eastern equine e.
  Economo's e.
  epidemic e.
  equine e.
  forest-spring e.
  Hayem's e.
  hemorrhagic e.
  hemorrhagic arsphenamine c.
  herpes simplex e.
  herpetic e.
  hyperplastica, e.
  Ilheus e.
  infantile e.
  influenzal e.
  Japanese B e.
  lead e.
  Leichtenstern's e.
  lethargic e.
  measles e.
  mumps e.
  Murray Valley e.
  neonatorum, e.
  periaxialis concentrica, e.

encephalitis (pl. encephalitides)
(continued)
  periaxialis diffusa, e.
  postinfectious e.
  postvaccinal e.
  Powassan e.
  purulent e.
  pyogenic e.
  Russian autumnal e.
  Russian endemic e.
  Russian autumn-spring e.
  Russian spring-summer e.
  Russian tick-borne e.
  Russian vernal e.
  St. Louis e.
  Schilder's e.
  Semliki Forest e.
  siderans, e.
  subacute inclusion body e.
  subcorticalis chronica, e.
  summer e.
  suppurative e.
  tick-borne e.
  toxoplasmic e.
  van Bogaert e.
  Venezuelan equine e.
  vernal e.
  vernoestival e.
  Vienna e.
  von Economo's e.
  western equine e.
  West Nile e.
  woodcutter's e.
encephalitogen
encephalitogenic
encephalization
encephaloarteriography
encephalocele
encephalocentesis
encephaloclastic
encephalocoele
encephalocystocele
encephalodialysis
encephalodysplasia
encephalofacial angiomatosis
encephalogram

encephalographic
  lead, e.
  tracing, e.
encephalography
encephaloid
encephalolith
encephalology
encephaloma
encephalomalacia
encephalomeningitis
encephalomeningocele
encephalomeningopathy
encephalomere
encephalometer
encephalomyelitis
  acute disseminated e.
  benign myalgic e.
  equine e.
  granulomatous e.
  parainfectious e.
  postinfectious e.
  postvaccinal e.
  toxoplasmic e.
  viral e.
  virus e.
encephalomyelocele
encephalomyeloneuropathy
encephalomyelopathy
  postinfection e.
  postvaccinial e.
  subacute necrotizing e.
encephalomyeloradiculitis
encephalomyeloradiculoneuritis
encephalomyeloradiculopathy
encephalomyocarditis
encephalon
encephalonarcosis
encephalopathia
  alcoholica, e.
encephalopathic
encephalopathy
  biliary e.
  bilirubin e.
  boxer's e.
  demyelinating e.
  dialysis e.

encephalopathy *(continued)*
  hepatic e.
  hypernatremic e.
  hypertensive e.
  hypoglycemic e.
  lead e.
  metabolic e.
  myoclonic e. of childhood
  portosystemic e.
  postanoxic e.
  posttraumatic e.
  progressive dialysis e.
  progressive subcortical e.
  punch-drunk e.
  saturnine e.
  spongiform e.
  subacute necrotizing e.
  subacute spongiform e.
  subcortical arteriosclerotic e.
  transmissible spongiform e.
  traumatic e.
  Wernicke's e.
encephalophyma
encephalopsy
encephalopsychosis
encephalopuncture
encephalopyosis
encephalorachidian
encephaloradiculitis
encephalorrhagia
encephalosclerosis
encephaloscope
encephaloscopy
encephalosepsis
encephalosis
encephalospinal
encephalothlipsis
encephalotome
encephalotomy
encephalotrigeminal angiomatosis
enchondroma
enchondromatosis
enchondromatous
enchondrosarcoma
enchondrosis
encopresis

encounter group
encounter therapy
encroachment
end-brush
end-bulb
end-feet
end-flake
end-gaze nystagmus
end-organ
end-plate
  potential (EPP), e.
end-point
  nystagmus, e.
  tremor, e.
endarterectomized
endarterectomy
endbrain
ending
  annulospiral e.
  club e. of Bartelmez
  encapsulated nerve e.
  epilemmal e.
  flower-spray e.
  free nerve e.
  grape e.
  nerve e.
endocarditis
endocranial
endocraniosis
endocranitis
endocranium
endocrinasthenia
endocrinotropic
endogenous
endomorph
endomorphic
endomorphy
endoneural
endoneurial
endoneuritis
endoneurium
endoneurolysis
endoperineuritis
endophasia
endorphin
endothelioma

endotracheal (ET)
enervation
ENG (electronystagmography)
English cane
engram
enhanced
enhancement
enissophobia
enkephalin
enkephalinergic
enomania
enosimania
enorphin
Enroth's sign
entasia
enteric cytopathogenic human orphan
   (ECHO) virus
enterovirus 70 and 71
entheomania
enthesitis
enthlasis
entorbital fissure
entrapment
   neuropathy, e.
enucleate
enucleation
enuresis
envious
environment
environmental stress
envy
EOG (electro-oculogram or electro-
   olfactogram)
EOM (extraocular muscles or movements)
EOMI (extraocular muscles or movements intact)
eonism
eosinophilia-myalgia syndrome (EMS)
EP (evoked potential)
epencephalic
epencephalon
ependopathy
ependyma
ependymal
ependymitis

ependymitis *(continued)*
   granularis, e.
ependymoblast
ependymoblastoma
ependymocyte
ependymocytoma
ependymoma
ependymopathy
ephapse
ephaptic
   transmission, e.
ephedrine sulfate
epi (epinephrine)
epicentral
epicoele
epicranial aponeurosis
epicranium
epicranius muscle
epicritic
   pain, e.
epidermoid
epidermoidoma
epidural
   bleed, e.
   blood patch, e.
   hematoma, e.
   hemorrhage, e.
   space, e.
epidurography
epilemma
epilemmal
epilepsia
   cursiva, e.
   gravior, e.
   major, e.
   minor, e.
   mitior, e.
   nutans, e.
   partialis continua, e.
   procursiva, e.
   rotatoria, e.
   tarda, e.
epilepsy
   abdominal e.
   acquired e.
   activated e.

epilepsy *(continued)*
    automatic e.
    Bravais-jacksonian e.
    catamenial e.
    cortical e.
    corticoreticular e.
    cryptogenic e.
    cursive e.
    diurnal e.
    essential e.
    focal e.
    gelastic e.
    generalized e.
    generalized flexion e.
    genetic e.
    grand mal e.
    haut mal e.
    hysterical e.
    idiopathic e.
    Jackson's e.
    jacksonian e.
    juvenile myoclonic e.
    Koshevnikoff's e.
    Lafora's type of e.
    larval e.
    laryngeal e.
    latent e.
    limbic e.
    localized e.
    major e.
    matutinal e.
    menstrual e.
    minor e.
    musicogenic e.
    myoclonus e.
    nocturnal e.
    organic e.
    petit mal e.
    photogenic e.
    photosensitive e.
    physiologic e.
    posttraumatic e.
    primary e.
    procursive e.
    progressive familial myoclonic e.
    psychic e.

epilepsy *(continued)*
    psychomotor e.
    reflex e.
    rolandic e.
    secondary e.
    sensory e.
    serial e.
    sleep e.
    spinal e.
    sylvian e.
    symptomatic e.
    tardy e.
    television e.
    temporal lobe e.
    thalamic e.
    tonic e.
    traumatic e.
    uncinate e.
    Unverricht-Lundborg type e.
epileptic
    equivalent, e.
    focus, e.
    fugue, e.
    seizure, e.
epileptiform
    convulsion, e.
    discharge, e.
    pattern, e.
epileptogenic
epileptogenous
epileptoid
    personality, e.
epileptologist
epileptology
epileptosis
epiloia
epimere
epinephrine
epinephros
epineural
    covering, e.
epineurial
    neurorrhaphy, e.
epineurium
epineurosis
epipial

episode
    acute schizophrenic e.
    hypomanic e.
    hypomanic schizophrenic e.
    major depressive e.
    manic e.
    psycholeptic e.
episodic
    dyscontrol, e.
    memory, e.
epispinal
epistemology
episthotonos
epistropheus
epitela
epithalamic
epithalamus
epithelioceptor
epithelioma
    myxomatodes psammosum, e.
epithelium
epitonic
EPP (end-plate potential)
EPSP (excitatory postsynaptic period)
Epstein curette
Epstein-Barr virus
Equanil
equilibration
equilibratory ataxia
equilibrium
    potential, e.
equine encephalomyelitis
equine gait
equinophobia
equivocal
ER (evoked response)
ERA (evoked response audiometry)
Erb's atrophy
Erb's disease
Erb's muscular dystrophy
Erb's palsy
Erb's paralysis
Erb's phenomenon
Erb's point
Erb's sign
Erb's syndrome

Erb's waves
Erb-Charcot disease
Erb-Duchenne palsy
Erb-Duchenne paralysis
Erb-Goldflam disease
Erb-Landouzy disease
Erb-Zimmerlin type
Erben's reflex
Erben's sign
erectile dysfunction
erection
erector muscle of spine
erector spinae
eremophobia
erethism
erethismic
erethisophrenia
erethistic
erethitic
ereuthrophobia
ERG (electroretinogram)
ergasia
ergasiatrics
ergasiatry
ergasiology
ergasiomania
ergasiophobia
ergasthenia
ergodynamograph
ergoesthesiograph
ergograph
ergomania
ergometer
ergonomics
ergophobia
ergostat
ergotamine tartrate
ergot poisoning
ergotism
Erhard's test
Erhard Seminars Training (EST)
Erichsen's sign
Erichsen's spine
erogenous
    zone, e.
erotic

erotic *(continued)*
  pyrolagnia, e.
  zoophilism, e.
eroticism
  anal e.
  oral e.
eroticomania
erotism
  anal e.
  muscle e.
  oral e.
erotize
erotogeneis
erotogenic
erotographomania
erotology
erotomania
erotomaniac
erotopath
erotopathy
erotophobia
erotopsychic
erotosexual
errors of commission
errors of omission
erythredema polyneuropathy
erythremia
erythromania
erythromelalgia
erythrophobia
erythroprosopalgia
escape phenomenon
escapist
eschar
Escala Inteligencia Wechsler Para Adultos (EIWA)
Escherich's sign
Eskalith
esophoria
esotericism
esotropia
ESP (extrasensory perception)
essential epilepsy
essential tremor
Essex-Lopresti axial fixation

EST (electric shock or electroshock therapy)
EST (Erhard Seminars Training)
Esterman visual function score
esthematology
esthesia
esthesic
esthesiogenic
esthesiology
esthesiomania
esthesiometer
esthesioneure
esthesioneuroblastoma
esthesioneurosis
esthesionosus
esthesiophysiology
esthesioscopy
esthesodic
esthetic
estheticokinetic
ET (endotracheal)
  catheter, E.
  tube, E.
etat vermoulu
ethanol
  abuse, e.
ethanolism
etheromania
ethyl alcohol (EtOH)
ethylene vinyl alcohol (EVAL)
EtOH (ethanol or ethyl alcohol)
  abuse, E.
  intake, E.
euadrenocorticism
euesthesia
eugnosia
eukinesia
eukinetic
Eulenberg's disease
Eulenberg's syndrome
eumetria
eunoia
eunuchoid habitus
euosmia
euphoretic
euphoria

euphoriant
euphoric
euphorigenic
euphoristic
eupnea
eupneic
eupractic
eupraxia
eupraxic
euryon
eusthenia
euthymism
euthyroid
euthyroidism
EVAL (ethylene vinyl alcohol)
evasion
eventration
eversion
eviration
evocation
evoked
evoked potential (EP)
    brain stem auditory e.
    scalp-recorded somatosensory e.
    somatosensory e.
    spinal somatosensory e.
    visual e.
evoked response (ER)
    auditory e.
    sensory e.
    visual e.
evoked response audiometry (ERA)
Ewing's sarcoma
exaltation
exanimation
excalation
excerebration
exchange transfusion
excitability
excitable
excitant
excitation
excitatory
    postsynaptic period (EPSP), e.
    postsynaptic potential (EPSP), e.
excitomotor

excitomotory
excitomuscular
excrescence
exencephalus
exencephaly
exercise tolerance
exertional vertigo
exhibitionism
exhibitionist
exhilarant
exhilaration
existential
    analysis, e.
    depression, e.
existentialism
Exner's plexus
exogenous
exophoria
exophthalmos
exophthalmos-macroglossia-gigantism
    syndrome
exophytic
exorcise
exorcism
exorcist
exostosis
exostotic
exotropia
expansive
    delusion, e.
    mood, e.
expansiveness
experential
experiences of alienation
experiences of influence
experiential
exploitation
exploitative
explosive
    personality, e.
    speech, e.
expressed skull fracture
expressive
    aphasia, e.
    apraxia, e.
    disorder, e.

expressive *(continued)*
    dysphasia, e.
    training, e.
exquisite pain
exsanguination
extended family
extensor
    lag, e.
    plantar response, e.
    posturing, e.
    tone, e.
exteriorize
external
    carotid artery, e.
    hydrocephalus, e.
    jugular vein, e.
    skeletal fixation device, e.
externalization
externalize
exteroceptive
exteroceptor
exterofection
exterofective
extinction
    phenomenon, e.
extra-axial
extrabulbar
extracampine
    hallucinations, e.
extracerebral
extracorticospinal
extracranial
extradural

extradural *(continued)*
    compression, e.
    defect, e.
    hematoma, e.
    hemorrhage, e.
extrahypothalamic
extramedullary
extrameningeal
extraocular muscles (EOM)
extrapsychic
extrapyramidal
extrasellar
extrasensory
    perception (ESP), e.
extrasexual
extravasation
extroversion
extrovert
extrude
extruded disk
extrusion
exuberant tissue
eye
    contact, e.
    -gaze communicator, e.
    grounds, e.
    lead, e.
    -minded, e.
    movement, e.
    muscle imbalance, e.
    tracking, e.
eyelid closure reflex
Eysenck Personality Questionnaire

Additional entries

Additional entries

F

fabere (flexion, abduction, external rotation, extension) sign
fabrication
Fabry's disease
fabulation
facet
   joint, f.
   rasp, f.
facetectomy
faceted
facetious
facetiousness
facial
   asymmetry, f.
   deceit, f.
   diplegia, f.
   droop, f.
   flattening, f.
   nerve (cranial nerve VII), f.
   palsy, f.
   symmetry, f.
   tic, f.
   weakness, f.
facies
   Hutchinson's f.
   Marshall Hall's f.
   myasthenic f.
   myopathic f.
   Parkinson's f.
   parkinsonian f.
   Potter f.
facile
facilitate
facilitation
   Wedensky f.
facilitator
facilitory
facility
faciocephalalgia
faciodigitogenital syndrome
facioplegia
facioscapulohumeral
   muscular dystrophy, f.

factitious
   tremor, f.
facultative
faculties
faculty
fadir (flexion, adduction, internal rotation) sign
failure to thrive
Fairbairn theory
Fajersztajn crossed sciatic sign
Fahersztajn iwell leg raising
falces (pl. of falx)
falcial
falcine region
falling to left
falling to right
Fallot's syndrome
Fallot's tetralogy
false joint
false pregnancy
falsification
   retrospective f.
falx (pl. falces)
   of cerebellum, f.
   of cerebrum, f.
   cerebri, f.
familial
   amaurotic idiocy, f.
   autonomic dysfunction, f.
   cerebellar ataxia, f.
   dysautonomia, f.
   myoclonic epilepsy, f.
   periodic paralysis, f.
   tremor, f.
Family APGAR (adaptability, partnership, growth, affection, resolve) Questionnaire
family sculpture
fan sign
FANA (fluorescent antinuclear antibody)
Fanana
   glia of F.
fantasize

fantasy
Fanconi's syndrome
FAPs (fibrillating action potentials)
Farabeuf's triangle
Farber disease
Farber lipogranulomatosis
far-field potential
far-field response
fascia (pl. fasciae)
   dentate f.
fasciae (pl. of fascia)
fascicle
fascicular
fasciculated
fasciculation
fasciculi (pl. of fasciculus)
fasciculus (pl. fasciculi)
   aberrans of Monokow, f.
   cuneatus, f.
   Foville, f. of
   Gowers, f. of
   gracilis, f.
   lenticularis, f.
   Rolando, f. of
   Schutz, f. of
fasciectomy
fasciodesis
fast component
fast wave activity
fastigial
fastigium
fat graft
fat pad
fatigability
fatigue
   battle f.
   combat f.
   pseudocombat f.
   stimulation f.
fatigue toxin
fausse reconnaissance
Fazio-Londe atrophy
Fazio-Londe syndrome
Fazio-Londe type
fearful
febrile

febrile *(continued)*
   convulsion, f.
   delirium, f.
   seizure, f.
   state, f.
febriphobia
Fechner's law
Federn theory
feebleminded
feeblemindedness
feedback
feeder
feeling
Feer's disease
Feingold diet
fellatio
felo-de-se
felt collar splint
Felton's paralysis
feltwork
   Kaes' f.
female intersex
feminism
feminist therapy
feminization
femoral nerve stretch test
fenestrated
   Drake clip, f.
   drape, f.
   tracheostomy tube, f.
fenestration
Fereol-Graux paralysis
Ferguson forceps
Ferguson scoliosis measuring method
Fergusson and Critchley's ataxia
Ferkel torticollis
Ferris Smith forceps
Ferris Smith-Halle bur
Ferris Smith-Kerrison rongeur
festinant
festinating gait
festination
fetal alcohol syndrome
fetal face syndrome
fetal hydantoin syndrome
fetish

fetishism
  transvestic f.
fetishist
fetishistic
Fevre-Languepin syndrome
FFC (fixed flexion contracture)
fiber of Remak
fibra (fibræ)
fibrae
  arcuate cerebri, f.
  arcuatae externae, f.
  arcuatae internae, f.
  cerebello-olivares, f.
  corticonucleares, f.
  corticospinales, f.
  pyramidales medullae, f.
fibrillating action potentials (FAPs)
fibrillation
fibrin glue
fibrinous
fibroblast
fibroblastic
  meningioma, f.
fibroblastoma
  perineural f.
fibrocalcific
fibrocartilage
fibrocartilagines
fibrocartilaginous
  disk, f.
fibrocartilago (fibrocartilagines)
fibrofascitis
fibroglioma
fibroma
fibromatosis
fibromuscular
  dysplasia (FMD), f.
fibromyositis
fibroneuroma
fibrosis
fibrositis
fibrotic
fibrous
  ankylosis, f.
  astrocytoma, f.
  hypertrophic pachymeningitis, f.

field
  cut, f.
  of vision, f.
fields of Forel
fifth cranial nerve
fight-or-flight reaction
figure
  fortification f.
figure-ground discrimination
fila (pl. of filum)
  olfactoria, f.
  radicularia nervorum spinalium, f.
filioparental
filling cells
filum (pl. fila)
  durae matris spinalis, f.
  of spinal dura mater, f.
  terminale, f.
fimbria hippocampi
fine
  -angled curette, f.
  movements, f.
  tremor, f.
finger
  agnosia, f.
  flexors, f.
  following, f.
  intrinsics, f.
  ladder, f.
  oximeter, f.
  phenomenon, f.
  sign, f.
  spelling, f.
  spreader, f.
  stall, f.
  -to-finger test, f.
  -to-nose (F to N) test, f.
  -to-nose-to-finger test, f.
fingeragnosia
fingerbreadth (pl. fingerbreadths)
fingerprint body myopathy
FIRDA (frontal irregular rhythm delta activity)
first cranial nerve (olfactory nerve)
fish poisoning
Fisher brace

fissula (pl. fissulae)
fissulae (pl. of fissula)
fissurae (pl. of fissura)
fissura (pl. fissurae)
  amygdaline f.
  basilar f.
  basisylvian f.
  Broca's f.
  callosal f.
  callosomarginal f.
  central f.
  cerebral f.
  cerebri lateralis, f.
  cerebrum, f's of
  craniofacial f.
  entorbital f.
  great horizontal f.
  hippocampal f.
  inferofrontal f.
  interparietal f.
  lateral f. of cerebrum
  longitudinal f.
  median f. of medulla oblongata
  median f. of spinal cord
  Monro, f. of
  occipital f.
  occipitosphenoidal f.
  Pansch's f.
  parieto-occipital f.
  petrobasilar f.
  petro-occipital f.
  posterolateral f. of cerebellum
  postpyramidal f.
  precentral f.
  prepyramidal f.
  presylvian f.
  Rolando, f. of
  sybsylvian f.
  subtemporal f.
  sylvian f.
  Sylvius, f. of
  tentorial f.
  transtemporal f.
  transverse f. of cerebrum
fissurae (pl. of fissura)
fissure

fissure *(continued)*
  Broca's f.
  calcarine f.
  dentate f.
  Pansch's f.
  Rolando's f.
  Sylvius, f. of
fit
five-minute memory
fix (take drugs)
fixating
fixation
  freudian f.
fixation device
fixation hook
fixation nystagmus
fixed
  dilated pupils, f.
  flexion contracture (FFC), f.
  gaze, f.
flaccid
  coma, f.
  hemiparesis, f.
  hemiplegia, f.
  paralysis, f.
flaccidity
flagellantism
flagellation
flail ankle
flail joint
flail limb
flailing
Flajani's disease
flame-shaped hemorrhage
flap
  raised, f.
  swung, f.
  turned, f.
flapping tremors
flash stimuli
flashback phenomenon
flasher
flashing
flat affect
flat-line EEG
flat-line EKG

Flatau's law
Flatau-Schilder disease
Flatt finger/thumb prosthesis
flattened affect
Flechsig's areas
Flechsig's field
Flechsig's primordial zones
Flechsig's tract
flex against gravity
flexibilitas cerea
flexibility
flexile
flexion
    and extension, f.
    contracture, f.
flexor
    apparatus, f.
    crease, f.
    plantar reflex, f.
    retinaculum, f.
    sheath, f.
    wad of five f.
flexorplasty
flexura
flexure
    basicranial f.
    cephalic f.
    cerebral f.
    cervical f.
    cranial f.
    lumbar f.
    mesencephalic f.
    nuchal f.
    pontine f.
flicker
    fusion threshold, f.
    phenomenon, f.
    photometer, f.
    test, f.
flight of ideas
flight of thoughts
flight reaction
flittering scotoma
float the brain
floccillation
floccitation

flocculonodular
    lobe, f.
flocculus
flooding
floppy infant syndrome
Florida cervical brace
Flourens' law
flow state
flower-spray endings
fluent aphasia
Fluhmann's test
flushing reservoir
flux
fly-catcher tongue
FMD (fibromuscular dysplasia)
F to N (finger-to-nose)
foam embolus
focal
    epilepsy, f.
    findings, f.
    lesion, f.
    motor signs, f.
    neurologic deficit, f.
    neurologic sign, f.
    seizure, f.
focality
Foix-Alajouanine syndrome
fold
    Veraguth's f.
folia (pl. of folium)
folie
    a deux, f.
    circulaire, f.
    du doute, f.
    du pourquoi, f.
    a famille, f.
    gemellaire, f.
    musculaire, f.
    raisonnante, f.
folium (pl. folia)
    cacuminis, f.
    cerebelli, f.
    cerebellum, f. of
    vermis, f.
follicle-stimulating hormone (FSH)

Folstein's Mini-Mental Status Examination
Foltz catheter
Fontana's markings
fontanel
fontanelle (pl. of fontanel)
fonticuli (pl. of fonticulus)
fonticulus (pl. fonticuli)
footboard
foot drop
foramen (pl. foramina)
    caecum medullae oblongatae, f.
    cecum ossis frontalis, f.
    interventricular, f.
    magnum, f.
    of Luschka, f.
    of Magendie, f.
    of Munro, f.
    of Vesalius, f.
    ovale ossis sphenoidalis, f.
    rotundum ossis sphenoidalis, f.
    spinosum, f.
foramen closure test
foramen-plugging forceps
foramina (pl. of foramen)
foraminal
    punch, f.
foraminotomy
foraminula (pl. of foraminulum)
foraminulum (pl. foraminula)
forced gaze
forced tremor
forceps
    Adson f.
    Bacon f.
    Bane f.
    bayonet f.
    Cairns' f.
    Chandler f.
    Cherry-Kerrison f.
    Crile f.
    Cushing f.
    Davis f.
    D'Errico f.
    DeVilbiss f.
    Ferguson f.

forceps *(continued)*
    Ferris Smith f.
    Gerald f.
    Gruenwald f.
    Hudson f.
    Hurd f.
    Leksell f.
    Lewin f.
    Love-Gruenwald f.
    Love-Kerrison f.
    Luer f.
    McKenzie f.
    Oldberg f.
    Raney f.
    Ruskin f.
    Schlesinger f.
    Schutz f.
    Scoville f.
    Sewall f.
    Smithwick f.
    Spence-Adson f.
    Spence f.
    Spurling f.
    Stevenson f.
    Stille-Liston f.
    Stille-Luer f.
    Sweet f.
    Wilde f.
forebrain
foreconscious
forefoot
Forel's decussation
foreleg
forensic
foresight
Forestier disease
forgetfulness
forgetting
form sense
formatio
    alba, f.
    grisea, f.
    reticularis pontis, f.
    vermicularis, f.
formation
    coffin f.

formation *(continued)*
   compromise f.
   gray reticular f.
   palisade f.
   reaction f.
   reticular f. of medulla oblongata
   reticular f. of mesencephalon
   reticular f. of pons
   reticular f. of spinal cord
   white reticular f.
formboard
forme fruste
formication
fornices (pl. of fornix)
fornix (pl. fornices)
   cerebri, f.
   of cerebrum, f.
Forrester head halter
Forrester-Brown head halter
Forssius-Eriksson syndrome
Forster-Penfield operation
Fort Bragg fever
fortification spectrum
49-er brace
forward flexion
fossa (pl. fossae)
   cerebellar , f.
   cerebral, f.
   cranial, f.
   cranii anterior, f.
   cranii media, f.
   cranii posterior, f.
   posterior, f.
fossae (pl. of fossa)
Foster bed
Foster frame
Foster Kennedy syndrome
Fothergill's disease
Fothergill's neuralgia
Fournier test
four-point cervical brace
four-point gait
four-point walker
four-poster cervical brace
fourth cranial nerve
fourth cranial nerve nucleus

Foville's fasciculus
Foville's syndrome
Foville's tract
Fowler maneuver
fractured background
fractured family
fragile-X syndrome
fragmentation
fragmented
fraise
Francheschetti syndrome
Francheschetti-Jadassohn syndrome
Francke's striae
Francois' syndrome
Frankel's sign
Frankfort horizontal plane
Frankl-Hochwart disease
Frazier cannula
Frazier dura elevator
Frazier dura hook
Frazier-Spiller operation
freckled adenoma
free association
free base
free-basing
free flap
free-floating anxiety
free fragment
free-swinging knee gait
Freeman-Sheldon syndrome
Freer elevator
freeze-dried bone
Fregoli syndrome
Freidreich's ataxia
Freidreich's disease
Frejka jacket
French S-shaped retractor
frenetic
frenzied
frenzy
Frenkel's movements
F response
fressreflex
Freud's cathartic method
Freud's theory
freudian

freudian slip
Frey's syndrome
fricative
Friderichsen-Waterhouse syndrome
Friedmann's vasomotor syndrome
Friedreich's ataxia
Freidreich's disease
Freidreich's tabes
Friedreich's foot
fright illness taxon
fright neuroses
frigid
frigidity
frigotherapy
frog breathing
Froin's syndrome
Frolich's syndrome
Froment's paper sign
Fromm theory
Frommann's lines
frons
    cranii, f.
frontal
    gyrus, f.
    horn, f.
    irregular rhythmic delta activity
      (FIRDA), f.
    lobe, f.
    lobe signs, f.
    lobe tumor, f.
    lobotomy, f.
    nerve, f.
    release sign, f.
    sinuses, f.
    sulcus, f.
    suture, f.
frontalis
frontocentral
fronto-occipital
frontoparietal
    operculum, f.
frontotemporal
    craniotomy, f.
frontozygomatic
    suture, f.
front-tap reflex

Froriep's induration
Froriep's law
frottage
frotteur
frotteurism
frozen shoulder
frustrated
frustration
Fryns syndrome
FSH (follicle-stimulating hormone)
FTA-ABS test
F to N (finger-to-nose) test
fucosidosis
fugue
    epileptic f.
    psychogenic f.
fugue state
Fukuyama congenital muscular dystrophy
full weight-bearing (FWB)
fullkorper
fulminant
fulminating
functional
    disease, f.
    encopresis, f.
    enuresis, f.
    level, f.
    overlay, f.
    psychosis, f.
    syncope, f.
functionalis
fund of information
fundi (pl. of fundus)
fundus (pl. fundi)
funduscope
funduscopic
funduscopy
fungal stain
funicular suture
funiculi (pl. of funiculus)
funiculitis
funiculus (pl. funiculi)
    cuneatus, f.
    cuneatus medullae oblongatae, f.
    gracilis medullae oblongatae, f.
    medulae spinalis, f.

funiculus (pl. funiculi) *(continued)*
   solitarius, f.
   teres, f.
   ventralis, f.
funiform
funny bone
FUO (fever of unknown origin)
furibund
furious
furor
   epilepticus, f.
Furstner's disease
fury
fused
fusiform
   gyrus, f.
fusimotor

fusion
   anterior spinal f.
   atlanto-occipital f.
   cervical interbody f.
   dowel spinal f.
   posterior spinal f.
   posterior cervical f.
   spinal f.
   symmetric vertebral f.
fusion faculty
fusion frequency
fusion of spine
fusional
Futura splint
F-wave
FWB (full weight-bearing)

Additional entries

G

GABA (gamma-aminobutyric acid)
GAD (glutamic acid decarboxylase)
Gaenslen's sign
GAF (Global Assessment of Functioning)
gag reflex
gain
gait
    antalgic g.
    apraxic g.
    ataxic g.
    athetotic g.
    calcaneous g.
    cerebellar g.
    Charcot's g.
    choreic g.
    cogwheel g.
    double-step g.
    drag-to g.
    drop-foot g.
    dystonic g.
    dystrophic g.
    equine g.
    festinating g.
    four-point g.
    free-swinging knee g.
    glue-footed g.
    gluteal g.
    heel-toe g.
    helicopod g.
    hemiplegic g.
    hysterical g.
    intermittent double-step g.
    listing g.
    Oppenheim's g.
    propulsion g.
    reeling g.
    scissor g.
    shuffling g.
    slipping-clutch g.
    spastic g.
    staggering g.
    steppage g.
    swaying g.

gait (continued)
    swing-through g.
    swing-to g.
    tabetic g.
    three-point g.
    Trendelenburg g.
    two-point g.
    waddling g.
gait analysis
gait and station
gait apraxia
gait ataxia
gait disturbance
gait training
gait unsteadiness
gaiter distribution
Galant's reflex
Galassi's pupillary phenomenon
galea
    aponeurotica, g.
    tendinous g.
galea forceps
galeaplasty
Galeazzi sign
Galen vein malformation
Galen's great cerebral vein
Galen's ventricle
galeophilia
galeophobia
Gallie atlantoaxial fusion technique
Galt trephine
Galton's whistle
galvanism
galvanocautery
galvanocontractility
galvanogustometer
galvanonervous
galvanopalpation
galvanosurgery
galvanotonus
Galveston Orientation and Amnesia Test
    (GOAT)
game leg

gamekeeper's thumb
gametophobia
gamma-aminobutyric acid (GABA)
Gamma Knife
gamma rigidity
gammacism
Gam-Mer bipolar cautery
gamophobia
Gamstorp's disease
Gandy clamp
ganglia (pl. of ganglion)
ganglial
gangliated
gangliectomy
gangliform
gangliitis
ganglioblast
gangliocyte
gangliocytoma
ganglioform
ganglioglioma
ganglioglioneuroma
gangliolytic
ganglion (pl. ganglia)
    blocker, g.
    cyst, g.
    hook, g.
    knife, g.
ganglionated
ganglionectomy
ganglioneure
ganglioneuroblastoma
ganglioneurofibroma
ganglioneuroma
ganglionic
    blockade, g.
ganglionitis
ganglionoplegia
ganglionoplegic
ganglionostomy
ganglioplegic
ganglioside
gangliosidoses (pl. of gangliosidosis)
gangliosidosis (pl. gangliosidoses)
gangliosympathectomy
ganja

Ganser symptom
Ganser syndrome
Ganslen's test
gap junction
Gapalan's syndrome
Garcin's syndrome
Gardner chair
Gardner headrest
Gardner meningocele repair
Gardner needle
Gardner syndrome
Gardner-Diamond syndrome
Gardner-Wells tong traction
Gardner-Wells tongs
gargalanesthesia
gargalesthesia
gargalesthetic
gargoylism
Garre's sclerosing osteomyelitis
GAS (general adaptation syndrome)
Gasser's ganglion
gasserectomy
gasserian
    ganglion, g.
    ganglion hook, g.
    ganglion syndrome, g.
    ganglionectomy, g.
Gastaut's syndrome
gastric feeding tube
gastric lavage
gastroc (slang for gastrocnemius)
gastrocnemius
    muscle, g.
    reflex, g.
Gatch bed
gatched bed
gate-control test
gate hypothesis
gatophobia
Gaucher disease
Gault reflex
Gault test
Gault's cochleopalpebral reflex
gauntlet
gay
Gaynor-Hart position

gaze
    palsy, g.
    preference, g.
Gee-Herter-Heubner syndrome
gegenhalten
Geigel reflex
gelasmus
Gelfoam cookie
Gelfoam-soaked pledgets
Gelfoam stamps
Gelineau's syndrome
Gelita B
Gelle's test
Gelocast
gelotherapy
Gel-Pad
Gelpi retractor
gemistocyte
gemistocytic
    astrocytoma, g.
    tumor, g.
Gemonil
gender
    dysphoria syndrome, g.
    identity disorder, g.
    role identify, g.
    testing, g.
gene
    mapping, g.
    therapy, g.
general adaptation syndrome (GAS)
General Electric CT/T 8800 scanner
generalization
    stimulus g.
generalize
generativity
genetic
    counseling, g.
    engineering, g.
    predisposition, g.
geniculate
    herpes, g.
    neuralgia, g.
    otalgia, g.
geniculum
genioglossus

genital retraction taxon
genitofemoral
    nerve, g.
    neuralgia, g.
genius
Gennari's line
genotype
genu (pl. genua)
    corpus callosum, g. of
    facial nerve, g. of
    internal capsule, g. of
    nervi facialis, g.
    recurvatum, g.
genua (pl. of genu)
geophagia
geophagist
Georgiade visor halo fixation apparatus
gephyrophobia
Gerald forceps
Gerdy's fontanelle
Gerhardt's disease
Gerhardt's syndrome
Gerhardt-Semon law
geriatric
Gerlach's network
Gerlier's disease
gerontophilia
gerontophobia
geropsychiatric
geropsychiatry
geropsychosis
Gerstmann's syndrome
Gesell developmental schedule
Gestalt theory
Gestalt therapy
gestaltism
geumophobia
GFAP (glial fibrillary acidic protein) test
Ghajar guide
Ghilarducci's reaction
ghost illness
ghost pain
ghost vessels
GIA stapler
Giacomini's band
giant-cell tumor

gibberish aphasia
gibbosity
gibbous deformity
Gibbs classification
gibbus
Gibney's perispondylitis
giddiness
Giemsa stain
Gifford reflex
Gifford retractor
Gifford sign
Gifford-Galassi reflex
gigantism
Gigli saw guide
Gigli wire saw
Gill-Manning decompression laminectomy
Gill-Manning-White spondylolithesis
    technique
gilded-boy story
Gill operation
Gilles de la Tourette syndrome
gimpy
ginger paralysis
Girard's treatment
girdle
    pain, g.
    sensation, g.
Girdlestone laminectomy
girdling
gitter cells
give-way phenomena
give-way weakness
giving up
giving way
glabbelad
glabella
glabellar
    reflex, g.
glabellum
Glanzmann's disease
Glasgow Coma Scale
Glasgow Outcome Scale
glass arm
glaucomflecken
glia
    ameboid g.

glia *(continued)*
    cytoplasmic g.
    Fanana, g. of
    fibrillary g.
gliacyte
glial
    cells, g.
    fibrillary acidic protein (GFAP), g.
glioblast
glioblastoma
    multiforme, g.
gliocyte
gliocytoma
gliofibrillary
gliogenous
glioma
    astrocytic g.
    endophytum, g.
    ependymal g.
    exophytum, g.
    ganglionic g.
    malignant g.
    mixed g.
    multiforme, g.
    nasal g.
    optic g.
    peripheral g.
    retinae, g.
    sarcomatosum, g.
    telangiectatic g.
glioma-polyposis syndrome
gliomatosis
gliomatous
gliomyoma
gliomyxoma
glioneuroma
gliophagia
gliopil
gliosa
gliosarcoma
gliosis
    basilar g.
    cerebellar g.
    diffuse g.
    hemispheric g.
    hypertrophic nodular g.

gliosis *(continued)*
    isomorphic g.
    lobar g.
    perivascular g.
    spinal g.
    unilateral g.
gliosome
glissade
glissadic
Glisson's sling
global
    amnesia, g.
    aphasia, g.
    Assessment of Functioning (GAF), g.
    Assessment Scale, g.
    hypotension, g.
    memory, g.
globoid
    cell, g.
    leukodystrophy, g.
globus
    hystericus, g.
    pallidus, g.
glomangioma
glomectomy
glomera (pl. of glomus)
glomerate
glomerulus
glomic
glomoid
glomus (pl. glomera)
glossalgia
glossectomy
glossitis
glossograph
glossokinesthetic
glossolalia
glossopexy
glossopharyngeal
    nerve (cranial nerve IX), g.
    neuralgia, g.
    neurotomy, g.
glossopharyngeus nerve
glossophobia
glossoplegia
glossopyrosis

glossospasm
glottal
glottis
glove and stocking distribution
glove anesthesia
glove area
glove distribution
glucocorticoid
glucocorticosteroid
glucose tolerance test
glue-footed gait
glue-sniffing
glutamic acid decarboxylase (GAD)
gluteal gait
glycogen debrancher deficiency
glycogen storage disease
glycogenosis
glycorrhachia
glycosuria
Gnathostoma spinigerum
gnostic sensation
goal-directed
goal-oriented
GOAT (Galveston Orientation and Amnesia Test)
Goggia's sign
goiter
Goldberg's syndrome
Goldenhar's syndrome
Goldflam's disease
Goldflam-Erb disease
Goldstein sign
Goldstein spinal fusion
Goldstein theory
Goldstein-Sheerer test
Goldthwait's brace
Goldthwait's sign
golf arm
Golgi body
Golgi bottle neuron
Golgi cells
Golgi's mixed method
Golgi's neuron
Golgi's theory
Goll's column
Goll's fasciculus

Goll's tract
Goltz's theory
Gombault's degeneration
Gombault's neuritis
Gombault-Philippe triangle
Gomori trichrome stain
gonad
gonadectomize
gonadectomy
gonadotherapy
gonadotropins
Gonda reflex
Good's syndrome
Goodenough Draw-a-Man test
Goodman syndrome
gooseneck rongeur
Gopalan's syndrome
Gordon's finger sign
Gordon's leg sign
Gordon's reflex
Gore-Tex
Gorlin's syndrome
Gorlin-Goltz syndrome
Gottron's sign
Gottstein's fibers
gouge
Gougerot-Nulock-Houwer syndrome
Gowers' column
Gowers' contraction
Gowers' disease
Gowers' fasciculus
Gowers' maneuver
Gowers' phenomenon
Gowers' sign
Gowers' syndrome
Gowers' tract
Gowers-type muscular dystrophy
gracile nucleus
graded response
Gradenigo's syndrome
Graefe's sign
Graefe's spot
Graefe's test
Graham nerve hook
Gram's stain
grand mal

grandiose
grandiosity
Grandry's corpuscles
Granger line
Granit loop
granulatio
    arachnoideales, g.
    cerebrales, g.
    pacchioni, g.
granulation
    arachnoidal g.
    pacchionian g.
    Virchow's g.
granulocytic brain edema
granulomatosis
granulomatous arteritis
grape endings
graphesthesia
graphokinesthetic
graphology
graphomotor
graphophobia
graphorrhea
graphospasm
Grashey's aphasia
grasp reflex
grass (marijuana)
Grasset's law
Grasset's phenomenon
Grasset's sign
Grasset-Bychowski sign
Grasset-Gaussel phenomenon
Grasset-Gaussel-Hoover sign
gratification
Graves' disease
gray
    central g.
    perihypoglossal g.
    silver g.
    steel g.
gray commissures
gray matter
    cerebral g.
    cervical spinal cord g.
    frontal lobe g.
    insula g.

gray matter *(continued)*
    lumbosacral spinal cord g.
    occipital lobe g.
    parietal lobe g.
    periventricular g.
    spinal cord g.
    temporal lobe g.
    thoracic spinal cord g.
gray scale ultrasound
gray spinal syndrome
gray substance
gray syndrome
gray tubercle
great toe push-off
Greenburg self-retaining retractor
Greenfield classification of spinocerebellar ataxia
Greenfield's disease
grenz ray
Greulich and Pyle skeletal maturation staging
grief
    reaction, g.
    process, g.
    therapy, g.
grieving
griffe des orteils
Griffith's sign
grimace
grinding
grip
    strength, g.
    tester, g.
Griscelli syndrome
griseotomy
grommet
groove
grooved director
groping
gross movements
Grotstein theory
group therapy
growth hormone
grubelsucht
Gruber's suture
Gruenwald forceps

grumous
grundplatte
Grunfelder's reflex
GSR (galvanic skin response)
guard
guarded chisel
guarding
Gubler's hemiplegia
Gubler's line
Gubler's paralysis
Gudden's atrophy
Gudden's commissure
Gudden's law
Gudden's tract
guide
    dog, g.
Guilford cervical brace
Guilford-Zimmerman personality test
Guillain-Barre polyneuritis
Guillain-Barre syndrome
Guilland's sign
guilt
    complex, g.
Guinon's disease
Gull's disease
Gull-Toynbee law
Gullstrand's law
gumma (pl. gummata)
gummata (pl. of gumma)
Gunn's phenomenon
Gunn's pupillary sign
Gunn's sign
Gunn's syndrome
gunnysacking
gustation
    colored g.
gustatism
gustatory
    audition, g.
    receptor, g.
    sweating , g.
gustolacrimal reflex
gustometer
gustometry
Guthrie test
gutter

gutter fracture
gutturotetany
Guyon's canal
gymnomania
gymnophobia
gynandrism
gynandroid
gynecomania
gynecomastia
gynecophonus
gynephobia
Gynergen
gynophobia
gyrate
   scalp, g.
gyre
gyrectomy
   frontal g.
gyrencephalic
gyri (pl. of gyrus)
   annectentes, g.
   breves insulae, g.
   cerebri , g.
   insulae, g.
   occipitales, g.
   operti, g.
   orbitales, g.
   profundi cerebri, g.
   transitivi cerebri, g.
gyrochrome
gyrometer
gyrose
gyrospasm
gyrous
gyrus (pl. gyri)
   angular g.
   angularis, g.
   annectant g.
   Broca's g.
   callosal g.
   callosus, g.
   central g.
   cerebrum, g. of
   cingulate g.
   cinguli, g.
   dentate g.

gyrus pl. (gyri) *(continued)*
   dentatus, g.
   fasciolaris, g.
   fornicatus, g.
   frontal g.
   fusiform g.
   fusiformis, g.
   geniculi, g.
   Heschl's g.
   hippocampal g.
   hippocampi, g.
   infracalcarine g.
   infracalcarinus, g.
   insulae, g.
   limbicus, g.
   lingual g.
   lingualis, g.
   long g. of insula
   marginal g.
   marginal g. of Turner
   marginalis, g.
   occipital g.
   occipitotemporal g.
   olfactorius, g.
   olfactory g.
   orbital g.
   paracentral g.
   parahippocampal g.
   parahippocampalis, g.
   paraterminal g.
   paraterminalis, g.
   parietal g.
   postcentral g.
   precentralis, g.
   preinsular g.
   quadrate g.
   rectus, g.
   short g. of insula
   subcallosal g.
   subcollateral g.
   supracallosal g.
   supramarginal g.
   temporal g.
   temporalis, g.
   uncinate g.
   uncinatus, g.

Additional entries

H

H disease
H graft
H reflex
Haab's reflex
Haas paralysis
habenula (pl. habenulae)
habenulae (pl. of habenula)
habenular
   commissure, h.
   trigone, g.
habit
   chorea h.
   masticory h.
   spasm h.
habit training
habitual
habituation
habitus
habromania
HACE (high-altitude cerebral edema)
Hachinski Ischemic Score
Haenel's symptom
Hahn's sign
hairline
Hajek chisel
Hajek mallet
Hajek punch
Hajek rongeur
Hajek-Ballenger elevator
Hajek-Koffler punch
Hajek-Skillern punch
Hakim shunt
Hakim syndrome
Hakim-Cordis pump
Haldol
halfway house
Hall drill
Hall neurosurgical craniotome
Hall neurotome
Hallerman-Streiff syndrome
Hallerman-Streiff-Francois syndrome
Hallervorden-Spatz disease
Hallervorden-Spatz syndrome

Hallpike caloric stimulation test
hallucinating
hallucination
   auditory h.
   autoscopic h.
   command h.
   depressive h.
   extracampine h.
   gustatory h.
   haptic h.
   hypnagogic h.
   hypnopompic h.
   kinesthetic h.
   kinetic h.
   lilliputian h.
   microptic h.
   mood-congruent h.
   mood-incongruent h.
   motor h.
   olfactory h.
   postdormital h.
   predormital h.
   reflex h.
   second-person h.
   somatic h.
   stump h.
   tactile h.
   third-person h.
   visual h.
hallucinative
hallucinatory
hallucinogen
hallucinogenesis
hallucinogenetic
hallucinogenic
hallucinosis
   acute alcoholic h.
   organic h.
hallucinotic
halo ring
halo sign
halo-pelvic traction
halo traction

halo vest
haloperidol
Halstead maneuver
Halstead-Wepman Aphasia Screening test
Halsted-Reitan test
halter
    Cerva Crane h.
    DePuy h.
    Diskard head h.
    Forrester head h.
    Forrester-Brown head h.
    head h.
    Redi head h.
    Repro head h.
    Upper 7 head h.
    Zimfoam head h.
    Zimmer head h.
hamartoma
hamartomania
hamartomatous
hamartophobia
Hamby retractor
Hamilton Anxiety Rating Scale
Hamilton Depression Rating Scale
hammer finger
hammer palsy
Hammerschlag's phenomenon
hammertoe
hammocking
Hammond's disease
hamstring muscle
hand
    ape h.
    claw h.
    cleft h.
    drop h.
    lobster-claw h.
    obstetrician's h.
    opera-glass h.
    writing h.
hand-flapping
hand intrinsics
Hand-Schuller-Christian disease
hand-shoulder syndrome
handedness
handfasted

handicap
handsock
Handtrol electrosurgical pencil
HANE (hereditary angioneurotic edema)
hangman's fracture
hangover
Hanhart's syndrome
Hansen's disease
haphalgesia
haphephobia
haptephobia
haptic
haptics
Harada's syndrome
Hardy microbipolar forceps
Hardy retractor
Hare's syndrome
harelip
harlequin sign
Harmon bone graft
harness
Harrington hook
Harrington hook driver
Harrington retractor
Harrington rod
Harrington spinal elevator
Harrington spinal fusion
Harris sling
Harris method
Harris migrainous neuralgia
Harris syndrome
Harris-Smith cervical fusion
Hartmann theory
Hartnup disease
harvest
Hashimoto's disease
hashish
Haslinger head rest
Hass' paralysis
haut mal epilepsy
Haynes cannula
Hayem's encephalitis
head
    banging, h.
    fracture frame, h.
    lag, h.

head *(continued)*
  trauma, h.
headache
  anemic h.
  anxiety h.
  bilious h.
  blind h.
  cluster h.
  congestive h.
  conversion h.
  cough h.
  depression h.
  dynamite h.
  emotional h.
  exertional h.
  functional h.
  helmet h.
  histamine h.
  Horton's h.
  hyperemic h.
  inflammatory h.
  lumbar puncture h.
  medicinal h.
  metabolic h.
  migraine h.
  miners' h.
  Monday morning h.
  occipital h.
  organic h.
  orgasmic h.
  postspinal h.
  psychogenic h.
  psychosis h.
  puncture h.
  pyrexial h.
  reflex h.
  rhinogenous h.
  sick h.
  spinal h.
  symptomatic h.
  tension h.
  thunderclap h.
  thundering h.
  toxic h.
  traumatic h.
  tumor h.

headache *(continued)*
  vacuum h.
  vascular h.
  vasomotor h.
headgear
headholder
headlight
headrest
hearing
  color h.
  double disharmonic h.
  monoaural g.
  visual h.
hearing aid
hearing distance
hearing hallucinations
hearing level
hearing loss
  Alexander's h.
  conductive h.
  pagetoid h.
  paradoxic h.
  sensorineural h.
  transmission h.
heat cramps
heat exhaustion
heat intolerance
heat stroke
heavy metal
heavy-particle irradiation
hebephrenia
hebephreniac
hebephrenic
  schizophrenia, h.
hebetic
hebetude
heboid
heboidophrenia
hedonia
hedonic
hedonism
hedonistic
hedonomania
hedonophobia
HEE (hemiconvulsion, hemiplegia, epilepsy) syndrome

Heelbo decubitus protector
heel-and-toe walking
heel-knee test
heel-to-shin test
heel-walking
Heffington lumbar seat spinal surgery
frame
Heidenhaim's syndrome
Heifitz clip
Heilbronner's sign
Heilbronner's thigh
Heimlich maneuver
Heimlich sign
Heine-Medin disease
Helbing's sign
helicopod
gait, h.
helicopodia
heliencephalitis
heliomania
heliophobia
heliotrope infraorbital discoloration
helmet headache
helplessness
Helsper laryngectomy button
Helweg's bundle
Helweg's tract
hemal
hemangioblastoma
hemangioma
hemarthrosis
hematencephalon
hematocephalus
hematoencephalic
hematoma
hematomyelia
hematomyelitis
hematomyelopore
hematorrhachis
hemeralopia
Hemholtz theory
hemiageusia
hemiageustia
hemialgia
hemiamblyopia
hemianacusia

hemianalgesia
hemianencephaly
hemianesthesia
alternate h.
cerebral h.
crossed h.
cruciata, h.
mesocephalic h.
pontile h.
spinal h.
hemianopia
absolute h.
altitudinal h.
bilateral h.
binasal h.
binocular h.
bitemporal h.
bitemporalis fugax, h.
complete h.
congruous h.
crossed h.
equilateral h.
heteronymous h.
homonymous h.
horizontal h.
incomplete h.
incongruous h.
lateral h.
nasal h.
quadrant h.
quadrantic h.
relative h.
temporal h.
true h.
unilateral h.
upper h.
vertical h.
hemianopic
hemianopsia
hemianoptic
hemianosmia
hemiapraxia
hemiasynergia
hemiataxia
hemiataxy
hemiathetosis

hemiatrophy
  facial h.
  progressive lingual h.
hemiaxial
hemiballism
hemiballismus
hemicentrum
hemicephalia
hemicerebrum
hemichorea
hemicorticectomy
hemicrania
hemicranial
hemicraniectomy
hemicraniosis
hemicraniotomy
hemidecortication
hemidepersonalization
hemidysergia
hemidysesthesia
hemidystrophy
hemiectromelia
hemiedema
hemiencephalus
hemiepilepsy
hemifacial
hemigeusia
hemigigantism
hemiglossal
hemihypalgesia
hemihyperesthesia
hemihypermetria
hemihyperplasia
hemihypertonia
hemihypertrophy
hemihypesthesia
hemihypoesthesia
hemihypometria
hemihypoplasia
hemihypotonia
hemilaminectomy
  blade, h.
  knife, h.
  prong, h.
  retractor, h.
hemilaminotomy

hemilateral
hemilesion
hemilingual
hemimelia
hemimyosthenia
hemineurasthenia
hemiopalgia
hemiopia
hemiopic
hemiparalysis
hemiparanesthesia
hemiparaplegia
hemiparesis
hemiparesthesia
hemiparetic
hemiparkinsonism
hemiplegia
  alternans hypoglossica, h.
  alternate h.
  alternating oculomotor h.
  ascending h.
  capsular h.
  cerebral h.
  contralateral h.
  crossed h.
  cruciata, h.
  facial h.
  faciobrachial h.
  faciolingual h.
  flaccid h.
  Gubler's h.
  infantile h.
  puerperal h.
  spastic h.
  spinal h.
  Wernicke's h.
hemiplegic
hemirachischisis
hemisacralization
hemiscotosis
hemisection
hemisensory
  loss, h.
hemiseptum
  cerebri, h.
hemisomatagnosia

hemispasm
hemisphere
   cerebellar h.
   cerebral h.
   dominant h.
hemispherectomy
hemispheric
   specialization. h.
hemispherium
   cerebelli, h.
hemisyndrome
hemisynergia
hemitetany
hemithermoanesthesia
hemithorax
hemitonia
hemitremor
hemivagotony
hemivertebra
hemlock poisoning
Hemoclip
hemoclipped
hemodialysis
hemodialyzed
hemodialyzer
hemofuscin
hemophobia
hemorrhage
hemorrhagic
   infarct, h.
hemostased
hemotympanum
Hemovac drain
Hemovac suction tube
Henke's space
Hennebert's sign
Henoch's chorea
Henoch-Schonlein syndrome
Henry paralysis
Henry-Geist spinal fusion
heparin
   flush, h.
   lock, h.
heparinization
heparinize
heparinized saline

hepatic
   coma, h.
   encephalopathy, h.
hepatitis
hepatitis panel
hepatojugular
hepatolenticular
   degeneration, h.
Hep-Lock
herd instinct
hereditary
   angineurotic edema (HANE), h.
hereditary sensory motor neuropathy
   (HSMN)
heredity
heredoataxia
heredodegeneration
heredodegenerative
heredodiathesis
heredofamilial
heredopathia
   atactica polyneuritoformis, h.
heredoretinopathia
   congenita, h.
Hering's law
Hering's nerve
Hering's test
Hering's theory
Hering-Breuer reflex
heritability
heritable
Hermansky-Pudlak syndrome
hermaphrodite
hermaphroditism
hermaphroditismus
herniate
herniated
   disk, h.
   intervertebral disk, h.
   nucleus pulposus (HNP), h.
herniation
   intervertebral disk, h. of
   nucleus pulposus, h. of
   transtentorial h.
   uncal h.
herniation syndrome

heroin
   toxicity, h.
heroinism
herpes
   zoster, h.
   encephalitis, h.
herpesvirus
herpetic
   neuralgia, h.
herpetophobia
Herring track
hersage
Hertwig-Magendie phenomenon
Herz (Hz)
Heschl's convolution
Heschl's gyrus
heteresthesia
heterodesmotic
heteroeroticism
heteroganglionic
heterogeneity
heterogeusia
heterography
heterolalia
heterolateral
heteroliteral
heteromeric
heteromerous
heteropathy
heterophasia
heterophemia
heterophoralgia
heterophoria
heteropsia
heteroptics
heterosexual
heterosexuality
heterosmia
heterosuggestion
heterotonia .
heterotopia
Heubner's endarteritis
Hewlett-Packard ear oximeter
hexing
Heyman's law
hiatus

Hibbs curette
Hibbs gouge
Hibbs periosteal elevator
Hibbs spinal fusion
Hibbs-Jones spinal fusion
Hibiclens scrub
hiccups
Hickman catheter
hierophobia
HIF (higher integrative functions)
high-altitude cerebral edema (HACE)
high-frequency deafness
high myope
high-speed drill
higher integrative functions (HIF)
Hilger facial nerve stimulator
hillock
Hilton's law
hindbrain
Hines and Brown test
hip flexors
Hippel's disease
Hippel-Landau disease
hippocampal
   commissure, h.
   fimbria, h.
   fissure, h.
   formation, h.
   gyrus, h.
   pressure groove, h.
hippocampus
   leonis, h.
   major, h.
   minor, h.
   nudis, h.
hippophobia
hippus
Hirano inclusion body
Hirschberg's reflex
Hirschberg's sign
Hirschsprung's disease
hirsutism
His' perivascular space
histamine headache
histaminic cephalalgia
histiocytosis X

histochemistry
histoneurology
histopathology
historrhexis
histrionic
    mania, h.
    personality disorder, h.
histrionism
hitchhiker sign
Hitzig test
HIVAGEN test
HNP (herniated nucleus pulposus)
Hoche's bandelette
Hochsinger's phenomenon
hockey-stick elevator
hod carrier's palsy
Hodgkin's disease
hodology
hodoneuromere
hodophobia
Hoen skull plate
Hoen ventricular needle
Hoffman reflex
Hoffmann's atrophy
Hoffmann's sign
Hoffmann-Werdnig syndrome
Hogg chair
Hoke lumbar brace
Hoke lumbar corset
holergasia
holergastic
holism
holistic
Hollenhorst plaque
hollow-back
Holmes' phenomenon
Holmes' sign
Holmes-Adie syndrome
Holmes-Rahe study
Holmes-Stewart phenomenon
Holmgren's test
holocenosis
holoprosencephaly
    familial alobar h.
holorachischisis
holotetanus

holotonia
Holscher root retractor
Holter monitor
Holter shunt
Holtzman Inkblot Technique
Holzknecht's space
Homans sign
Homen's syndrome
home assessment
homeostatic function
Homer-Wright rosette
homesickness
homicidal
    ideation, h.
    intent, h.
    precautions, h.
homicide
homicidomania
homilophobia
homocystinuria
homodesmotic
homoerotic
homoeroticism
homolateral
homonymous
    anopsia, h.
    hemianopia, h.
    hemianopsia, h.
homophile
homophobia
homosexual
    panic, h.
homosexuality
hook bundle of Risien Russell
Hoorweg's law
Hoover's sign
hopelessness
horizontal gaze
hormion
horn
    Ammon, h. of
    lateral ventricles, h. of
    spinal cord, h. of
Horner's law
Horner's syndrome
Horner-Bernard syndrome

horse (heroin)
horseshoe
   flap, h.
   headholder, h.
   incision, h.
Horsley bone wax
Horsley dura separator
Horsley trephine
Horsley's operation
Horsley's sign
Hortega cells
Hortega method
Horton's cephalalgia
Horton's disease
Horton's headache
Horton's syndrome
hospitalism
hostile
hostility
hot flashes
hot spot
hotline
hottentotism
Houghton's law
hourglass tumor
Houston halo cervical support
Howship-Romberg sign
Hoyne's sign
HPA (hypothalamic-pituitary-adrenal)
   system
H reflex
HSA (hypersomnia-sleep apnea)
HSA syndrome
HSMN (hereditary sensory motor neurop-
   athy)
HSV (herpes simplex virus)
HSV encephalitis
Hubbard physical therapy tank
Huber needle
Hudson brace
Hudson bur
Hudson cranial drill
Hueter's sign
Huguenin's edema
Hughston-Losee jerk test
humanistic

Human's sign
humpback
humpbacked spinal curvature
hunchback
Hunt's atrophy
Hunt's disease
Hunt's paradoxical phenomenon
Hunt's striatal syndrome
Hunt's tremor
Hunt and Hess neurological classification
Hunter's syndrome
Hunter-Hurler syndrome
Huntington's chorea
Huntington's dementia
Huntington's disease
Huntington's sign
Hurd dissector
Hurd forceps
Hurler's syndrome
Hurler-Scheie syndrome
Hutchinson's facies
Hutchinson's mask
Hutchinson's sign
Hutchinson's teeth
Hutchinson's triad
Hutchinson-Gilford disease
Hutchinson-Gilford syndrome
hutchinsonian
Hutchison type
H-wave
hyaline membrane syndrome
hydranencephaly
hydrargyromania
Hydra-Cadence gait control unit
hydrencephalocele
hydrencephalomeningocele
hydrencephalus
hydrencephaly
hydrocephalic
hydrocephalocele
hydrocephaloid
hydrocephalus
   communicating h.
   congenital h.
   ex vacua, h.
   noncommunicating h.

hydrocephalus *(continued)*
  normal-pressure h.
  normal-pressure occult h.
  obstructive h.
  occult normal-pressure h.
  otitic h.
  secondary h.
hydrocephaly
Hydrocollator
hydrocortisone
hydrodipsia
hydrodipsomania
hydroencephalocele
hydrogymnastics
hydrokinesitherapy
hydrokinetic
hydromania
hydromelia
hydromeningitis
hydromeningocele
hydromicrocephaly
hydromyelia
hydromyelocele
hydromyelomeningocele
hydrophobia
hydrophobophobia
hydrophorograph
hydrophthalmos
hydrorachis
hydrorachitis
hydrosyringomyelia
hydroxyapatite
Hyfrecator
hygroma
hygromatous
hypalgesia
hypalgesic
hypalgetic
hypalgia
hypanakinesia
hypanakinesis
hypaphrodisia
hypaxial
hypegiaphobia
hypencephalon
hyperabduction

hyperacousia
hyperactive
  child syndrome, h.
hyperactivity
hyperacusia
hyperacusis
hyperadrenalism
hyperadrenocorticism
hyperaffectivity
hyperakusis
hyperalertness
hyperalgesia
hyperalgesic
hyperalgetic
hyperalgia
hyperalimentation
hyperammonemia
hyperanacinesia
hyperanakinesia
hyperaphia
hyperaphic
hyperargininemia
hyperarousal
hyperbaric chamber
hyperbaric oxygen
hyperbarism
hyperbeta-alaninemia
hypercathexis
hypercryalgesia
hypercryesthesia
hyperdipsia
hyperdynamia
hyperdynamic
hyperechema
hyperencephalus
hyperenergia
hypereosinophilic
hyperequilibrium
hypererethism
hyperergasia
hyperergia
hyperesthesia
  acoustic h.
  auditory h.
  cerebral h.
  gustatory h.

hyperesthesia *(continued)*
   muscular h.
   olfactory h.
   oneiric h.
   optic h.
   sexualis, h.
   tactile h.
hyperesthetic
hyperexplexia
hyperextend
hyperextension
hyperflex
hyperflexion
hypergasia
hypergeusia
hypergnosia
hypergnosis
hypergonadism
hypergraphia
hyperhedonia
hyperhedonism
hyperinsulinism
hyperirritability
hyperisotonia
hyperisotonic
hyperkalemia
hyperkinesia
hyperkinesis
hyperkinetic
   reaction, h.
   syndrome, h.
hyperlordosis
hyperlysinemia
hypermania
hypermetamorphosis
hypermetria
hypermetropia
hypermimia
hypermnesia
hypermnesic
hypermobility
hypermyotonia
hypermyotrophy
hypernasality
hypernatremia
hypernea

hyperneic
hyperneurotization
hypodipsic
hypernatremic
hypernephroma
hypernormal
hypernyctohemeral syndrome
hyperopia
hyperorality
hyperorexia
hyperosmia
hyperosmolality
hyperosmolar
hyperosphresia
hyperostosis
   ankylosing spinal h.
   corticalis deformans juvenilis, h.
   corticalis generalisata, h.
   cranii, h.
   diffuse idiopathic skeletal h.
   flowing h.
   frontalis interna, h.
   infantile cortical h.
   Morgagni's h.
   senile ankylosing h. of spine
hyperpallesthesia
hyperparathyroidism
hyperparesthesia
hyperparesthetic
hyperpathia
hyperphagia
hyperphasia
hyperphonia
hyperphoria
hyperphrenia
hyperphysics
hyperponesis
hyperponetic
hyperpragic
hyperpraxia
hyperprosexia
hyperpselaphesia
hyperptyalism
hyperreact
hyperreactive
hyperreflexia

hyperreflexia *(continued)*
   autonomic h.
hyperreflexic
hyperreligiosity
hyperreligious
hypersensibility
hypersensitivity
hypersexual
hypersexuality
hypersomia
hypersomnia
   -bulimia syndrome, h.
   -sleep apnea (HSA), h.
   -sleep apnea syndrome, h.
hypersomnolence
hypersthenia
hypersympathicotonus
hypertarachia
hypertelorism
hypertension
hypertensive
   encephalopathy, h.
   retinopathy, h.
hyperthermalgesia
hyperthermesthesia
hyperthermia
hyperthymergasia
hyperthymia
hyperthymic
hyperthymism
hyperthyroid
hyperthyroidism
hypertonia
hypertonic
   solution, h.
hypertonicity
hypertonus
hypertrophia
hypertrophy
hypertryptophanemia
hypervalinemia
hyperventilation
   syndrome, h.
hyperventilate
hyperviscosity
   syndrome, h.

hypervolemia
hypesthesia
   acoustic h.
   auditory h.
   gustatory h.
   tactile h.
   thermal h.
hyphedonia
hypnagogic
   hallucinations, h.
   hypersynchrony, h.
hypnagogue
hypnalgia
hypnic
   jerk, h.
hypnoanalysis
hypnoanesthesia
hypnobatia
hypnocinematograph
hypnodontics
hypnogenetic
hypnogenic
hypnogenous
hypnoid
hypnoidal
hypnoidization
hypnolepsy
hypnology
hypnomania
hypnonarcoanalysis
hyponarcosis
hypnopedia
hypnophobia
hypnopompic
   hallucinations, h.
   postdormital hallucinations, h.
hypnosia
hypnosis
hypnosophy
hypnotherapist
hypnotherapy
hypnotic
   state, h.
   suggestion, h.
   trance, h.
hypnotism

hypnotist
hypnotization
hypnotize
hypnotoxin
hypoactive
   reflex, h.
hypoactivity
hypoacusis
hypoadrenalism
hypoadrenocorticism
hypoaffective
hypoaffectivity
hypoaldosteronism
hypoalgesia
hypobaropathy
hypochondria
hypochondriac
hypochondriacal
   neurosis, h.
   reflex, h.
hypochondriasis
hypocinesia
hypodense
hypodensity
hypodipsia
hypodynamia
hypoechoic
hypoequilibrium
hypoergasia
hypoergic
hypoergy
hypoesophoria
hypoesthesia
hypoesthetic
hypoevolutism
hypoexophoria
hypofunction
hypogenitalism
hypogeusesthesia
hypogeusia
hypoglossal
   alternating hemiplegia, h.
   nerve (cranial nerve XII), h.
hypoglossia-hypodactyly syndrome
hypoglossohyoid triangle
hypoglossus nerve

hypoglycemia
hypoglycemic
   coma, h.
   shock, h.
   shock therapy, h.
hypoglycorrhachia
hypogonadism
hypogonadotrophic hypogonadism
hypohypnotic
hypoinsulinism
hypokalemia
hypokalemic periodic paralysis
hypokinesia
hypokinesis
hypokinetic
hypolemmal
hypoliquorrhea
hypomagnesemia
hypomania
hypomaniac
hypomanic
   attack, h.
hypomelancholia
hypomelanosis of Ito
hypomere
hypometria
hypomnesis
hypomotility
hypomyotonia
hyponatremia
hyponoia
hypo-osmolality
hypopallesthesia
hypoparathyroidism
hypoperfusion
hypophonia
hypophoria
hypophosphatasia
hypophosphatemia
hypophrenia
hypophrenic
hypophrenosis
hypophyseal
hypophysectomize
hypophysectomy
hypophysial

hypophysioprivic
hypophysiotropic
hypophysiotropic hormones
hypophysis
  cerebri, h.
hypophysitis
hypopinealism
hypopituitarism
hypopnea
hypoponesis
hypopotassemia
hypopotentia
hypopraxia
hypoprosody
hypopselaphesia
hyporeactive
hyporeflexia
hyposensitive
hyposexual
hyposexuality
hyposmia
hyposomnia
hyposphresia
hypostatic pneumonia
hyposthenia
hypostheniant
hyposthenic
hyposuprarenalism
hyposympathicotonus
hyposynergia
hypotaxia
hypotelorism
hypotension
  orthostatic h.
hypotensive
  response, h.
hypotensor
hypothalamic
  -pituitary-adrenal (HPA) system, h.
  sulcus, h.
  syndrome, h.
  thermostat, h.
hypothalamicohypophyseal
hypothalamicothalamic
hypothalamopituitary
hypothalamotomy

hypothalamus
  caudal nucleus of h.
  dorsal nucleus of h.
  dorsomedial nucleus of h.
  infundibulum of h.
  medial nucleus of h.
  nucleus intercalatus of h.
  periventricular gray matter of h.
  supraoptic region of h.
  tuberous nucleus of h.
  ventromedial nucleus of h.
hypothermia
  endogenous h.
hypothermia blanket
hypothymia
hypothymic
hypothymism
hypothyroid
hypothyroidism
hypothyrosis
hypotonia
  benign congenital h.
hypotonic
hypotonicity
hypotonus
hypotony
hypotropia
hypoventilation
hypovolemia
hypovolemic
hypoxemia
hypoxia
hypoxic
  hypoxia, h.
hypsarrhythmia
hypsokinesis
hypsonosus
Hyrtl's law
hysteria
  anxiety h.
  canine h.
  conversion h.
  dissociative h.
  fixation h.
  libidinosa, h.
  major, h.

hysteria *(continued)*
    malingering h.
    minor, h.
    monosymptomatic h.
hysteric
    angina, h.
hysterical
    blindness, h.
    conversion, h.
    neurosis, h.
    personality, h.
    seizures, h.
hystericism
hystericoneuralgic

hysterics
hysteriform
hysteroepilepsy
hysteroepileptogenic
hysteroerotic
hysterogenic
hysteroid
hysteromania
hysteronarcolepsy
hysteroneurasthenia
hysteroneurosis
hysteropia
hysteropsychosis
Hz (Herz)

Additional entries

I

ianthinopsia
iatrogenic
    disorder, i.
    dural tear, i.
iatrogeny
I band
ICA (internal carotid artery)
ICAO (internal carotid artery occlusion)
ICB (Incomplete Sentence Blank) test
ice (street drug)
iced calorics
Iceland disease
icewater calorics
icewater reflex
icewater test
ichthyophobia
ichthyosis
iconolagny
ICP (intracranial pressure)
    catheter, I.
    monitor, I.
ICT (insulin coma therapy)
ictal
icteric
ictus
    epilepticus, i.
    paralyticus, i.
    sanguinis, i.
    solis, i.
id
    anxiety, i.
IDDM (insulin-dependent diabetes)
idea
    association, i.'s of
    autochthonous i.
    compulsive i.
    impulsive i.
    dominant i.
    fixed i.
    flight of i's
    imperative i.
    influence, i. of
    reference, i. of

idea *(continued)*
    referential i.
ideal
    ego i.
idealistic
idealization
ideation
    incoherent i.
ideational
    agnosia, i.
    dyspraxia, i.
idee
    fixe, i.
identity
    core i.
    gender i.
    ego i.
    gender i.
identification
identity crisis
ideodynamism
ideogenetic
ideogenous
ideoglandular
ideokinetic
    apraxia, i.
ideology
ideometabolic
ideometabolism
ideomotion
ideomotor
    apraxia, i.
    dyspraxia, i.
ideomuscular
ideophrenic
ideoplastia
ideovascular
idiocracy
idiocratic
idiocy
    absolute i.
    amaurotic i.
    amaurotic familial i.

idiocy *(continued)*
   athetotic i.
   Aztec i.
   complete i.
   cretinoid i.
   developmental i.
   diplegic i.
   eclamptic i.
   epileptic i.
   erethistic i.
   genetous i.
   hemiplegic i.
   hydrocephalic i.
   intrasocial i.
   Kalmuk i.
   microcephalic i.
   mongolian i.
   moral i.
   paralytic i.
   paraplegic i.
   plagiocephalic i.
   profound i.
   scaphocephalic i.
   sensorial i.
   spastic amaurotic axonal i.
   torpid i.
   traumatic i.
   xerodermic i.
idiogenic
   osmoles, i.
idiogenesis
idioglossia
idioglottic
idiographic
idiohypnotism
idio-imbecile
idiolalia
idiolog
idiologism
idiomuscular
   contraction, i.
idioneural
idioneurosis
idiopathic
   CNS hypersomnolence, :
   epilepsy, i.

idiopathic *(continued)*
   orthostatic hypotension, i.
   scoliosis, i.
   thrombocytopenic purpura (ITP), i.
   thrombocytosis, i.
idiophrenic
idiopsychologic
idioreflex
idioretinal
idiospasm
idiosyncrasy
idiosyncratic
idiot
   erethistic i.
   mongolian i.
   pithecoid i.
   profound i.
   -savant, i.
   superficial i.
   torpid i.
idiotic
idiotropic
   type, i.
Ilheus encephalitis
iliac
   crest, i.
iliolumbar
iliopsoas muscle
iliosacral
iliosciatic
iliospinal
iliotibial
Ilizarov system
illicit
illegitimacy
illegitimate
illness
   compressed-air i.
   emotional i.
   high-altitude i.
   manic-depressive i.
   mental i.
   psychosomatic i.
illuminism
illusion
illusional

IM (intramuscular)
image
   accidental i.
   body i.
   eidetic i.
   false i.
   heteronymous i.
   homonymous i.
   incidental i.
   inverted i.
   memory i.
   mental i.
   mirror i.
   motor i.
   negative i.
   sensory i.
image intensification
image intensifier
imagery
   auditory i.
   smell i.
   tactile i.
   taste i.
   visual i.
imagination
imagine
imagines (pl. of imago)
imaging
imago (pl. imagines)
imbalance
   autonomic i.
   binocular i,
   sympathetic i.
   vasomotor i.
imbecile
imbecility
   moral i.
   phenylpyruvic i.
IMED infusion device
imipramine
imitative synkinesis
immature
immaturity
immediate memory
immediate recall
immobile

immobilization
immobilized
immunocompromised
immunocytochemical
immunodeficiency
immunodepression
immunodepressive
immunoelectrophoresis
immunosuppression
immunosuppressive
immunosympathectomy
immunotherapy
imperception
imperforate
imperforation
imperious acts
impingement
impinging
implosion
   flooding, i.
impostor syndrome
impotence
impotency
   anatomic i.
   atonic i.
   functional i.
   organic i.
   psychic i.
   symptomatic i.
   vasculogenic i.
impotent
impoverished
impoverishment
impression
impressionable
imprinting
impulse
   enteroceptive i.
   excitatory i.
   exteroceptive i.
   inhibitory i.
   irresistible i.
   nerve i.
   nervous i.
   neural i.
   proprioceptive i.

impulsion
 wandering i.
impulsive
impulsivity
in extremis
INAD (infantile neuroaxonal dystrophy)
inadequacy
inadequate
inanition
inappetence
inarticulate
inborn
 error of metabolism, i.
inbreeding
incallosal
incest
 family, i.
incestuous
incidence
incident
incisura (pl. incisurae)
 cerebelli, i.
 clavicularis sternii, i.
 frontalis, i.
 temporalis, i.
 tentorii cerebelli, i.
incisurae (pl. of incisura)
incisure
incitogram
incoagulability
incoagulable
incoherence
incoherent
 ideation, i.
 speech, i.
incommitance
incompatibility
incompatible
incompetence
incompetency
incompetent
Incomplete Sentence Blank (ICB) Test
incontinence
 giggle i.
 intermittent i.
 paralytic i.

incontinence *(continued)*
 urinary stress i.
incontinent
incontinentia
 pigmenti, i.
 pigmenti achromians, i.
incoordinate
incoordination
incorrigible
increased density
increased flexion reflex
increased stretch reflex
incubus
independent living
independent living skills
index (pl. indices)
Indian bow paralysis
indicanorachia
indices (pl. of index)
indifference
indifferent
individuation
Indoklon convulsive therapy
induced allergic encephalomyelitis
induced allergic neuritis
induction
 spinal i.
indusium griseum
indwelling catheter
INE (infantile necrotizing encephalomyelopathy)
inebriant
inebriated
inebriation
inebriety
inertia
infantile
 amaurotic familial idiocy, i.
 muscular atrophy, i.
 necrotizing encephalomyelopathy
  (INE), i.
 neuroaxonal dystrophy (INAD), i.
 paralysis, i.
 progressive spinal muscular dystrophy, i.
infantilism

infantilism *(continued)*
   angioplastic i.
   Brissaud's i.
   cachectic i.
   celiac i.
   dysthyroidal i.
   hepatic i.
   hypophyseal i.
   idiopathic i.
   intestinal i.
   myxedematous i.
   pituitary i.
   renal i.
   sex i.
   symptomatic i.
   universal i.
infant stimulation
infarct
infarctectomy
infarcted
infarction
   brain stem i.
   cerebral i.
   lacunar i.
   watershed i.
infection
inferior
   cerebral vein, i.
   cervical ganglion, i.
   frontal gyrus, i.
   frontomarginal sulcus, i.
   fronto-occipital sulcus, i.
   horn, i.
   occipital gyrus, i.
   olivary nucleus, i.
   olive, i.
   parietal lobule, i.
   petrosal sinus, i.
   preoptic nucleus, i.
   sagittal sinus, i.
   temporal gyrus, i.
   temporal sulcus, i.
   tubercle of Humphrey, i.
inferiority
   complex, i.
inferolateral

inferomedian
inferonasal
inferoposterior
inferotemporal
inflammatory headache
infolding
information
   retrieval, i.
infraclavicular
infraisthmal
infraoccipital
   nerve, i.
infraorbital
   nerve, i.
infrapsychic
infraspinatus
   muscle, i.
infraspinous
   muscle, i.
infratemporal
infratentorial
infundibula
infundibular
   stem, i.
infundibuloma
infundibulum (infundibula)
   hypothalami, i.
Infuse-a-port
Ingram-Withers-Speltz motor test
inherent
inheritance
inhibit
inhibited
inhibition
inhibitor
inhibitory
   interneuron, i.
   postsynaptic potential (IPSP), i.
   response, i.
iniencephaly
inion
   bump, i.
initis
inkblot test
inlay graft
inner child

inner self
inner table
innervated
innervation
   collateral i.
   double i.
   reciprocal
innervatory
   dyspraxia, i.
innominate
INO (intranuclear ophthalmoplegia)
inoccipitia
inomyositis
inophragma
inosclerosis
inotagma
inotropic
inotropism
in-positional jerks
inriding
insane
insanity
   adolescent i.
   affective i.
   alcoholic i.
   alternating i.
   anticipatory i.
   choreic i.
   circular i.
   climacteric i.
   communicated i.
   compound i.
   compulsive i.
   consecutive i.
   cyclic i.
   doubting i.
   emotional i.
   hereditary i.
   homicidal i.
   homochronous i.
   hysteric i.
   idiophrenic i.
   impulsive i.
   manic-depressive i.
   moral i.
   perceptional i.

insanity *(continued)*
   periodic i.
   polyneuritic i.
   primary i.
   puerperal i.
   recurrent i.
   senile i.
   simultaneous i.
   toxic i.
insanoid
insatiable
insecure
insecurity
insenescence
insensate
insensibility
insensible
insight
insightful
insolation
   hyperpyrexial i.
insomnia
insomniac
insomnic
inspectionism
instant Zen (LSD)
instinct
   aggressive i.
   death i.
   ego i.
   herd i.
   life i.
   mother i.
   sexual i.
instinctive
institutionalize
instrumental activities of daily living
instrumentation
insula
insular
insulin
   coma, i.
   coma therapy (ICT), i.
   coverage, i.
   -dependent diabetes mellitus (IDD), i.
   shock, i.

insulin *(continued)*
   shock therapy (IST), i.
insult
insultus
   hystericus, i.
intact
   neurologically, i.
   neurovascularly, i.
   reflexes, i.
intake and output (I&O)
integrate
integration
intellect
intellectual
intellectualization
intellectualize
intelligence
   quotient (IQ), i.
   test, i.
intelligent
intelligible
intemperance
intention tremor
interaccessory
interannular
interarticular
interbody
   fusion, i.
   ligament, i.
interbrain
intercalary
intercalate
intercalated disk
intercentral
intercerebral
intercoccygeal
intercostobrachial nerve
intercourse
intercristal
interest checklist
interfamilial
intergranular
intergyral
interhemicerebral
interhemispheric
interictal

interiorization
interlaminar
interligamentary
interligamentous
intermeningeal
intermittency
intermittent claudication
intermuscular
internal
   capsule, i.
   carotid artery (ICA), i.
   carotid artery occlusion (ICAO), i.
   hydrocephalus, i.
   jugular vein, i.
   rotation in extension (IRE), i.
   rotation in flexion (IRF), i.
internalization
internalize
International Symbol of Access
International 10-20 system
interneuron
internuclear ophthalmoplegia
internuncial neuron
interoceptive
interoceptor
interparenchymal
interparietal
interparoxysmal
interpediculate
interpeduncular
interpersonal
   behavior, i.
   maladaptation, i.
   relations, i.
interpial
Interpore
interposition
interpret
interpretation
interpretive
intersciatic
intersex
intersexual
intersexuality
interspace
interspinal

interspinous
   pseudoarthrosis, i.
interstice
interstitial
intertransverse
intervene
intervention
interventricular
intervertebral
   body, i.
   disk, i.
   disk narrowing, i.
   disk space, i.
   fibrocartilage, i.
   joint, i.
   punch, i.
   space, i.
interwave latency
intima
intimacy
intimal
intimate
intoeing
intoxicant
intoxicated
intoxication
   alcohol i.
   idiosyncratic i.
   pathological i.
   water i.
intra-arachnoid
intra-articular
intracanal
intracarpal
intracephalic
intracerebellar
intracerebral
intracisternal
intracranial
   arachnoid, i.
   hypertension, i.
   pressure (ICP), i.
   pressure catheter, i.
   pressure monitor, i.
   subdural space, i.
intracristal

intracristal *(continued)*
   space, i.
intradural
intrafamilial
   pedophilia, i.
intrafissural
intrafusal
intragemmal
intragyral
intraictal
intraligamentous
intralimbic
   gyrus, i.
intralobar
intramedullary
intrameningeal
intramural
intramuscular (IM)
intraneural
intranuclear ophthalmoplegia (INO)
intraocular
   pressure, i.
intraorbital
intraosseous
intraparietal
intrapial
intrapontine
intrapsychic
intrapyramidal
   fissure, i.
intrarachidian
intrasellar
intraspinal
intrastitial
intrathecal
intrathenar
intravascular
   coagulation, i.
intravenous (I.V.)
intraventricular
intravertebral
Intrel II spinal cord stimulation system
intrinsic
   minus deformity, i.
   muscles, i.
   plus deformity, i.

intrinsics
introjection
introspection
introspective
introversion
introvert
introverted
intuition
intuitive
invagination
inventory
inversion
    sexual i.
    -recovery technique, i.
invert
invertors
invocation
invoke
involuntary
involuntomotory
involutional
    melancholia, i.
    psychosis, i.
inward feelings
iodoventriculography
iophobia
iotacism
Iowa pressure articulation test
ipsilateral
ipsiversion
    ocular i.
IPSP (inhibitory postsynaptic potential)
IQ (intelligence quotient)
irascible
irascibility
IRE (internal rotation in extension)
IRF (internal rotation in flexion)
iris bombe
irisopsia
irradiation
irrational
irreversibility of conduction
irritable
irritability
irritation
    cerebral i.

irritation *(continued)*
    direct i.
    functional i.
    nerve root i.
    spinal i.
Isaacs' syndrome
ISB (Incomplete Sentence Blank) test
ischemia
    brain stem i.
    cerebral i.
    transient carotid i.
ischemic
    claudication, i.
    infarct, i.
    insult, i.
ischial
ischialgia
ischiodynia
ischioneuralgia
ischiovertebral
ischium
ischogyria
Ishihara plates
Ishihara test
island
    Calleja, i. of
    Reil, i. of
islet cell
isoadrenocorticism
isobaric
isobolism
isobutylnitrite
isochronia
isochronous
isocoria
isocortex
isodense
isoechoic
isoeffect
isoelectric
isoelectric EEG
isoenergetic
isokinetic exercise
isolation
isolation of affect
isolative

isolophobia
isometric
    contraction, i.
    contraction phase, i.
    exercise, i.
    muscle, i.
    relaxation, i.
isotonic
    exercise, i.
isotonicity
isovaleric acidemia
Isovue
IST (insulin shock therapy)
isthmectomy
isthmi (pl. of isthmus)
isthmic
isthmoparalysis

isthmoplegia
isthmospasm
isthmus (pl. isthmi)
    of cingulate gyrus, i.
Itard-Cholewa sign
ITE (in-the-ear) hearing aid
iter
    Sylvius, i. of
iteral
ithylordosis
ithyokyphosis
ITP (idiopathic thrombocytopenic pur-
    pura)
IV (intravenous)
IVDA (intravenous drug abuse)
ivory bones
ixomyelitis

Additional entries

J

jacket
  flexion body j.
  Frejka j.
  halo body j.
  Kydex body j.
  Minerva cervical j.
  orthoplast j.
  plaster-of-Paris j.
  Risser j.
  Royalite body j.
  Sayre's j.
  strait j.
Jackson Personality Inventory
Jackson's epilepsy
Jackson's law
Jackson's rule
Jackson's safety triangle
Jackson's syndrome
jacksonian
  epilepsy, j.
  march, j.
  motor seizure, j.
Jacobson theory
Jacquet's biokinetic treatment
jactatio
  capitis nocturna, j.
jactation
jactitation
Jadelot's lines
Jaffe-Lichtenstein disease
Jahnke's syndrome
jake neuritis
jake paralysis
Jakob's disease
Jakob-Creutzfeldt disease
Jamaica ginger paralysis
Jamaica ginger polyneuritis
jamais entendu
jamais pense
jamais vu
Jamar dynamometer
Jamar grip tester
Janet's disease

Janet's test
Janet's theory
Janin's tetanus
Jannetta bayonet forceps
Jannetta procedure
Jannetta retractor
Jansen retractor
Jansky-Bielschowsky disease
Japanese B encephalitis
jargon
  agraphia, j.
  aphasia, j.
Jarisch-Herxheimer fever reaction
Jarjavay's muscle
Javid clamp
Javid shunt
jaw claudication
jaw jerk
jaw winking
jealousy
Jefferson fracture
Jellinek's sign
Jendrassik maneuver
Jendrassik sign
jerk
  Achilles j.
  ankle j.
  biceps j.
  elbow j.
  jaw j.
  knee j.
  quadriceps j.
  tendon j.
  triceps surae j.
jerk nystagmus
Jervell and Lange-Nielsen syndrome
jet lag
Jevity isotonic liquid nutrition
jeweler forceps
Jewett brace
jitteriness
jitters
jittery

Jobst pressure garment
Jobst stockings
Jocasta complex
Joffroy's reflex
Joffroy's sign
Johnson-Zuck-Wingate motor test
joint (marijuana)
joint
    approximation, j.
    disease, j.
    heat, j.
    motion, j.
    position sense (JPS), j.
    redness, j.
    space, j.
    space narrowing, j.
    stiffness, j.
    warmth, j.
joints of Luschka
Jolly's myasthenic reaction
Jolly's position
Jolly's test
Joseph disease
joule
JPS (joint position sense).
judgment
    affect, j. and

judgmental
jugular
    ganglion, j.
    glossopharyngeal nerve, j.
    tenth cranial nerve, j.
    vagus nerve, j.
    vein, j.
jugum
    cerebralia ossium cranii, j.
jumped process complex
jumper disease of Maine
jumping disease
Jumping Frenchmen of Maine
jungian
Jung's method
Jung's theory
Juri flap
jury-mast
Juster reflex
juvenile
    pilocytic astrocytoma, j.
juxta-articulation
juxtallocortex
juxtaposition
juxtaspinal
juxtaspinal

Additional entries

_____

_____

_____

_____

_____

_____

_____

_____

_____

_____

K

K-ABC
Kaes' feltwork
Kaes' line
Kaes-Bekhterev layer
Kahler's law
kaif
kakke
kakosmia
Kalischer's disease
kallikrein-kinin (KK) system
Kalmuk idiocy
Kalmuk type
Kanavel brain-exploring cannula
Kanavel cannula
Kanavel conductor
Kanavel sign
Kanner syndrome
Kaposi's sarcoma
Karnofsky index
Karnofsky rating scale
Kartagener syndrome
Kashida's sign
Kashin-Beck disease
Kast syndrome
kathisophobia
katophoria
katotropia
katzenjammer
Kaufman Assessment Battery for Children
kava
Kayser-Fleischer ring
K-complex
Kearns-Sayre syndrome
KED (Kendrick extrication device)
Keen's point
Kehrer's reflex
Keith-Wagener (KW)
Keith-Wagener changes
Keith-Wagener classification
Keith-Wagener retinopathy
Keith-Wagener-Barker (KWB)
Kellogg-Speed lumbar spinal fusion
Kelly hemostat

Kendrick extrication device (KED)
Kennedy's syndrome
Kenny treatment
kenophobia
kenotoxin
Kent mental test
Kerandel's sign
kerasin
keratitis
keraunoneurosis
Kernberg theory
kernicterus
Kernig's sign
Kernohan grading (I, II, etc)
Kernohan's notch
kernschwund
Kerr's sign
Kerrison curette
Kerrison punch
Kerrison rongeur
Kestenbaum operation
Kestenbaum sign
ketoacidosis
ketoacidotic
ketosis
ketotic
Kety-Schmidt method
Key elevator
Key-Retzius connective tissue sheath
Khodadad clip
Kienbock's disease
Killgren treatment
Kiloh-Nevin syndrome
Kimberly sign
kinanesthesia
kineplasty
kinesalgia
kinesialgia
kinesiatrics
kinesics
kinesi-esthesiometer
kinesimeter
kinesiodic

kinesiology
kinesiometer
kinesioneurosis
kinesiotherapy
kinesis
kinesitherapy
kinesodic
kinesthesia
kinesthesiometer
kinesthesis
kinesthetic
kinetic
kinetism
kinetogenic
kinetographic
kinetoscope
kinetoscopy
kinetosis
kinetotherapy
King brace
kinky-hair disease
kinky-hair syndrome
kinohapt
kinology
kinomometer
Kinsbourne syndrome
kinship
kinsomania
Kirlian photography
Kirmisson periosteal raspatory
Kisch's reflex
kissing facets
kissing spine
kite apparatus
KK (kallikirein-kinin or knee kick)
Klapp's creeping treatment
kleeblattschadel
Klein's theory
Kleine-Levin syndrome
kleinian
Kleinert-Kutz micro
Kleist's hooking
Kleist's sign
Klemme laminectomy retractor
kleptolagnia
kleptomania

kleptomaniac
kleptophobia
Kleig eye
Klinefelter's syndrome
Klippel's disease
Klippel-Feil sign
Klippel-Feil syndrome
Klippel-Feldstein syndrome
klismaphilia
Klonopin
Klove-Matthews Motor Steadiness Battery
Klumpke's palsy
Klumpke's paralysis
Klumpke-Dejerine paralysis
Klumpke-Dejerine syndrome
Kluver-Barrera method
Kluver-Bucy syndrome
Knapp's law
knee jerk
knee kick (KK)
knemometry
Knie's sign
Knight back brace
Knight-Taylor thoracic brace
knismogenic
Knodt rod spinal fusion
Kocher's point
Kocher's reflex
Kocher's sign
Kocher-Debre-Semelaigne syndrome
Koerber-Salus-Elschnig syndrome
Kohnstamm phenomenon
koilorrhachic
Kolmer test
Koln clip
Kolodny scalp hemostat
kolytic
koniocortex
Kontrast-U
kopf-tetanus
kophemia
kopiopia
Koplik's spot
kopophobia
Koranyi's sign

koro
Korsakoff's amnesia
Korsakoff's psychosis
Korsakoff's syndrome
Korte-Ballance operation
Koshevnikoff's disease
Koshevnikoff's epilepsy
Kostmann's syndrome
Kovalevsky's canal
Krabbe's disease
Krabbe's leukodystrophy
Krabbe-Weber-Dimitri disease
Kraepelin classification
Kraepelin theory
kraepelinian schema
Kraske's position
kratometer
krauomania
Krause's bulbs
Krause's end-bulbs
Krause's denervation
Krause's operation
Krause's syndrome
Krause's ventricle
Kretschmer type
Krishaber's disease
Kronecker's puncture
Krukenberg's chopsticks
Krukenberg's spindle
kubisagari
Kufs' disease
Kugelberg-Welander disease
Kuhlmann's test
Kuhne's muscular phenomenon
Kuhne's spindle
Kuhne's terminal plates

Kulmuk idiocy
Kummell's disease
Kummell's spondylitis
Kummell-Verneuil disease
Kupressoff's center
Kurtzke disability score
kuru
Kussmaul aphasia
Kussmaul coma
Kussmaul paralysis
Kussmaul sign
Kussmaul-Kien respiration
Kussmaul-Landry paralysis
KW (Keith-Wagener)
 classification, K.
kwashiorkor
kwaski shakes
KWB (Keith-Wagener-Barker)
 classification, K.
Kyasanur Forest disease
Kydex body jacket
kymatism
kymograph
kyphoarachitis
kyphos
kyphoscoliosis
kyphoscoliotic
kyphosis
 juvenile k.
 lumbar k.
 lumbosacral k.
 Scheuerman's k.
 Scheuerman's juvenile k.
kyphotic
kyrtorrhachic

Additional entries

Additional entries

L

la belle indifference
labialism
labile
    affect, l.
lability
    emotional l.
labiochorea
labiochoreic stuttering
Laborde's method
labyrinth
labyrinthectomy
labyrinthine reflex
labyrinthitis
lack-of-check reflex
lacrimation
lactic acidosis
lactic dehydrogenase (LDH)
lactulose
lacuna (pl. lacunae)
lacunae (pl. of lacuna)
lacunar
    disease, l.
    infarct, l.
lacunes
lacunule
Ladd-Franklin theory
Lafora body
Lafora's disease
Lafora's epilepsy
Lafora's sign
lag
    phase, l.
lagophthalmos
laliatry
laliophobia
lallation
lalognosis
lalomania
laloneurosis
lalopathology
lalopathy
lalophobia
laloplegia

lalorrhea
lambdacism
lambdacismus
lambdoid suture
Lambert-Eaton syndrome
Lambotte's osteotome
lame
lameness
lamina (pl. laminae)
    dura, l.
    hypothalamus, l. of
    inferior l. of sphenoid bone
    medullaris lateralis corporis striati, l.
    medullaris medialis corposis striati, l.
    ossium cranii, l.
    propria, l.
    vertebral arch, l. of
lamina dissector
lamina elevator
lamina gouge
laminae (pl. of lamina)
    albae cerebelli, l.
    medullares cerebelli, l.
    medullares thalami, l.
laminagram
laminography
laminal
    arch, l.
laminaplasty
laminar
laminectomy
    chisel, l.
    frame, l.
    punch, l.
    raspatory, l.
    retractor, l.
    rongeur, l.
laminitis
laminogram
laminography
laminotomy
lamprophonia
lamprophonic

lancinating
   pain, l.
Lancisi's nerves
Lancisi's stria
Laundau color test
Landau reflex
landmark
   bony l.
   cephalometric l.
   craniometric l.
   orbital l.
   radiographic l.
Landolt pituitary speculum
Landouzy's disease
Landouzy's dystrophy
Landouzy's type
Landouzy-Dejerine atrophy
Landouzy-Dejerine muscular dystrophy
Landouzy-Dejerine type
Landouzy-Grasset law
Landry's disease
Landry's palsy
Landry's paralysis
Landry's syndrome
Langdon Down's disease
Lange's test
Langenbeck periosteal elevator
Langer's muscle
languor
Lanterman's incisures
Lanterman-Schmidt incisures
lantern test
lap board
Lapicque's law
LaPort triangle
lapsus
   calami, l.
   linguae, l.
   memoriae, l.
Larodopa
Larsen's syndrome
laryngeal
   reflex, l.
   vertigo, l.
laryngectomee
laryngectomize

laryngography
laryngoparalysis
laryngopharyngectomy
laryngophony
laryngoplegia
laryngoscopy
laryngospasm
laryngostroboscope
laryngotracheotomy
lascivia
LaSegue's disease
Lasegue's sign
Lasegue's test
laser (light amplification by stimulated
   emission of radiation)
   cane, l.
   speckle, l.
lassitude
latah
late infantile amaurotic familial idiocy
latency
   of response, l.
latency period
latent
   content, l.
laterad
lateral
   aperture, l.
   approach, l.
   cerebral fissure, l.
   column, l.
   corticospinal tract, l.
   decubitus position, l.
   gaze, l.
   gray column, l.
   gutter, l.
   horn, l.
   lemniscus, l.
   lemniscus nucleus, l.
   mammillary nucleus of Rose, l.
   medullary lamina, l.
   occipital gyrus, l.
   occipital sulcus, l.
   recess, l.
   sinus, l.
   spinorubral tract, l.

lateral *(continued)*
    spinothalamic tract, l.
    ventricle, l.
lateralis
laterality
    crossed l.
    dominant l.
lateralization
lateralizing
    finding, l.
    sign, l.
laterodeviation
lateroduction
lateroflexion
lateroposition
lateropulsion
laterotorsion
lateroversion
latex agglutination test
lathyrism
lathyrogen
latissimus
    dorsi muscle, l.
LATS (long-acting thyroid stimulator)
laughter
    compulsive l.
laughter reflex
Launois syndrome
Launois-Cleret syndrome
Laurence Biedl syndrome
Laurence-Moon-Biedl syndrome
Lauth's ligament
law
    all-or-none l.
    Aran's l.
    avalanche, l. of
    Babinski's l.
    Bastian's l.
    Bastian-Bruns l.
    Bell's l.
    Bell-Magendie l.
    Bowditch's l.
    contrary innervation, l. of
    Cushing's l.
    denervation, l. of
    Desmarres' l.

law *(continued)*
    diffusion, l. of
    diminishing returns, l. of
    Donders' l.
    Edinger's l.
    Elliott's l.
    Ewald's l.
    excitation, l. of
    facilitation, l. of
    fatigue, l. of
    Fechner's l.
    Flatau's l.
    Flourens' l.
    Froriep's l.
    Gerhardt-Semon l.
    Grasset's l.
    Gudden's l.
    Gull-Toynbee l.
    Gullstrand's l.
    Hering's l.
    Heyman's l.
    Hilton's l.
    Hook's l.
    Hoorweg's l.
    Horner's l.
    isochronism, l. of
    isolated conduction l. of
    Jackson's l.
    Kahler's l.
    Knapp's l.
    Landouzy-Grasset l.
    Laplcque's l.
    Magendie's l.
    Meltzer's l.
    Muller's l.
    myelogenetic l.
    Nernst's l.
    Pfluger's l.
    Prevost's l.
    psychophysical l.
    referred pain, l. of
    refreshment, l. of
    relativity, l. of
    Ritter-Valli l.
    Schroeder van der Kolk's l.
    Semon's l.

law *(continued)*
  Semon-Rosenbach l.
  Sherrington's l.
  specific irritability, l. of
  specificity of nervous energy, l. of
  Stokes' l.
  Toynbee's l.
  Valli-Ritter l.
  van der Kolk's l.
  Waller's l.
  wallerian l.
  Weber's l.
  Weber-Fechner l.
  Wundt-Lamansky l.
Lawen-Roth syndrome
Lawford's syndrome
lawn tennis arm
Lawrence-Moon syndrome
laxator
laxity
  ligament, l. of
LDH (lactic dehydrogenase)
L-dopa
LE (lupus erythematosus)
lead
  encephalopathy, l.
  pipe contraction, l.
  pipe rigidity, l.
  placement, l.
  poisoning, l.
leading edge
leakage headache
leaping atrophy
learned behavior
learning
  latent l.
  sight l.
learning disability
learning disorder
leash
Leatherman child spinal hook
leaves of dura
Leber's disease
lecherous
lechery
Lectron II electrode gel

Leeds Scale
Leeuwenhoek's disease
LeFort III fracture
left-hand dominant
left-handed
leg lag
leg-length discrepancy
Legal's disease
Legg-Calve-Perthes syndrome
legionnaires' disease
LeGrand-Geblewics phenomenon
leiasthenia
Leichtenstern's encephalitis
Leichtenstern's phenomenon
Leichtenstern's sign
Leichtenstern's type
Leigh disease
Leigh syndrome
leiodystonia
Lejeune's syndrome
Leksell forceps
Leksell laminectomy punch
Leksell rongeur
Leksell stereotactic frame
lemniscal
lemnisci (pl. of lemniscus)
lemniscus (pl. lemnisci)
  acoustic l.
  lateral l.
  medial l.
  optic l.
  sensory l.
  spinal l.
  trigeminal l.
lemoparalysis
lemostenosis
Lennox syndrome
Lennox-Gastaut syndrome
Lenox-Hill brace
lens
lenticular
  ansa, l.
  capsule, l.
  opacity, l.
lenticulo-optic
lenticulostriate

lenticulothalamic
lentivirus
Lenz's syndrome
leonine facies
leontiasis
leopard syndrome
leprechaun facies
leprechaunism
leprosy
leptocephalia
leptomeningeal
  cyst, l.
leptomeninges (pl. of leptomeninx)
leptomeningioma
leptomeningitis
  interna, l.
  sarcomatous l.
leptomeningopathy
leptomeninx (pl. leptomeninges)
leptophonia
Leri's sign
Leriche's disease
Leriche's operation
Leriche's syndrome
Lermoyez's syndrome
LeRoy scalp clip applying forceps
lesbian
lesbianism
Lesch-Nyhan syndrome
lesser splanchnic nerve
lesser superficial petrosal nerve
lethargic
lethargy
  hysteric l.
  induced l.
  lucid l.
lethe
letheomania
lethologica
Letterer-Siwe disease
Leudet's sign
Leudet's tinnitus
leu-enkephalin
leukencephalitis
leukodystrophy
  globoid l.

leukodystrophy *(continued)*
  globoid cell l.
  hereditary cerebral l.
  Krabbe's l.
  metachromatic l.
  spongiform l.
  sudanophilic l.
leukoencephalitis
  acute hemorrhagic l.
  periaxialis concentrica, l.
  van Bogaert's sclerosing l.
leukoencephalomalacia
leukoencephalopathy
  metachromatic l.
  multifocal l.
  progressive l.
  progressive multifocal l.
  subacute sclerosing l.
leukoencephaly
  metachromatic l.
leukoerythroblastosis
leukokoria
leukomyelitis
leukomyelopathy
leukotome
leukotomy
  transorbital l.
levator (pl. levatores)
  nerve, l.
levatores (pl. of levator)
LeVeen peritoneal shunt
LeVeen valve
level
  activity, l. of
  consciousness, l. of
Levi-Lorain type
Levin thermocouple cordotomy electrode
Levinson test
levitation
levoclination
levocycloduction
levodopa
levoduction
levogyration
levophobia
levorotation

levorotatory
levoscoliosis
levothyroxine
levotorsion
Lewin forceps
Lewin theory
Lewy inclusion body
Lex-Ton frame
Leyden's ataxia
Leyden-Mobius dystrophy
Leyden-Mobius syndrome
Leyden-Mobius type
Leyla retractor
Leyla-Yasargil retractor
Leyton Obsessional Inventory
Lezak's Malingering Test
Lhermitte's sign
Lhermitte and McAlpine syndrome
Lhermitte-Duclos disease
liberomotor
libidinal
libidinous
libido
    bisexual l.
    ego l.
Librium
Lichtheim's aphasia
Lichtheim's disease
Lichtheim's plaques
Lichtheim's sign
Lichtheim's syndrome
Lichtheim's test
lid
    drop, l.
    lag, l.
    reflex, l.
Liddell and Sherrington reflex
lidocaine
Lidone
Lidz theory
lie detector
Liepmann's apraxia
life support
lifestyle
Liga clip
liga-clipped

ligament
ligamenta (pl. of ligamentum)
    flava, l.
ligamentous
    instability, l.
    laxity, l.
    strain, l.
ligamentum (pl. ligamenta)
    denticulatum, l.
    flavum, l.
light
    -dark discrimination, l.
    -headed, l.
    microscopy, l.
    perception, l.
    reflex, l.
    sense, l.
    touch sensation, l.
Light headrest
Light-Veley apparatus
Light-Veley drill
Light-Veley headrest
lilliputian hallucination
limb
    -kinetic apraxia, l.
    -kinetic dyspraxia, l.
    salvage, l.
    threat, l.
limbi (pl. of limbus)
limbic
    system, l.
limbus (pl. limbi)
limen (pl. limina)
    insula, l. of
    twoness, l. of
    vestibuli, l.
limina (pl. of limen)
liminal
    stimulus, l.
    value, l.
liminometer
limitation
    extension, l. of
    flexion, l. of
    motion, l. of
limosis

Lindau's syndrome
Linder's sign
line
  Baillarger, l. of
  Gennari, l. of
linear
  skull fracture, l.
lingual
  titubation, l.
linguistics
lingula (pl. lingulae)
  cerebelli, l.
lingulae (pl. of lingula)
lip
  reading, l.
  reflex, l.
  smacking, l.
Lipiodol
lipochrome
lipohyalinosis
lipoma
lipomatous
lipomeningocele
lipoprotein
lipoproteinemia
lipothymia
lipping
Lisch's nodule
lisping
Lissauer's marginal zone
Lissauer's paralysis
Lissauer's tract
lissencephalia
lissencephalic
lissencephaly
lissive
list
Listeria monocytogenes
listhesis
listing gait
literal paraphasia
Lithane
lithium
Lithobid
Lithonate
Lithotabs

Little's disease
livedo reticularis
liver flap
Livierato's sign
LMN (lower motor neuron)
loading dose
lobar
  cerebral atrophy, l.
lobate
lobe
  hypophysis, anterior l. of
  pituitary gland, anterior l. of
  cerebrum, caudate l. of
  cerebellar l.
  cerebellum, l. of
  crescentic l. of cerebellum
  flocculonodular l.
  frontal l.
  gracile l. of cerebellum
  limbic l.
  neural l.
  neural l. of neurohypohysis
  neural l. of pituitary gland
  occipital l.
  olfactory l.
  optic l.
  parietal l.
  posterior l. of hypophysis
  posterior l. of pituitary gland
  prefrontal l.
  quadrangular l. of cerebellum
  quadrate l. of cerebral hemisphere
  semilunar l.
  temporal l.
  temporosphenoid l. of cerebral hemi-
    sphere
lobectomy
lobi (pl. of lobus)
lobite
lobotomy
  frontal l.
  prefrontal l.
  transorbital l.
lobotomy electrode
lobotomy needle
Lobstein's disease

Lobstein's syndrome
lobule
   cerebellum, l. of
   pituitary gland, l. of
   thymus, l. of
lobulus
   centralis cerebelli, l.
   paracentralis, l.
   parietalis, l.
   quadrangularis cerebelli, l.
   semilunaris, l.
lobus (pl. lobi)
   frontalis, l.
   occipitalis, l.
   olfactorius, l.
   parietalis, l.
   temporalis, l.
local circuit theory
localization
   cerebral l.
localizer
localizing neurological sign
Locan theory
loci (pl. of locus)
locked-in syndrome
locker-room syndrome
lockjaw
locomotion
locomotive
locomotor
   ataxia, l.
locomotorial
locomotorium
locomotory
locus (pl. loci)
   ceruleus, l.
   control, l. of
   ferrugineus, l.
Loew-Terry-Machiachan syndrome
logagnosia
logagraphia
logamnesia
logaphasia
logasthenia
logoclonia
logoklony

logokophosis
logomania
logoneurosis
logopathy
logopedia
logopedics
logoplegia
logorrhea
logospasm
Lombard's test
Lombardi's sign
loneliness
lonely
long-acting thyroid stimulator (LATS)
long memory
long tract
   signs, l.
longing
longiradiate
longissimus muscle
longitudinal
   cerebral fissure, l.
   fasciculi of pons, l.
longsightedness
longus
loop
   gamma l.
   Granit l.
   hypoglossal nerve, l. of
   Hyrtl's l.
   Mcyer's l.
   spinal nerves, l's of
loose association
loosening of associations
Lorain type
Lorain's disease
Lorain's infantilism
lorazepam
lordoscoliosis
lordosis
   cervical l.
   lumbar l.
   thoracic l.
lordotic
   curve, l.
   view, l.

loss
    consciousness, l. of
    memory, l. of
    motion, l. of
    muscle tone, l. of
    sensation, l. of
    sphincter control, l. of
Lou Gehrig disease
Louis-Bar syndrome
Louisville Fear Survey
loupe
    magnification, l.
Love leukotome
Love root retractor
Love-Adson elevator
Love-Gruenwald rongeur
Love-Kerrison rongeur
Loven reflex
low voltage fast activity
Lowe's disease
Lowe's oculocerebrorenal syndrome
Lowenthal's tract
lower motor neuron (LMN)
    lesion, l.
Lowman balance board
loxia
Loxitane
loxotic
LP (lumbar puncture)
LS (lumbosacral)
LSD (lysergic acid diethylamide)
L-spine (lumbar spine)
LSU reciprocation gait orthosis
L-thyroxine
L-tryptophan myopathy
Lucae bone mallet
lucency
lucent
Luciani's triad
lucid
    interval, l.
lucidity
luckenschadel
Luer forceps
lues
luetic

Luft's disease
lumbago
lumbar
    aortogram, l.
    arteriogram, l.
    curvature, l.
    disk, l.
    disk herniation, l.
    kyphosis, l.
    laminectomy, l.
    lordosis, l.
    lordotic curve, l.
    myelogram, l.
    myotome, l.
    nerve, l.
    nerve block, l.
    plexus, l.
    puncture (LP), l.
    puncture headache, l.
    puncture needle, l.
    reflex, l.
    region, l.
    scoliosis, l.
    spinal cord, l.
    spine (L-spine), l.
    splanchnic nerve, l.
    spondylosis, l.
    spurring, l.
    sympathectomy, l.
    sympathetic nervous system, l.
    vertebrae, l.
    vertebral disk, l.
    vertebral joint, l.
lumbarization
lumbocostal
lumbocrural
lumbodorsal
lumbodynia
lumboiliac
lumbosacral (LS)
    fusion, l.
    joint, l.
    plexus, l.
    spinal cord, l.
    spine (LS spine), l.
    sprain, l.

lumbosacral (LS) *(continued)*
   strain, l.
   trunk, l.
   vertebra, l.
lumbus
lumen (pl. lumina)
lumina (pl. of lumen)
luminal
Luminal
Lumiwand
Lumsden's center
lunacy
lunatic
lunatism
Lundvall's blood crisis
lupus
   erythematosus (LE), l.
lupus panel
Luque instrumentation
Luque rod fixation
lura
lural
Luria-Nebraska Neuropsychological Battery
Luschka's foramen
Lust's phenomenon
Lust's reflex

Lust's sign
luxatio
luxation
Luys' body
lycanthropy
lycorexia
Lyme disease
lymphangioma
lymphatic
lymphatomatosis
lymphogranuloma
lymphogranulomatosis
lymphoma
lymphomatous
lymphopathy
lymphoproliferative
lyophilization
lyse
lysergic acid diethylamide (LSD)
lysergide
Lysholm's line
lysis
Lyssa body
lyssavirus
lyssophobia
lytic lesion

Additional entries

M

MacAusland lumbar brace
MacAusland procedure
macerated
Macewen's sign
Machado test
Machado-Guerreiro test
Machado-Joseph disease
Machover test
Mackenzie's syndrome
macrencephaly
MA (mental age)
macrocephalous
macrocephaly
macrocrania
macrodystrophia
macroencephaly
macroglia
macrography
macrogyria
macromania
macromelia
    paresthetica, m.
macroprosopia
macropsia
macrosmatic
macrosomatia
macrostereognosia
macrovesicular
macula
macular
    cherry-red spot myoclonus
      syndrome, m.
    sparing, m.
maculocerebral
maculopapular
mad
Maddox rod test
madness
madreporic coral
Maffucci's syndrome
Magendie's foramen
Magendie's law
Magendie's sign

Magendie's space
Magendie-Hertwig sign
magic mushrooms
magical thinking
Magnan's movement
Magnan's sign
Magnan's symptom
magnesium
magnesemia
magnetic
    gait, m.
    resonance imaging (MRI), m.
    resonance spectroscopy (MRS), m.
    stimulation, m.
magnetism
magnetoencephalography (MEG)
magnetometer
Magnevist
magnification
magnifying loupe
Magnus and de Kleijn neck reflexes
Mahler theory
main
    accoucheur, m.
    en crochet, m.
    en griffe, m.
    en pince, m.
    en singe,m.
    fourche, m.
    succulente, m.
mainstreaming
Make-a-Picture-Story Test
mal
    de mer, m.
    grand m.
    haute m.
    petit m.
    rouge, m.
Malacarne's space
malacia
malacic
maladaptation
maladaptive

maladie
  des tics, m.
maladjusted
maladjustment
malaise
malangulation
malaria
malarial
male intersex
malformation
malformed
malignancy
malignant
  hypertension, m.
  hyperthermia, m.
  lymphocytoma, m.
  meningioma, m.
mali-mali
malinger
malingerer
malingering
Malis angled-up bipolar forceps
Malis bipolar electrocautery
Malis CMC-II bipolar coagulator
Malis irrigation forceps
malleation
mallet finger
mallet toe
malposed
malposition
malrotation
malum
  vertebrale suboccipitale, m.
malunion
malunited
mamillary body
mamillopeduncular
mamillothalamic
mandibular reflex
maneuver
  Adson m.
  Allen m
  Crede m.
  Fowler m.
  Gowers' m.
  Halstead m.

maneuver *(continued)*
  Heimlich m.
  Jendrassik m.
  Phalen's m.
  Schreiber's m.
  Sellick m.
  soldier's m.
  Valsalva m.
manganese poisoning
mania
  acute m.
  acute hallucinatory m.
  akinetic m.
  a potu, m.
  Bell's m.
  dancing m.
  doubting m.
  epileptic m.
  hysterical m.
  mitis, m.
  periodical m.
  puerperal m.
  Ray's m.
  reasoning m.
  religious m.
  secandi, m.
  transitory m.
  unproductive m.
maniac
maniacal
maniaphobia
manic
  attack, m.
  -depressive, m.
  episode, m.
  syndrome, m.
manifest
  squint, m.
manifestation
maniloquism
manipulate
manipulation
manipulative
Mann's sign
mannerism
mannitol

Mannkopf's sign
mannosidosis
manometer
manometrics
manometry
mantle
    layer, m.
mantra
    meditation, m.
manual
    muscle test, m.
manudynamometer
MAO (monoamine oxidase)
MAOI (monoamine oxidase inhibitor)
maple syrup urine disease (MSUD)
mapping of defect
marantic
    thrombosis, m.
marantology
marasmic
marasmoid
marasmus
marble bone disease
marble state
Marburg virus disease
March's disease
marche a petit pas
Marchesani's syndrome
Marchi's balls
Marchi's method
Marchi's reaction
Marchi's tract
Marchiafava-Bignami disease
Marcus Gunn jaw-winking syndrome
Marcus-Gunn phenomenon
Marcus-Gunn pupil
Marcus-Gunn's pupillary sign
Marfan disease
Marfan syndrome
marginal
    gyrus, m.
    layer, m.
    sulcus, m.
Marie's ataxia
Marie's disease
Marie's quadrilateral space

Marie's sclerosis
Marie's sign
Marie-Bamberger disease
Marie-Foix sign
Marie-Robinson syndrome
Marie-Strumpell disease
Marie-Strumpell spondylitis
Marie-Tooth disease
marijuana
Marinesco's sign
Marinesco's succulent hand
Marinesco-Radovici reflex
Marinesco-Sjogren syndrome
Marinol
Mariotte's spot
marital
Marlow's test
Maroteaux-Lamy syndrome
marriage encounter
marrowbrain
Marsh's disease
Marshall and Tanner pubertal staging
Marshall Hall's facies
marsupialization
marsupialize
Martinotti's cells
Martorell's syndrome
Mary Jane (marijuana)
masculation
masculinization
masculinize
mask
    ecchymotic m.
    Hutchinson's m.
    Parkinson's m.
    tabetic m.
mask facies
masked depression
masking
Maslow theory
masochism
masochist
masochistic
mass
    effect, m.
    lesion, m.

mass *(continued)*
    psychogenic illness, m.
    reflex, m.
massa
    intermedia, m.
Masserman theory
masseter muscle
masseteric sling
Masson method
MAST (medical OR military antishock
    trousers)
masturbate
masturbation
Mata's triangle
matchsticked
mater
    dura m.
    pia m.
maternal deprivation syndrome
matriarch
matriarchal
matrilineal
matroclinous
matrocliny
matter
    gelatinous m.
    gray m. of nervous system
    white m. of nervous system
Mattis Dementia Rating Scale
matutinal
Mauchart's ligament
Maudsley Obsessional-Compulsive In-
    ventory
Mauthner's membrane
Mauthner's test
maxillofacial
Mayer's reflex
Mayer's sign
Mayerhofer's test
Mayerson's sign
Mayfield clip
Mayfield-Kees headrest
Mayo's sign
MBD (minimal brain dysfunction)
MBP (myelin basic protein)
M-bur

MCA (middle cerebral artery)
McAndrews Alcoholism Scale
McArdle's disease
McCarthy Scales of Children's Abilities
McCarthy's reflex
McCarthy's sign
McCormac's reflex
McCune-Albright syndrome
McFadden clip
McKenzie bur
McKenzie clip
McKenzie drill
McNaught keel
MCP (metacarpophalangeal)
    joint, M.
MCTC (metrizamide CT cisternogram)
MCTD (mixed connective tissue disease)
MD (muscular dystrophy)
MDAC (multiple-dose activated charcoal)
MEA (multiple endocrine adenopathies)
Means' sign
Mears sacroiliac plate
measles
    encephalitis, m.
Mebaral
mechanism
    defense m.
    neutralizing m.
mechanoreceptor
mechanotherapy
Meckel's band
Meckel's cave
Meckel's cavity
Meckel's ganglion
Meckel's space
Meckel's syndrome
Meckel-Gruber syndrome
mecocephalic
mecystasis
mediad
medial
    frontal sulcus of Eberstaller, m.
    longitudinal fasciculus, m.
medialis
median
    eminence, m.

median *(continued)*
   forebrain, m.
   nerve, m.
   nerve compression, m.
   nerve decompression, m.
   nerve entrapment, m.
   sulcus, m.
medianis
mediate
mediation
mediator
medication effect
medicephalic
medicerebellar
medicerebral
medicopsychology
medicosocial
medifrontal
Medin's disease
medioccipital
mediolateral
MediPort
meditate
meditation
Mediterranean disease
medium
medius
Medtronic Pulsor Intrasound pain reliever
medulla (pl. medullae)
   adrenal m.
   oblongata, m.
   spinal m.
   spinalis m.
   thymi, m.
   thymus, m.
medullae (pl. of medulla)
medullary
   cystic disease, m.
   lamina, m.
medullated
   nerve fiber, m.
medullation
medullectomy
medulliadrenal
medullispinal
medullitis

medullization
medulloadrenal
medulloarthritis
medulloblast
medulloblastoma
   Cushing's m.
medulloencephalic
medulloepithelioma
medullosuprarenoma
medullotherapy
Mees' lines
MEG (magnetoencephalography)
megalencephalon
megalencephaly
megalgia
megalocephaly
megalomania
megalomaniac
megaphagia
megavitamin
megophthalmos
mehlnahrschaden
Meige's syndrome
Meissner's tactile corpuscles
melagra
melalgia
melancholia
   affective m.
   agitata, m.
   agitated m.
   attonita, m.
   climacteric m.
   flatuous m.
   hypochondriaca, m.
   hypochondriacal m.
   involutional m.
   panphobic m.
   religiosa, m.
   sexual m.
   simplex, m.
   stuporosa, m.
   stuporous m.
   suicidal m.
melancholiac
melancholic
melancholy

melanin
melanoma
melissophobia
Melkersson's syndrome
Melkersson-Rosenthal syndrome
melomania
melosalgia
Meltzer's law
membrane of Liliequist
memory
   affect m.
   anterograde m.
   echoic m.
   eye m.
   five-minute m.
   iconic m.
   immunologic m.
   kinesthetic m.
   long-term m.
   retrograde m.
   screen m.
   short-term m.
   visual m.
memory deficit
memory-impaired
memory impairment
memory loss
memory trace
MEN (multiple endocrine neoplasia)
menarche
Mendel's dorsal reflex of foot
Mendel's reflex
Mendel-Bekhterev reflex
Mendel-Bekhterev sign
Mengert's shock syndrome
Meniere's disease
Meniere's syndrome
meningeal
   artery, m.
   cry, m.
   field, m.
   hemorrhage, m.
   hydrops, m.
   inflammation, m.
   irritation, m.
   plague, m.

meningeal *(continued)*
   sarcoma, m.
   sarcomatosis, m.
   signs, m.
   spaces, m.
meningematoma
meningeocortical
meningeoma
meningeorrhaphy
meninges (pl. of meninx)
meninghematoma
meningina
meninginitis
meningioma
   angioblastic m.
   fibroblastic m.
   malignant m.
   meningothelial m.
   mesodermal m.
   olfactory groove m.
   psammomatous m.
meningiomatosis
meningism
meningismus
meningitic
meningitides (pl. of meningitis)
meningitis (pl. meningitides)
   acute aseptic m.
   African m.
   bacterial m.
   basilar m.
   benign lymphocytic m.
   carcinomatosa, m.
   cerebral m.
   cerebrospinal m.
   cryptococcal m.
   eosinophilic m.
   epidermic cerebrospinal m.
   external m.
   granulomatous m.
   gummatous m.
   internal m.
   listeria m.
   lymphocytic m.
   meningococcal m.
   metastatic m.

meningitis (pl. meningitides) *(continued)*
    Mollaret's m.
    mumps m.
    mycotic m.
    necrotoxica reactiva, m.
    occlusive m.
    ossificans, m.
    otitic m.
    parameningococcus m.
    plague m.
    pneumococcal m.
    posterior m.
    purulent m.
    pyogenic m.
    Quincke's m.
    septicemic m.
    serosa circumscripta, m.
    serosa circumscripta cystica, m.
    serous m.
    simple m.
    spinal m.
    sterile m.
    sympathetica, m.
    syphilitic m.
    torula m.
    torular m.
    traumatic m.
    tubercular m.
    tuberculous m.
    viral m.
meningitophobia
meningoarteritis
meningoblastoma
meningocele
    spurious m.
meningocephalitis
meningocerebritis
meningococcal polysaccharide vaccine
    group A and C
meningococcemia
    acute fulminating m.
meningococci
meningococcidal
meningococcin
meningococcosis
meningococcus (pl. meningococci)

meningocortical
meningocyte
meningoencephalitis
    due to Naegleria and Acanthamoeba,
      m.
    eosinophilic m.
    mumps m.
    primary amebic m.
    syphilitic m.
meningoencephalocele
meningoencephalomyelitis
meningoencephalomyelopathy
meningoencephalopathy
meningoexothelioma
meningofibroblastoma
meningogenic
meningoma
meningomalacia
meningomyelitis
meningomyelocele
meningomyeloencephalitis
meningomyeloradiculitis
meningomyelorrhaphy
meningo-osteophlebitis
meningopathy
meningopneumonitis
meningorachidian
meningoradicular
meningoradiculitis
meningorecurrence
meningorrhagia
meningorrhea
meningosis
meningothelial meningioma
meningothelioma
meningotyphoid
meningovascular
    syphilis, m.
meninx (pl. meninges)
    fibrosa, m.
    serosa, m.
    tenuis, m.
    vasculosa, m.
Menkes' disease
Menkes' syndrome
Mennell's sign

menopausal
menopause
  artificial m.
  male m.
  premature m.
  surgical m.
menses
menstrual
menstruation
mental
  aberration, m.
  age (MA), m.
  anesthesia, m.
  blind spot, m.
  chemistry, m.
  clouding, m.
  confusion, m.
  deficiency, m.
  disorder, m.
  disturbance, m.
  dullness, m.
  faculties, m.
  fog, m.
  function, m.
  healing, m.
  health, m.
  hygiene, m.
  lapse, m.
  linking, m.
  Measurements Yearbook, M.
  process, m.
  retardation, m.
  status, m.
  subnormality, m.
  telepathy, m.
mentalia
mentality
mentally
  competent, m.
  deranged, m.
  ill, m.
  incompetent, m.
  retarded, m.
mentation
menticide
menton

mentulomania
MEP (motor evoked potential or multimodality evoked potential)
meralgia
  paresthetica, m.
mercurial palsy
merergastic
merinthophobia
Merkersson-Rosenthal syndrome
Merke's discs
merocoxalgia
merocrania
meroergasia
meropia
merorachischisis
merosmia
Merzbacher-Pelizaeus disease
mesaxon
mescal
  bean, m.
  button, m.
mescaline
mescalism
mesencephal
mesencephalic
mesencephalitis
mesencephalohypophyseal
mesencephalon
mesencephalotomy
mesenchyma
mesenchymal
  tumor, m.
  villous core, m.
mesenchymoma
mesioinferior
mesmerism
mesmerize
mesodermal
mesoglia
mesoglioma
mesoneurium
mesopia
mesorachischisis
mesothenar
Mestinon
metabolic

metabolic *(continued)*
  acidosis, m.
  alkalosis, m.
  disorder, m.
  encephalopathy, m.
  headache, m.
metabolimetry
metabolism
metabolite
metacarpophalangeal (MCP)
metachromasia
metachromatic leukodystrophy
metadromic progression
metal plate
metal rod
metallesthesia
metallic coil embolization
metallophilia
metallophobia
metameric syndrome
metamorphopsia
metaphrenia
metaphysical
metaphysics
metaplexus
metapsyche
metapsychics
metapsychism
metapsychology
metapsychosis
metastases (pl. of metatasis)
metastasis (pl. metastases)
metastasize
metatela
metathalamus
metencephal
metencephalic
metencephalon
metencephalospinal
met-enkephalin
metepencephalon
methadone
methamphetamine
methionine malabsorption syndrome
methomania
methyl alcohol poisoning

methyl methacrylate
methyl metolazone
methylene blue
methysergide maleate
metonymy
metopic
  suture, m.
metopion
metopism
metopodynia
Metrazol shock therapy
metrizamide
  cisternography, m.
  CT cisternogram (MCTC), m.
  myelography, m.
metrostasis
Meyer cervical orthosis
Meyer loop
Meyer theory
Meyer-Betz disease
Meyer-Schwickerath and Weyers syndrome
Meyerding chisel
Meyerding curette
Meyerding gouge
Meyerding osteotome
Meynert's bundle
Meynert's cell
Meynert's commissure
Meynert's decussation
Meynert's tract
MGBG
MI (myocardial infarction)
MIBG (metaiodobenzylguanidine)
mication
Michaelis' rhomboid
Michel clip
Michel deafness
Michel deformity
micrencephalon
micrencephalous
micrencephaly
microadenoma
microaneurysm
microarousal
microbipolar cautery

microbipolar forceps
microbrenner
microcephalic
microcephalous
microcephalus
microcephaly
microcrania
microcystic
microdissection
microembolus
microglia
microglial
microgliocyte
microglioma
microgliomatosis
micrographia
microgyri
microgyria
microgyrus
microinfarct
microinstrumentation
microinvasive
microlumbar
   diskectomy, m.
micromegalopsia
micromelia
micromyelia
microneedle
microneurosurgery
micropathology
microperfusion
microphobia
micropoint cautery
microprobe
micropsia
micropsychotic
microscissors
microscopy
microsleep
microsmatic
microsurgery
microsurgical
   DREZ-otomy, m.
   technique, m.
microtechnique
MicroTeq belt-worn device

microtia
microtus
microwave diathermy (MWD)
micturition syncope
MID (multi-infarct dementia)
Midas Rex drill
Midas Rex pneumatic instruments
midaxillary line
midbrain
middle cerebral artery (MCA)
midfrontal
midlife crisis
midline
   shift, m.
   structures, m.
midoccipital
mid-pons
Midrin
midsagittal
   plane, m.
midtegmentum
Miege's syndrome
Mierzejewski effect
migraine
   abdominal m.
   acute confusional m.
   cluster m.
   fulgurating m.
   hemiplegic m.
   ophthalmic m.
   ophthalmoplegic m.
migraine headache
migraineur
migrainoid
migrainous
   hemiplegia, m.
migrate
migration
migratory pain
Mikulicz's disease
Mikulicz's syndrome
miliary
milieu
   ward m.
milieu therapy
milkmaid grip

Millard-Gubler paralysis
Millard-Gubler syndrome
Miller-Fisher syndrome
Milligan's trichrome stain
millipore filter technique
millivolt (mv)
Millon Clinical Multiaxial Inventory
Mills' disease
Milontin
Mils bipolar cautery
Miltown
Milwaukee brace
Milwaukee cervicothoracolumbosacral orthosis
mimesis
mimicking
mimicry
mimmation
mimocausalgia
mind
    -altering, m.
    -blowing, m.
    control, m.
    cure, m.
    -expanding, m.
    set, m.
mineralization
mineralocorticoids
Minerva cervical jacket
mini-arousals
minimal brain damage
minimal brain dysfunction (MBD)
minimal cerebral dysfunction
Minimata disease
Mini-Mental State Examination
minimum
    audibile, m.
    audible m.
    cognoscibile, m.
    legibile, m.
    light m.
    sensibile, m.
    separabile, m.
    visibile, m.
Minnesota Multiphasic Personality Inventory (MMPI)

Minnesota Preschool Scale
Minor's disease
Minor's sign
minuthesis
miophone
miopragia
miosis
mirror focus
mirror movement
mirror writing
mirroring
miryachit
misaction
misandria
misanthropist
misanthropy
misocainia
misogamy
misogyny
misologia
misoneism
misopedia
Mitchell's disease
Mitchell's treatment
Mitmachen
mitochondrial
Mittlemeyer's test
mittor
mixed apnea
mixed connective tissue disease (MCTD)
MixEvac
mixoscopia
Mixter clamp
MMPI (Minnesota Multiphasic Personality Inventory)
MNCV (motor nerve conduction velocity)
mnemasthenia
mnemic
mnemonic
Moban
Moberg's ninhydrin
mobile
    arm support, m.
    spasm, m.
mobility
    -impaired, m.

mobility *(continued)*
   Inventory for Agoraphobia, M.
   training, m.
mobilization
mobilize
Mobius' disease
Mobius' sign
Mobius' syndrome
modality
model
modeling
MODY (maturity-onset diabetes of the
   young)
Moe-style spinal hook
Moebius' sign
Moebius' syndrome
mogiarthria
mogilalia
mogiphonia
Mohr syndrome
molder's sign
molecular genetics
molilalia
Mollaret's meningitis
mollis chorea
molysmophobia
Monakow's fasciculus
Monakow's syndrome
Monakow's theory
Monakow's tract
monathetosis
monaural hearing loss
monaxon
monaxonic
Monckeberg's sclerosis
Mondini's deafness
Mondonesi reflex
monesthetic
Monge's disease
mongolian
   idiocy, m.
   idiot, m.
   spot, m.
mongolism
   translocation m.
mongoloid

monkey paw
monoamine oxidase (MAO)
monoamine oxidase inhibitory (MAOI)
monoaminergic
monoanesthesia
monoblepsia
monochorea
monochromatism
   cone m.
   rod m.
monocular diplopia
monomania
monomeuric
monomoria
monomyoplegia
monomyositis
mononeural
mononeuric
mononeuritis
   multiplex, m.
mononeuropathy
   multiplex, m.
mononoea
monoparesis
monoparesthesia
monophasia
monophasic
monoplegia
monoplegic
monopolar coagulation
monopolar electrocautery
monopsychosis
monorecidive
monosomy
monospasm
monospastic
monosynaptic
monotherapy
Monro's foramen
Monro's sulcus
Montgomery-Asberg Scale
monticulus
   cerebelli, m.
mood
   -altering, m.
   -congruent, m.

mood *(continued)*
   disorder, m.
   disturbance, m.
   incongruent, m.
   shift, m.
   swing, m.
moon face
moon facies
Moon's molars
Moore's syndrome
moral
   judgment, m.
morale
moralistic
morbid
morcellated
morcellation
morcellement
morcellize
Morel syndrome
Morel-Kraepelin disease
mores
Morgagni's disease
Morgagni's hyperostosis
Morgagni-Stewart-Morel syndrome
moria
moribund
Morita therapy
Morley's peritoneocutaneous reflex
morning glory seeds
morning glory syndrome
Moro embrace reflex
Moro reflex
Moro test
moron
moronity
morphine sulfate
morphinism
morphinomania
morphology
Morquio's disease
Morquio's sign
Morquio's syndrome
Morquio-Ullrich disease
morsicatio buccarum
mortise

mortised
Morton's neuralgia
Morton's toe
Morton-Horwitz nerve cross-over sign
Morvan's chorea
Morvan's disease
Morvan's syndrome
mosaicism
Moschcowitz's disease
mosquito hemostat
Mosso's ergograph
motion
   active m.
   passive m.
   range of m.
motion sickness
motivated
motivation
motive
   achievement m.
   aroused m.
motoceptor
motofacient
motoneuron
   alpha m.
   gamma m.
   heteronymous m.
   homonymous m.
   lower m.
   peripheral m.
   upper m.
motor
   activity, m.
   and sensory changes, m.
   aphasia, m.
   area, m.
   ataxia, m.
   behavior, m.
   blocking, m.
   branch, m.
   cell, m.
   cortex, m.
   discriminative acuity, m.
   disturbance, m.
   endplate, m.
   evoked potential (MEP), m.

motor *(continued)*
   fibers, m.
   hyperactivity, m.
   impersistence, m.
   nerve, m.
   nerve conduction velocity
      (MNCV), m.
   neuron, m.
   nucleus, m.
   phenomenon, m.
   plate, m.
   points, m.
   root, m.
   sense, m.
   skills, m.
   speech area, m.
   strength, m.
   unit, m.
   weakness, m.
motorgraphic
motoricity
motorium
   commune, m.
motorius
motorogerminative
motorpathy
Mott's law of anticipation
mottling
mounding phenomenon
mountain fever
mountain sickness
mourning
mouse-tooth forceps
mouth and hand synkinesis
mouthstick
movement
   active m.
   angular m.
   artifact m.
   associated m.
   athetoid m.
   automatic m.
   autonomic m.
   choreic m.
   choreiform m.
   circus m.

movement *(continued)*
   conjugate eye m.
   contralateral associated m.
   dystonic m.
   forced m.
   Frenkel's m.
   Magnan's m.
   nonrapid eye (NREM) m.
   passive m.
   rapid eye (REM) m.
   saccadic m.
   scissors m.
   spontaneous m.
   synkinetic m.
movement artifact
movement disorder
movement perseveration
moyamoya disease
Moynahan syndrome
Mozer's disease
MRI (magnetic resonance imaging)
MRS (magnetic resonance spectroscopy)
MS (multiple sclerosis)
MSLT (multiple sleep latency test)
MSUD (maple syrup urine disease)
Mu rhythm
Muckle-Wells syndrome
mucocele
mucolipidosis
mucopolysaccharidase
mucopolysaccharide
mucopolysaccharidoses (pl. of
      mucopolysaccharidosis)
mucopolysaccharidosis (pl.
      mucopolysaccharidoses)
mucormycosis
Muehr craniotome
MUGA (multiple gated acquisition) scan
Mulder's angle
mulibrey nanism
Muller's fibers
Muller's law
multifactorial
multifocal
multifocal leukoencephalopathy
multiganglionic

multi-infarct dementia (MID)
Multilingual Alphabet Examination
multimodality evoked potential (MEP)
multiple
  -dose activated charcoal (MDAC), m.
  endocrine adenomatosis, m.
  endocrine adenopathies (MEA), m.
  endocrine neoplasia (MEN), m.
  gated acquisition (MUGA) scan, m.
  lentigines syndrome, m.
  meningiomas, m.
  myeloma, m.
  neurofibromatosis, m.
  neuroma, m.
  personality, m.
  sclerosis (MS), m.
  sleep latency test (MSLT), m.
  spike complex, m.
  spike foci, m.
  sulfatase deficiency, m.
  tic syndrome, m.
Multipoise headrest
multisynaptic
mumps
  meningitis, m.
  meningoencephalitis, m.
Munchausen syndrome
Munchmeyer's disease
Munson's sign
murdering while asleep
Murphy theory
Murray theory
Murray Valley disease
Murray Valley encephalitis
muscle
  abductor m.
  adductor m.
  agonistic m.
  antagonistic m.
  antigravity m.
  biceps m.
  brachioradial m.
  Chassaignac's axillary m.
  coccygeal m.
  congenerous m.
  coracobrachial m.

muscle *(continued)*
  cremaster m.
  deltoid m.
  depressor m.
  detrusor m.
  diaphragmatic m.
  emergency m.
  epicranial m.
  epimeric m.
  erector m. of spine
  extensor m.
  extraocular m.
  extrinsic m.
  facial expression, m's of
  facial m.
  femoral m.
  fixation m.
  fixator m.
  flexor m.
  frontal m.
  gastrocnemius m.
  gemellus m.
  gluteal m.
  hamstring m.
  hypaxial m.
  hypomeric m.
  iliac m.
  iliococcygeal m.
  iliocostal m.
  infraspinous m.
  intercostal m.
  interspinal m.
  intertransverse m.
  intraocular m.
  intrinsic m.
  involuntary m.
  Jarjavay's m.
  Langer's m.
  latissimus dorsi m.
  levator m.
  longissimus m.
  mesothenar m.
  nonstriated m.
  oblique m.
  obturator m.
  occipital m.

muscle *(continued)*
   ocular m.
   oculor m.
   otatory m.
   opposing m.
   palmar m.
   piriform m.
   platysma m.
   postaxial m.
   preaxial m.
   pronator m.
   pubococcygeal m.
   quadrate m.
   quadriceps m.
   rectococcygeus m.
   rhomboid m.
   ribbon m.
   rotator m.
   sacrococcygeal m.
   sacrospinal m.
   semispinal m.
   semitendinous m.
   serratus m.
   skeletal m.
   smooth m.
   soleus m.
   somatic m.
   sphincter m.
   spinal m.
   sternocleidomastoid m.
   sternomastoid m.
   sternothyroid m.
   strap m.
   striated m.
   striped m.
   subclavius m.
   subcostal m.
   suboccipital m.
   subvertebral m.
   supraspinous m.
   synergic m.
   synergistic m.
   tarsal m.
   temporoparietal m.
   tensor m.
   teres major m.

muscle *(continued)*
   teres minor m.
   thenar m.
   tibial m.
   transverse m.
   transversospinal m.
   trapezius m.
   triceps m.
   unipennate m.
   unstriated m.
   vestigial m.
   vocal m.
   voluntary m.
   yoked m.
muscle-action potential
muscle artifact
muscle atrophy
muscle contraction headache
muscle cramps
muscle fiber
muscle fiber types, fast twitch and slow
   twitch
muscle group
muscle guarding
muscle mass
muscle palsy
muscle relaxant
muscle-setting exercises
muscle soreness
muscle spindle
muscle stamp
muscle strength
muscle stretch reflex
muscle tension
muscle testing
muscle tone
muscle tonus
muscle wasting
muscle weakness
muscular
muscular atrophy
   Charcot-Marie-Tooth m.
   hypertrophic polyneuritic-type m.
   infantile m.
   peroneal m.
   post-poliomyelitis m.

muscular atrophy *(continued)*
   progressive m.
muscular contractions
muscular dystrophy (MD)
   Becker m.
   distal-type m.
   Duchenne-type m.
   facioscapulohumeral-type m.
   Landouzy-Dejerine progressive m.
   limb-girdle-type m.
   ophthalmoplegic-type m.
muscular fibrillation
muscular rigidity
muscularis
muscularity
muscularize
musculature
musculi (pl. of musculus)
   abductor digiti minimi manus, m.
   abductor digiti minimi pedis, m.
   abductor digiti quinti manus, m.
   abductor digiti quinti pedis, m.
   abductor hallucis brevis, m.
   abductor hallucis longus, m.
   abductor pollicis brevis, m.
   abductor pollicis longus, m.
   adductor brevis, m.
   adductor hallucis, m.
   adductor longus, m.
   adductor magnus, m.
   adductor minimus , m.
   adductor pollicis, m.
   biceps brachii, m.
   biceps femoris, m.
   bipennatus, m.
   brachialis, m.
   brachioradialis, m.
   capitis, m.
   coccygeus, m.
   colli, m.
   coracobrachialis, m.
   cremaster, m.
   cruciatus, m.
   cutaneus, m.
   deltoideus, m.
   depressor, m.

musculi (pl. of musculus) *(continued)*
   detrusor, m.
   dorsi, m.
   epicranius, m.
   erector spinae, m.
   extensor carpi radialis brevis, m.
   extensor carpi radialis longus, m.
   extensor carpi ulnaris, m.
   extensor digiti minimi, m.
   extensor digit quinti proprius, m.
   extensor digitorum, m.
   extensor digitorum brevis, m.
   extensor digitorum longus, m.
   extensor hallucis brevis, m.
   extensor hallucis longus, m.
   extensor indicis proprius, m.
   extensor pollicis brevis, m.
   extensor pollicis longus, m.
   flexor carpi radialis, m.
   flexor carpi ulnaris, m.
   flexor digiti minimi brevis, m.
   flexor digiti quinti, m.
   flexor digitorum, m.
   flexor hallucis brevis, m.
   flexor hallucis longus, m.
   flexor pollicis brevis, m.
   flexor pollicis longus, m.
   frontalis, m.
   fusiformis, m.
   gastrocnemius, m.
   gemellus, m.
   gluteus maximus, m.
   gluteus medius, m.
   gluteus minimus, m.
   gracilis, m.
   iliacus, m.
   iliococcygeus, m.
   iliocostalis, m.
   infraspinatus, m.
   intercostales, m.
   interossei dorsales manus, m.
   interossei dorsales pedis, m.
   interossei palmares, m.
   interossei plantares, m.
   interspinales, m.
   intertransversarii, m.

musculi (pl. of musculus) *(continued)*
latissimus capitis, m.
latissimus dorsi, m.
levator, m.
longissimus, m.
longissimus cervicis, m.
longissimus dorsi, m.
longissimus thoracis, m.
longus capitis, m.
longus colli, m.
lumbricales manus, m.
lumbricales pedis, m.
membri inferioris, m.
membri superioris, m.
mentalis, m.
multifidi, m.
multipennatus, m.
obliquus, m.
obliquus capitis inferior, m.
obturator, m.
occipitalis, m.
occipitofrontalis, m.
oculi, m.
opponens digiti minimi, m.
opponens pollicis, m.
orbicularis, m.
orbitalis, m.
palmaris brevis, m.
palmaris longus , m.
pectoralis major, m.
pectoralis minor, m.
peroneus, m.
piriformis, m.
plantaris, m.
popliteus, m.
pronator quadratus, m.
pronator teres, m.
psoas, m.
pubococcygeus, m.
puborectalis, m.
pubovaginalis, m.
quadratus, m.
quadriceps, m.
rectococcygeus, m.
rectus abdominis, m.
rectus femoris, m.

musculi (pl. of musculus) *(continued)*
rectus inferior, m.
rectus lateralis, m.
rectus medialis, m.
rectus superior, m.
rhomboideus major, m.
rhomboideus minor, m.
risorius, m.
rotatores breves, m.
rotatores cervicis, m.
rotatores lumborum, m.
rotatores thoracis, m.
sacrococcygeus, m.
sacrospinalis, m.
sartorius, m.
scalenus anterior, m.
scalenus medius, m.
scalenus minimus, m.
scalenus posterior, m.
semimembranosus, m.
semispinalis capitis, m.
semispinalis cervicis, m.
semispinalis thoracis, m.
semitendinosus, m.
serratus posterior inferior, m.
serratus posterior superior, m.
skeleti, m.
soleus, m.
sphincter, m.
spinalis, m.
spinalis capitis, m.
spinalis cervicis, m.
spinalis thoracis, m.
splenius capitis, m.
sternocleidomastoideus, m.
styloglossus, m.
subclavius, m.
suboccipitales, m.
supinator, m.
supraspinatus, m.
tarsalis, m.
temporalis, m.
temporoparietalis, m.
tensor fascia lata, m.
teres major, m.
teres minor, m.

musculi (pl. of musculus) *(continued)*
  thoracis, m.
  tibialis anterior, m.
  tibialis posterior, m.
  transversospinalis, m.
  trapezius, m.
  triceps brachii, m.
  triceps surae, m.
  unipennatus, m.
  uvulae, m.
  vastus intermedius, m.
  vastus lateralis, m.
  zygomaticus, m.
musculoaponeurotic
musculocutaneous
musculoelastic
musculofascial
musculomembranous
musculophrenic
musculoskeletal
musculospiral
musculospiralis
musculotendinous
musculotonic
musculotropic
musculus (pl. musculi)
mushroom overlap
music therapy
musical alexia
musicogenic
  epilepsy, m.
musicomania
musicotherapy
mussitation
mutacism
mutant
mutation
mute
  reflexes, m.
mutilatation
mutilate
mutism
  akinetic m.
  deaf m.
  elective m.
mv (millivolt)

MWD (microwave diathermy)
myalgia
  abdominis, m.
  capitis, m.
  cervicalis, m.
  epidemic m.
  lumbar m.
myasthenia
  angiosclerotic m.
  gravis, m.
  gravis pseudoparalytica, m.
  laryngis, m.
  neonatal m.
myasthenic
  smile, m.
myatonia
  congenita, m.
myatony
myatrophy
myautonomy
mycetismus
  cerebris, m.
  nervosus, m.
mycosis
mycotic
  aneurysm, m.
mydriasis
  alternating m.
  bounding m.
  paralytic m.
  spasmodic m.
  spastic m.
  spinal m.
  springing m.
mydriatic
myectomy
myectopia
myectopy
myelacephalus
myelanosis
myelalgia
myelapoplexy
myelasthenia
myelatelia
myelatrophy
myelauxe

myelencephalitis
myelencephalon
myelencephalospinal
myelencephalous
myeleterosis
myelin
  basic protein (MBP), m.
  degeneration, m.
  sheath, m.
myelinated
myelination
myelinic
myelinization
myelinoclasis
  acute perivascular m.
  central pontine m.
  postinfection perivenous m.
myelinogenesis
myelinogenetic
  field, m.
myelinogeny
myelinolysis
  central pontine m.
myelinopathy
myelinosis
myelinotoxic
myelinotoxicity
myelitic
myelitis
  acute m.
  apoplectiform m.
  ascending m.
  bulbar m.
  cavitary m.
  central m.
  chronic m.
  compression m.
  cornual m.
  descending m.
  diffuse m.
  disseminated m.
  foudroyant m.
  hemorrhagic m.
  interstitial m.
  neuro-optic m.
  parenchymatous m.

myelitis *(continued)*
  periependymal m.
  sclerosing m.
  systemic m.
  transverse m.
  traumatic m.
  vaccinia, m.
myeloarchitecture
myelocele
myeloclast
myelocoele
myelocone
myelocyst
myelocystic
myelocystocele
myelocystomeningocele
myelocyte
myelocythemia
myelocytic
myelocytoma
myelocytosis
myelodiastasis
myelodysplasia
myelodysplastic
myeloencephalic
myeloencephalitis
  eosinophilic m.
  epidemic m.
myelofibrosis
myelofugal
myelogenesis
myelogenetic law
myelogenic
myelogenous
myelogeny
myelogram
  cervical m.
  gas m.
  lumbar m.
  metrizamide m.
  oxygen m.
  positive contrast m.
  radionuclide m.
  thoracic m.
myelography
  air m.

myeloid
myeloidin
myeloidosis
myelokentric
myelolipoma
myelolysis
myelolytic
myeloma
myelomalacia
myelomatoid
myelomatosis
myelomenia
myelomeningitis
myelomeningocele
myelomere
myelomyces
myelon
myeloneuritis
myelonic
myelo-opticoneuropathy
myeloparalysis
myelopathic
   muscular atrophy, m.
myelopathy
   ascending m.
   descending m.
   focal m.
   sclerosing m.
   transverse m.
   traumatic m.
myelopetal
myelophage
myelophthisis
myeloplegia
myelopoiesis
   extramedullary m.
myelopore
myeloproliferative
myeloradiculitis
myeloradiculodysplasia
myeloradiculopathy
myelorrhagia
myelorrhaphy
myelosarcoma
myelosarcomatosis
myeloschisis

myeloscintogram
myelosclerosis
myelosis
   funicular m.
myelospasm
myelospongium
myelosuppression
myelosuppressive
myelosyphilis
myelosyphilosis
myelotherapy
myelotome
myelotomy
   commissural m.
Myers-Briggs Type Indicator
Myerson's sign
myesthesia
myiodesopsia
myitis
myoarchitectonic
myoasthenia
myoatrophy
myoblast transfer
Myobock artificial hand
myobradia
myocardial infarction (MI)
myocellulitis
myoceptor
myocerosis
myocervical collar
myochorditis
myoclonia
   epileptica, m.
   fibrillaris multiplex, m.
   fibrillary m.
   pseudoglottic m.
myoclonic
   epilepsy, m.
   jerk, m.
   seizures, m.
myoclonus
   ocular m.
   multiplex, m.
   palatal m.
   spinal m.
myocomma

myocrismus
myocyte
myocytolysis
myocytoma
myodegeneration
myodemia
myodiastasis
myodynamia
myodynamic
myodynamometer
myodynia
myodystonia
myodystony
myodystrophia
   fetalis, m.
myodystrophy
myoedema
myoelastic
myoelectric
   arm, m.
   prosthesis, m.
myoelectrical
myofascial
   pain dysfunction, m.
myofasciitis
myofibril
myofibrilla (pl. myofibrillae)
myofibrillae (pl. of myofibrilla)
myofibrillar
myofibroblast
myofibroma
myofibrosis
myofibrositis
myofilament
myofunctional
myogelosis
myogen
myogenesis
myogenetic
myogenic
myoglia
myoglobin
myoglobinuria
myogram
myography
myohypertrophia

myohypertrophia *(continued)*
   kymoparalytica, m.
myoid
myoidism
myoischemia
myokerosis
myokinase
myokinesimeter
myokinesis
myokinetic
myokymia
myolemma
myolin
myolipoma
myologia
myology
myolysis
myomalacia
myomelanosis
myomere
myometer
myonecrosis
myoneural
   junction, m.
myoneuralgia
myoneurasthenia
myoneure
myoneurectomy
myoneuroma
myonosus
myonymy
myopachynsis
myopalmus
myoparalysis
myoparesis
myopathia
   infraspinata, m.
myopathic
   facies, m.
myopathy
   alcoholic m.
   centronuclear m.
   corticosteroid m.
   cortisone m.
   distal m.
   endocrine m.

myopathy *(continued)*
   facial m.
   fingerprint body m.
   glucocorticoid-induced m.
   hypertrophic branchial m.
   hypothyroid m.
   infiltrative m.
   L-tryptophan m.
   megaconial m.
   metabolic m.
   mitochondrial m.
   multicore m.
   myotubular m.
   nemaline m.
   ocular m.
   rod m.
   thyrotoxic m.
myope
myophage
myophagism
myophone
myopia
myopic
myoplasm
myoplastic
myoplasty
myopolar
myopotential
myoprotein
myopsychic
myopsychopathy
myoreceptor
myorrhaphy
myorrhexis
myosalgia
myosarcoma
myoschwannoma
myosclerosis
myoscope
myoseism
myosin
myosinase
myosinogen
myosinose
myositis
   acute disseminated m.

myositis *(continued)*
   acute progressive m.
   a frigore, m.
   clostridial m.
   epidemic m.
   fibrosa, m.
   infectious m.
   interstitial m.
   ischemic m.
   multiple m.
   orbital m.
   ossificans, m.
   parenchymatous m.
   primary multiple m.
   progressive ossifying m.
   purulenta, m.
   rheumatoid, m.
   serosa, m.
   spontaneous bacterial m.
   traumatic m.
   trichinous m.
myospasia
myospasm
myospasmia
myosthenic
myosthenometer
myostroma
myostromin
myosuture
myosynizesis
myotactic
   paranomia, m.
myotasis
myotatic
   reflex, m.
myotenontoplasty
myotenositis
myotenotomy
myothermic
myotility
myotomal
myotome
   caudal m.
   cervical m.
   lumbar m.
   occipital m.

myotome *(continued)*
   sacral m.
   thoracic m.
myotomic
myotomy
myotone
myotonia
   congenita, m.
myotonic
   discharge, m.
   dystrophy, m.
myotonoid
myotonometer
myotonus
myotony
myotrophic
myotrophy
myotropic
myotube
myotubular

myotubule
myovascular
Mysoline
mysophilia
mysophobia
mysticism
mytacism
mythomania
mythophobia
mythoplasty
myxasthenia
myxedema
   coma, m.
   madness, m.
myxoglioma
myxoma
myxomatous
myxovirus
myoneuroma

Additional entries

Additional entries

N

Nadbath akinesia
Naegeli syndrome
Naffziger's syndrome
Naffziger's test
Nagel's test
Nageotte's bracelets
Nageotte's cells
Nager's acrofacial dysostosis
nail biting
naked axon
Naloxone
nanism
   mulibrey n.
   pituitary n.
   renal n.
   senile n.
   symptomatic n.
nanocephaly
nanocormia
nanoid
nanophthalmos
nanosomia
nanus
napex
Narcan
narcism
narcissism
narcissistic
   object choice, n.
narcoanalysis
narcodiagnosis
narcohypnia
narcohypnosis
narcolepsy
narcolepsy-cataplexy syndrome
narcoleptic
   tetrad, n.
narcolysis
narcoma
narcomania
narcomatous
narcophobia
narcose

narcosis
   basal n.
   basis n.
   carbon dioxide n.
   insufflation n.
   intravenous n.
   medullary n.
narcosomania
narcostimulant
narcosynthesis
narcotherapist
narcotherapy
narcotic
   addict, n.
   addiction, n.
   agent, n.
   antagonist, n.
   blockade, n.
   poisoning, n.
narcotism
narcotize
narcous
narrow-angle glaucoma
Nardil
nasal cannula
Nashold TC electrode
nasioiniac
nasion
nasociliary
nasofrontal
nasogastric tube
nasolabial
   crease, n.
   droop, n.
   fold, n.
nasonnement
naso-oral
nasopharyngeal
   electrode, n.
nasoseptal
nasospinale
natatory ligament
nausea anesthesia

Navane
NCV (nerve conduction velocity)
Nd:YAG laser (neodymium: yttrium-aluminum-garnet laser)
near-death experience
near-field response
near drowning
near-miss SIDS
near-sighted
near-syncope
nearthrosis
neck
    conformer, n.
    extension, n.
    dorsal head of spinal cord, n. of
    posterior horn of spinal cord, n. of
    vertebra, n. of
    vertebral arch, n. of
    precautions, n.
    preference, n.
    -righting reflex, n.
    sign, n.
    stiffness, n.
    supple, n.
Neck-Trac
necrencephalus
necromancy
necromania
necromimesis
necrophagia
necrophagous
necrophile
necrophilia
necrophilic
necrophilism
necrophilous
necrophobia
necrosadism
needle
    abscess, n.
    aspiration, n.
    biopsy, n.
    tracks, n.
needlepoint electrocautery
neencephalon
negation

negative
    attitude, n.
    pressure, n.
negativism
negativistic
neglect
Negri body
Negro phenomenon
Negro sign
Neisser's reaction
Neisseria meningitidis
neisserial
Nelson's syndrome
nemaline myopathy
neocerebellum
neocortex
neoencephalon
Neoflex bendable knife
neoglottis
neokinetic
NeoKnife
neolalia
neolalism
neologism
neopallium
neophilism
neophobia
neophrenia
neoplasm
neoplastic
neoplastigenic
neostigmine
neostriatal syndrome
neostriatum
neothalamus
neovascularization
nepenthic
nephelopsychosis
nephrosialidosis
Neri's sign
Nernst equation
Nernst's law
nerval
nerve
    abducent n.
    accessory n.

nerve *(continued)*
    acoustic n.
    afferent n.
    anabolic n.
    Andersch's n.
    Arnold's n.
    articular n.
    auditory, n.
    auricular n.
    autonomic n.
    axillary n.
    Bell's n.
    carotid n.
    celiac n.
    centrifugal n.
    centripetal n.
    cerebral n.
    cervical n.
    ciliary n.
    coccygeal n.
    cochlear n.
    cranial n.
    crotaphitic n.
    cubital n.
    cutaneous n.
    depressor n.
    diaphragmatic n.
    digastric n.
    digital n.
    efferent n.
    eight cranial n.
    eleventh cranial n.
    encephalic n.
    esodic n.
    exciter n.
    excitoreflex n.
    exodic n.
    facial n.
    femoral n.
    fifth cranial n.
    first cranial n.
    fourth cranial n.
    frontal n.
    furcal n.
    fusimotor n.
    gangliated n.

nerve *(continued)*
    hypogastric n.
    hypoglossal n.
    ilioinguinal n.
    infraoccipital n.
    inhibitory n.
    intercostal n.
    intercostobrachial n.
    Jacobson's n.
    Langley's n.
    laryngeal n.
    lingual n.
    longitudinal n's of Lancisi
    lumbar n.
    lumboinguinal n.
    Luschka, n. of
    mandibular n.
    maxillary n.
    median n.
    medullated n.
    meningeal n.
    mental n.
    motor n.
    musculocutaneous n.
    musculospiral n.
    myelinated n.
    mylohyoid n.
    nasociliary n.
    nasopalatine n.
    ninth cranial n.
    nonmedullated n.
    obturator n.
    occipital n.
    oculomotor n.
    olfactory n.
    ophthalmic n.
    optic n.
    pain n.
    palatine n.
    parasympathetic n.
    parotid n.
    pectoral n.
    perineal n.
    peripheral n.
    peroneal n.
    petrosal n.

nerve *(continued)*
  phrenic n.
  pilomotor n.
  piriform n.
  plantar n.
  pneumogastric n.
  popliteal n.
  presacral n.
  pressor n.
  pterygoid n.
  pudendal n.
  pudic n.
  radial n.
  recurrent n.
  recurrent laryngeal n.
  sacral n.
  sciatic n.
  second cranial n.
  secretory n.
  sensory n.
  seventh cranial n.
  sinuvertebral n.
  sixth cranial n.
  somatic n.
  spinal n.
  splanchnic n.
  subclavian n.
  subcostal n.
  sublingual n.
  suboccipital n.
  subscapular n.
  sudomotor n.
  supraclavicular n.
  supraorbital n.
  suprascapular n.
  sural n.
  sympathetic n.
  temporal n.
  tenth cranial n.
  terminal n.
  third cranial n.
  thoracic n.
  thoracodorsal n.
  tibial n.
  Tiedemann's n.
  trigeminal n.

nerve *(continued)*
  trochlear n.
  trophic n.
  twelfth cranial n.
  tympanic n.
  ulnar n.
  unmyelinated n.
  vagus n.
  vasoconstrictor n.
  vasodilator n.
  vasomotor n.
  vasosensory n.
  vertebral n.
  vestibulocochlear n.
  visceral n.
  Willis, n. of
  Wrisberg, n. of
  Wrisberg's n.
  zygomaticofacial n.
  zygomaticotemporal n.
nerve action
nerve-action current
nerve block
nerve cell
nerve center
nerve compression
nerve conduction
  deafness, n.
  defect, n.
  study, n.
  velocity (NCV), n.
nerve cord
nerve deafness
nerve decompression
nerve ending
nerve entrapment
nerve fiber
nerve fibril
nerve gas
nerve growth factor
nerve head
nerve hook
nerve impingement
nerve impulse
nerve net
nerve plexus

nerve root
  compression, n.
  decompression, n.
  irritability, n.
  irritation, n.
  rhizotomy, n.
nerve separator
nerve stimulation
nerve stretching
nerve trunk
nervi (pl. of nervus)
nervimotility
nervimotion
nervimotor
nervimuscular
nervomuscular
nervone
nervonic acid
nervosity
nervous
  bladder, n.
  breakdown, n.
  debility, n.
  energy, n.
  exhaustion, n.
  impulse, n.
  mannerism, n.
  pregnancy, n.
  prostration, n.
  spasm, n.
nervous system
  autonomic n.
  central n.
  peripheral n.
  vegetative n.
nervous tension
nervous tic
nervous tissue
nervous twitch
nervousness
nervus (pl. nervi)
  abducens, n.
  accessorius, n.
  acusticus, n.
  alveolaris inferior, n.
  alveolares superior, n.

nervus (pl. nervi) *(continued)*
  anococcygei, n.
  articulares anteriores, n.
  auricularis magnus, n.
  auricularis posterior, n.
  auriculotemporalis, n.
  axillaris, n.
  cardiaci thoracici, n.
  caroticotympanici, n.
  carotici externi, n.
  caroticus internus, n.
  cerebrales, n.
  cervicales, n.
  ciliares breves, n.
  ciliares longi, n.
  coccygeus, n.
  cochlearis, n.
  craniales , n.
  cutaneus, n.
  digitales dorsales, n.
  digitales plantares, n.
  digitales volares, n.
  dorsalis scapulae, n.
  encephalici, n.
  ethmoidalis anterior, n.
  ethmoidalis posterior, n.
  facialis, n.
  femoralis, n.
  fibularis communis, n.
  fibularis profundus, n.
  fibularis superficialis, n.
  frontalis, n.
  genitofemoralis, n.
  glossopharyngeus, n.
  gluteus, n.
  hypogastricus, n.
  hypoglossus, n.
  iliohypogastricus, n.
  ilio-inguinalis, n.
  infraorbitalis, n.
  infratrochlearis, n.
  intercostobrachiales, n.
  intermediofacialis, n.
  intermedius, n.
  interosseus anterior, n.
  interosseus cruris, n.

nervus (pl. nervi) *(continued)*
  interosseus dorsalis, n.
  interosseus posterior, n.
  interosseus volaris, n.
  ischiadicus, n.
  jugularis, n.
  labiales, n.
  lacrimalis, n.
  laryngeus inferior, n.
  laryngeus recurrens, n.
  laryngeus superior, n.
  lingualis, n.
  lumbales, n.
  mandibularis, n.
  massetericus, n.
  maxillaris, n.
  meatus acustici externi, n.
  medianus, n.
  mentalis, n.
  mixtus, n.
  musculi quadrati femoris, n.
  musculi tensoris tympani, n.
  musculocutaneus, n.
  mylohyoideus, n.
  nasociliaris, n.
  nasopalatinus, n.
  obturatorius, n.
  obturatorius accessorius, n.
  obturatorius internus, n.
  occipitalis major, n.
  occipitalis minor, n.
  occipitalis tertius, n
  oculomotorius, n.
  olfactorii, n.
  ophthalmicus, n.
  opticus, n.
  palatinus, n.
  pectoralis lateralis, n.
  pectoralis medialis, n.
  perineales, n.
  peroneus profundus accessorius, n.
  petrosus major, n.
  petrosus profundus, n.
  phrenicus, n.
  phreni accessorii, n.
  piriformis, n.

nervus (pl. nervi) *(continued)*
  plantaris lateralis, n.
  plantaris medialis, n.
  presacralis, n.
  pterygoideus, n.
  pterygopalatini, n.
  pudendus, n.
  quadratus femoris, n.
  radialis, n.
  rectales inferiores, n.
  recurrens, n.
  saccularis, n.
  sacrales, n.
  saphenus, n.
  sensorius, n.
  spinales, n.
  spinosus, n.
  splanchnici lumbales, n.
  splanchnici pelvini, n.
  splanchnici sacrales, n.
  splanchnicus thoracicus imus, n.
  splanchnicus thoracicus major, n.
  splanchnicus thoracicus minor, n.
  subclavisu
  subcostalis, n.
  sublingualis, n.
  suboccipitalis, n.
  subscapularis, n.
  supraclaviculares intermedii, n.
  supraclaviculares laterales , n.
  supraclaviculares mediales, n.
  supraorbitalis, n.
  suprascapularis, n.
  supratrochlearis, n.
  suralis, n.
  temporales profundi, n.
  tentorii, n.
  terminales, n.
  thoracici, n.
  thoracicus longus, n.
  thoracodorsalis, n.
  tibialis, n.
  transversus colli, n.
  trigeminus, n.
  trochlearis, n.
  tympanicus, n.

nervus (pl. nervi) *(continued)*
   ulnaris, n.
   vagus, n.
   vertebralis, n.
   vestibularis, n.
   vestibulocochlearis, n.
   zygomaticus, n.
nest of veins
net
Netherton's syndrome
Nettleship-Falls type ocular albinism
network
   Gerlach's n.
   Gesvelst, n. of
   idiotype-anti-idiotype n.
neuradynamia
neuragmia
neu
neurad
neuragmia
Neurain drill
Neurairtome drill
neural
   arch, n.
   cell, n.
   crest, n.
   fold, n.
   foramina, n.
   nevus, n.
   plate, n.
   segment, n.
   spine, n.
   stalk, n.
   tube, n.
   tube defect, n.
neuralgia
   cardiac n.
   cervicobrachial n.
   cervico-occipital n.
   cranial n.
   degenerative n.
   facial n.
   facialis vera, n.
   Fothergill's n.
   geniculate n.
   glossopharyngeal n.

neuralgia *(continued)*
   hallucinatory n.
   Harris' n.
   migrainous n.
   Hunt's n.
   idiopathic n.
   intercostal n.
   mammary n.
   mandibular joint n.
   migrainous n.
   Morton's n.
   nasociliary n.
   occipital n.
   otic n.
   peripheral n.
   postherpetic n.
   red n.
   reminiscent n.
   sciatic n.
   Sluder's n.
   sphenopalatine n.
   stump n.
   supraorbital n.
   symptomatic n.
   trifacial n.
   trigeminal n.
   vidian n.
   visceral n.
neuralgic
   amyotrophy, n.
neuralgiform
neuramebimeter
neuraminic acid
neuranagenesis
neurangiosis
neurapophysis
neurapraxia
neurarchy
neurarthropathy
neurasthenia
   acoustic n.
   traumatic n.
neurastheniac
neurasthenic
   neurosis, n.
neurataxia

neurataxy
neuratrophia
neuratrophic
neuratrophy
neuraxial
neuraxis
neuraxitis
neuraxon
neure
neurectasia
neurectasis
neurectoderm
neurectomy
  presacral n.
neurectopia
neurectopy
neurenteric
  canal, n.
  cyst, n.
neurepithelial
neurepithelium
neurergic
neurexeresis
neuriatry
neuridine
neurilemma
neurilemmal
neurilemmitis
neurilemmoma
  acoustic n.
  ameloblastic n.
  malignant n,
  trigeminal n.
neurility
neurimotility
neurimotor
neurinoma
  acoustic n.
neurinomatosis
neurite
neuritic
  atrophy, n.
neuritis
  adventitial n.
  alcoholic n.
  ascending n.

neuritis *(continued)*
  axial n.
  brachial n.
  central n.
  degenerative n.
  descending n.
  dietetic n.
  diphtheritic n.
  disseminated n.
  endemic n.
  fallopian n.
  Gombault's n.
  interstitial n.
  interstitial hypertrophic n.
  intraocular n.
  jake n.
  latent n.
  lead n.
  leprous n.
  malarial n.
  migrating n.
  migrans, n.
  multiple n.
  multiple malarial n.
  multiplex endemica, n.
  nodosa, n.
  optic n.
  orbital n.
  optic n.
  parenchymatous n.
  periaxial n.
  peripheral n.
  porphyric n.
  postfebrile n.
  postocular n.
  pressure n.
  puerperalis traumatica, n.
  radiation n.
  radicular n.
  retrobulbar n.
  rheumatic n.
  saturnina, n.
  sciatic n.
  segmental n.
  senile n.
  shoulder-girdle n.

neuritis *(continued)*
  sympathetic n.
  syphilitic n.
  tabetic n.
  toxic n.
  traumatic n.
neuroallergy
neuroamebiasis
neuroanastomosis
neuroanatomy
neuroarthritism
neuroarthropathy
neuroastrocytoma
neurobehavioral
Neurobehavioral Cognitive Status Examination
neurobiology
neurobiotaxis
neuroblast
neuroblastoma
neurobrucellosis
neurobuccal
neurocanal
neurocardiac
neurocele
neurocentral
neurocentrum
neuroceptor
neuroceratin
neurochemical
neurochemistry
neurochitin
neurochondrite
neurochorioretinitis
neurochoroiditis
neurocirculatory
  asthenia, n.
neurocladism
neuroclonic
neurocoele
neurocommunications
neurocranial
neurocranium
neurocrine
neurocrinia
neurocristopathy

neurocutaneous
  marking, n.
neurocyte
neurocytology
neurocytolysin
neurocytolysis
neurocytoma
neurodealgia
neurodeatrophia
neurodegenerative
neurodendrite
neurodendron
neuroderm
neurodermatitis
  disseminated n.
neurodermatosis
neurodermatophia
neurodevelopmental
neurodiagnosis
neurodiagnostic
neurodin
neurodynamic
neurodynia
neuroectoderm
neuroeffector
neuroelectricity
neuroelectrotherapeutics
neuroelectrotherapy
neuroencephalomyelopathy
  optic n.
neuroendocrine
  transducer, n.
neuroendocrinology
neuroenteric
neuroepidermal
neuroepithelial
neuroepithelioma
neuroepithelium
neurofiber
  afferent n.
  association n.
  commissural n.
  efferent n.
  postganglionic n.
  preganglionic n.
  projection n.

neurofiber *(continued)*
    somatic n.
    tangential n.
    visceral n.
neurofibra (pl. neurofibrae)
neurofibrae (pl. of neurofibra)
neurofibril
neurofibrilla (pl. neurofibrillae)
neurofibrillae (pl. of neurofibrilla)
neurofibrillar
neurofibrillary tangles
neurofibroma
    plexiform n.
neurofibromatosis
neurofibrosarcoma
neurofibrositis
neurofilament
neurofixation
neurogangliitis
neuroganglion
neurogastric
neurogen
neurogenesis
neurogenetic
neurogenic
    bladder, n.
    claudication, n.
    fracture, n.
    muscular atrophy, n.
    sarcoma, n.
    shock, n.
    ulcer, n.
neurogenous
neuroglia
neurogliacyte
neuroglial
neurogliar
neurogliocyte
neurogliocytoma
neuroglioma
    ganglionare, n.
neurogliomatosis
neurogliosis
neuroglycopenia
neurogram
neurography

neurohematology
neurohistology
neurohormonal
neurohormone
neurohumor
neurohumoral
neurohumoralism
neurohypnology
neurohypophysectomy
neurohypophysial
neurohypophysis
neuroid
    nevus, n.
neuroimmunologic
neuroimmunology
neuroinduction
neuroinidia
neurokeratin
neurokinet
neurokyme
neurolabyrinthitis
neurolathyrism
neurolemma
neurolemmoma
neuroleptanalgesic
neuroleptanesthetic
neuroleptic
    agent, n.
    anesthesia, n.
    drug, n.
    malignant syndrome, n.
neurolinguistics
neurolipomatosis
    dolorosa, n.
neurologia
neurologic
    deficit, n.
neurological
neurologist
neurology
neurolues
neuroluetic
neurolymph
neurolymphomatosis
    gallinarum, n.
neurolysin

neurolysis
neurolytic
neuroma
  acoustic n.
  amputation n.
  amyelinic n.
  appendiceal n.
  cutis, n.
  cystic n.
  false n.
  fascicular n.
  ganglionar n.
  ganglionated n.
  ganglionic n.
  malignant n.
  medullated n.
  Morton's n.
  mucosal n.
  multiple n.
  myelinic n.
  nevoid n.
  plexiform n.
  telangiectodes, n.
  traumatic n.
  true n.
  Verneuil's n.
neuromagnetometer
neuromalacia
neuromalakia
neuromatosis
neuromatous
neuromechanism
neuromelanin
neuromeningeal
neuromere
neuromessenger
neuromimesis
neuromimetic
neuromittor
neuromodulation
neuromotor
neuromuscular
  junction, n.
  transmission, n.
neuromyal
neuromyasthenia

neuromyasthenia *(continued)*
  epidemic n.
neuromyelitis
  optica, n.
neuromyic
neuromyon
neuromyopathic
neuromyositis
neuromyotonia
neuron
  afferent n.
  associative n.
  bipolar n.
  central n.
  commissural n.
  connector n.
  correlation n.
  efferent n.
  Golgi type I n.
  Golgi type II n.
  intercalary n.
  internuncial n.
  long n.
  lower motor n.
  motor n.
  multiform n.
  multipolar n.
  peripheral n.
  sensory n.
  polymorphic n.
  postganglionic n.
  preganglionic n.
  premotor n.
  projection n.
  pseudounipolar n.
  pyramidal n.
  sensory n.
  short n.
  unipolar n.
  upper motor n.
neuron doctrine
neuronagenesis
neuronal
  ceroid lipofuscinosis, n.
  specificity, n.
neuronatrophy

neurone
neuronephric
neuronevus
neuronic
neuronin
neuronitis
neuronopathic
neuronopathy
neuronophage
neuronophagia
neuronosis
neuronotropic
neuronymy
neuro-ophthalmology
neuro-optic
neuro-otic
neuro-otology
neuropacemaker
neuropapillitis
neuroparalysis
neuroparalytic
neuropathic
neuropathic fracture
neuropathogenesis
neuropathogenicity
neuropathology
neuropathy
    alcohol-nutritional n.
    alcoholic n.
    amblyopia n.
    amyloid n.
    ascending n.
    brachial plexus n.
    compression-entrapment n.
    compressive n.
    demyelination n.
    descending n.
    diabetic n.
    entrapment n.
    focal n.
    granulomatous n.
    hereditary sensory motor n.
    hereditary sensory radicular n.
    hypertrophic mono- n.
    infectious n.
    ischemic n.

neuropathy *(continued)*
    multifocal n.
    optic n.
    periaxial n.
    peripheral n.
    progressive hypertrophic interstitial n.
    retrobulbar n.
    segmental n.
    selective autonomic n.
    serum n.
    serum sickness n.
    trigeminal n.
    vincristine n.
neuropeptide
neurophage
neuropharmacology
neurophilic
neurophonia
neurophthalmology
neurophthisis
neurophysin
neurophysiologic treatment approach
neurophysiology
neuropil
neuropilem
neuroplasm
neuroplasty
neuroplexus
neuropodia (pl. of neurapodium)
neuropodion
neuropodium (pl. neuropodia)
neuropore
neuropotential
neuropraxia
neuroprobasia
neuropsychiatric
neuropsychiatrist
neuropsychiatry
neuropsychic
neuropsychology
neuropsychopathy
neuropsychopharmacology
neuropsychosis
neuropyra
neuropyretic
neuroradiology

neurorecidive
neurorecurrence
neuroregulation
neurorelapse
neuroretinitis
neuroretinopathy
   hypertensive n.
neuroroentgenography
neurorrhaphy
   epineurial n.
   perineurial n.
neurorrheuma
neurosarcocleisis
neurosarcokleisis
neurosarcoma
neuroscience
neurosclerosis
neuroscope
neurosecretion
neurosecretory
NeuroSectOR
neurosegmental
neurosensory
neuroses (pl. of neurosis)
neurosis (pl. neuroses)
   accident n.
   actual n.
   anxiety n.
   association n.
   cardiac n.
   character n.
   combat n.
   compensation n.
   compulsion n.
   conversion n.
   craft n.
   depersonalization n.
   depressive n.
   expectation n.
   experimental n.
   fatigue n.
   fixation n.
   gastric n.
   homosexual n.
   hypochondriacal n.
   hysterical n.

neurosis (pl. neuroses) *(continued)*
   intestinal n.
   neurasthenic n.
   obsessional n.
   obsessive-compulsive n.
   occupational n.
   pension n.
   phobic n.
   posttraumatic n.
   professional n.
   rectal n.
   regression n.
   sexual n.
   torsion n.
   transference n.
   traumatic n.
   vegetative n.
   war n.
neurosism
neuroskeletal
neuroskeleton
neurosome
neurospasm
neurosplanchnic
neurospongioma
neurospongium
neurostatus
neurosthenia
neurostimulation
neurosurgeon
neurosurgical
   bur, n.
   headrest, n.
neurosurgery
   microvascular n.
   stereotaxic n.
neurosuture
neurosyphilis
   asymptomatic n.
   congenital n.
   ectodermogenic n.
   meningeal n.
   meningovascular n.
   mesodermogenic n.
   parenchymatous n.
   paretic n.

neurosyphilis *(continued)*
   tabetic n.
neurosystemitis
   epidemica, n.
neurotabes
   diabetica, n.
neurotagma
neurotendinous
neurotensin
neurotension
neuroterminal
neurothecitis
neurothele
neurotherapeutics
neurotherapy
neurothlipsis
neurotic
neurotica
neuroticism
neurotigenic
neurotization
neurotmesis
neurotology
neurotome
neurotomography
neurotomy
   radiofrequency n.
   retrogasserian n.
neurotonia
neurotonic
neurotonometer
neurotony
neurotoxia
neurotoxic
neurotoxicity
neurotoxin
Neuro-Trace
neurotransducer
neurotransmission
neurotransmitter
Neurotrast
neurotrauma
neurotripsy
neurotrophasthenia
neurotrophic
   ulcer, n.

neurotrophy
neurotropic
neurotropism
neurotropy
neurotrosis
neurotubule
neurovaccine
neurovaricosis
neurovariola
neurovascular
   bundle, n.
   island graft, n.
   status, n.
neurovascularly intact
neurovegetative
neurovirulence
neurovirulent
neurovirus
neurovisceral
neurula
neurulation
neururgic
neutral
   position, n.
   warmth, n.
nevi (pl. of nevus)
Neville prosthesis
nevus (pl. nevi)
   flammeus, n.
Nevyas drape retractor
New Age
New Consciousness
New's needle
nicking
Nicolau's septineuritis
Nicolet C-wave
Nicolet Nerve Integrity Monitor-2
   (NIM-2)
nicotine
   poisoning, n.
nicotinism
nictitating spasm
nictitation
NIDDM (noninsulin-dependent diabetes
   mellitus)
nidus

nidus *(continued)*
   avis cerebelli, n.
Niemann disease
Niemann-Pick disease
night sweat
night terrors
night vision
nightmare
nightwalking
nigra
nigral
nigricans
nigrosin
nigrostriatal
nihilism
nihilistic
nikethamide
NIM-2 (Nicolet Nerve Integrity
   Monitor-2)
nimodipine
Nimotop
ninth cranial nerve
niphablepsia
niphotyphlosis
Nipride
Nissl bodies
Nissl granules
Nissl method
Nissl stain
Nissl substance
nitric acid poisoning
nitrites
nitritoid
   crisis, n.
nitrogen narcosis
NMR (nuclear magnetic resonance)
NMRI (nuclear magnetic resonance
   imaging)
Noack's syndrome
nociassociation
nociceptive
   impulses, n.
   reflex, n.
nociceptor
   polymodal n.
nociebo effect

nocifensor
noci-influence
nociperception
noctambulation
noctambulic
noctimania
noctiphobia
nocturnal
   emission, n.
   enuresis, n.
   headache, n.
   myoclonus, n.
   penile tumescence (NPT), n.
   polysomnography (NPSG), n.
nodding
   spasm, n.
node
   Ranvier, n. of
nodi (pl. of nodus)
nodular
nodule
noduli (pl. of nodulus)
nodulus (pl. noduli)
nodus (pl. nodi)
noematachograph
noematachometer
noematic
noesis
noetic
noise
   level, n.
   pollution, n.
nomadism
nominal aphasia
nomothetic
non compos mentis
non sequitur
nonadaptive
nonauthoritarian
noncommunicating hydrocephalus
nonconfrontational
nondepolarizer
nondisjunction
nonendocrine
nonfluent aphasia
non-Hodgkin's lymphoma

noninsulin-dependent diabetes mellitus (NIDD)
nonjudgmental
nonmedullated
nonmyelinated
Nonne's syndrome
Nonne-Apelt reaction
non-neoplastic
nonrapid eye movement (NREM or non-REM)
non-REM (nonrapid eye movement) sleep, n.
nonrestraint
nonsedative
nonsense syndrome
nonsensical
nonsexual
nonsteroidal anti-inflammatory drugs (NSAIDs)
nonthymomatous
nonus
nonviable
nookleptia
noopsyche
noradrenaline
noradrenergic
norepinephrine
norm
norma
    anterior, n.
    basilaris, n.
    facialis, n.
    frontalis, n.
    inferior, n.
    lateralis, n.
    occipitalis, n.
    sagittalis, n.
    superior, n.
    ventralis, n.
    verticalis, n.
normal pressure hydrocephalus (NPH)
normalcy
normalization
normergic
normoactive
normotension

normotensive
normotonia
normotonic
Norpramin
Norrie's disease
nortriptyline hydrochloride
nose candy (cocaine)
nosebrain
nosegay
nosencephalus
NOSIE (Nurse Observation Scale for Inpatient Evaluation)
nosomania
nosophilia
nosophobia
nostalgia
nostalgic
nostomania
nostril reflex
notalgia
notancephalia
notanencephalia
notch
    intervertebral n.
    sciatic n.
    spinoglenoid n.
note blindness
notencephalocele
Nothnagel's acroparesthesia
Nothnagel's sign
Nothnagel's syndrome
Nothnagel's type
notochord
notogenesis
notomyelitis
noumenal
noumenon
Novafil suture
novelty potential
noxa
noxious
    imagery, n.
    stimulus, n.
NPH (normal pressure hydrocephalus)
NPSG (nocturnal polysomnography)
NPT (nocturnal penile tumescence)

NREM (nonrapid eye movement)
  sleep, N.
NSAIDs (nonsteroidal anti-inflammatory
  drugs)
nuchal
  rigidity, n.
nuclear
  bag fiber, n.
  bag region, n.
  chain fiber, n.
  family, n.
  magnetic resonance (NMR), n.
  magnetic resonance imaging
    (NMRI), n.
nuclectomy
nuclei (pl. of nucleus)
Nucleotome system
nucleus (pl. nuclei)
  accumbens, n.
  ambiguuus, n.
  basalis, n.
  cuneate n.
  Darkschewitsch, n. of
  Darkschewitsch's n.
  gracilis, n.
  Gudden, n. of
  hypoglossal n.
  lateralis of Le Gros Clark, n.
  lateralis medullae oblongatae, n.
  Luys, n. of
  Perlia, n. of
  proprius, n. of
  pulposus, n. of
  red n.
  reticular, n. of
  root of cerebellum, n. of
  Rose, n. of
  ruber, n.
  thalamus, n., of
  vestibular n.
nude
nudism
nudity
nudomania
nudophobia
NuKO knee orthosis

numb
number writing
numbness
nunnation
Nurolon suture
Nurse Observation Scale for Inpatient
    Evaluation (NOSIE)
nurturance
nurture
nurturing
nutation
nutatory
nyctalgia
nyctalope
nyctalopia
nyctaphonia
nycterine
nycterohemeral
nyctophilia
nyctophobia
nyctophonia
nyctotyphlosis
Nylen-Barany maneuver
Nylen-Barany test
nympholepsy
nymphomania
nymphomaniac
nystagmic
nystagmiform
nystagmograph
nystagmoid
nystagmus
  amaurotic n.
  amblyopic n.
  ataxic n.
  aural n.
  caloric n.
  central n.
  Cheyne's n.
  Cheyne-Stokes n.
  congenital n.
  hereditary n.
  convergence n.
  convergence-retraction n.
  disjunctive n.
  dissociated n.

nystagmus *(continued)*
  downbeat n.
  electrical n.
  end-gaze n.
  end-point n.
  end-position n.
  fixation n.
  galvanic n.
  gaze n.
  jerk n.
  jerky n.
  labyrinthine n.
  latent n.
  lateral n.
  miner's n.
  ocular n.
  opticokinetic n.
  optokinetic n.
  oscillating n.
  palatal n.
  paretic n.
  pendular n.

nystagmus *(continued)*
  periodic alternating n.
  positional n.
  railroad n.
  resilient n.
  retraction n.
  rhythmical n.
  rotatory n.
  secondary n.
  see-saw n.
  spontaneous n.
  uldulatory n.
  unilateral n.
  upbeat n.
  vertical n.
  vestibular n.
  vibratory n.
  visual n.
  voluntary n.
nystagmus-myoclonus
nystaxis

Additional entries

O

1 1/2 syndrome
OA (occipital artery)
OAS (orthopedic antibiotic solution)
OAV (oculoauriculovertebral)
   dysplasia, O.
   syndrome, O.
obcecation
obdormition
obducent
obeliac
obeliad
obelion
Ober's test
Ober-Barr procedure
Obermayer's test
Obersteiner-Redlich area
obesity
   hypothalamic o.
obex
obfuscation
object
   blindness, o.
   relations, o.
obliquus reflex
obliteration
   cortical o.
Oblomov syndrome
oblongata
oblongatal
obmutescence
obnubilation
OBS (organic brain syndrome)
obsess
obsession
   impulsive o.
   inhibitory o.
obsessional neurosis
obsessive
obsessive-compulsive
   neurosis, o.
   personality, o.
   psychoneurosis, o.
obsessive neurotic

obsessive personality
obsessive rumination
obstructive
   hydrocephalus, o.
   neuropathy, o.
   sleep apnea (OSA), o.
obtund
obtundation
obtunded
obtundent
obturator
   muscle, o.
   nerve, o.
   sign, o.
   test, o.
obtuse
obtusion
occipital
   bone, o.
   fontanelle, o.
   foramen, o.
   gyrus, o.
   headache, o.
   horn, o.
   lobe, o.
   lobe tumor, o.
   muscle, o.
   myotome, o.
   nerve, o.
   pole, o.
   sulcus, o.
occipitalis
occipitalization
occipitoanterior
occipitoatlantoid articulation
occipitoatloid
occipitoaxoid
occipitobasilar
occipitobregmatic
occipitocalcarine
occipitocervical
occipitofacial
occipitofrontal

occipitomastoid
occipitomental
occipitoparietal
occipitoposterior
occipitotemporal
occipitothalamic
occiput
    cranium, o. of
occlude
occluding
occlusion
occlusive lesion
occult
occultism
occupation neurosis
occupational therapist
occupational therapy (OT)
ochlomania
ochlophobia
octopus test
ocular
    bobbing, o.
    dysmetria, o.
    flutter, o.
    palsy, o.
    pressure, o.
oculinium
oculocephalic
    reflex, o.
oculocephalogyric
    reflex, o.
oculocerebral-hypopigmentation syndrome
oculocerebromucormycosis
oculocerebrorenal syndrome
oculodento-osseous syndrome
oculogyration
oculogyric
    crisis, o.
oculomandibulofacial syndrome
oculomotor
    nerve (cranial nerve III), o.
    nucleus, o.
    paralysis, o.
oculomotorius
oculoplethysmography (OPG)

oculoplethysmography/carotid
    phonoangiography (OPG/CPA)
oculoreaction
oculospinal
oculovestibular reflex
oculozygomatic
    line, o.
OD (overdose)
OD'd (overdosed)
odaxesmus
odaxetic
odontoid process
odontophobia
odontoprisis
odynacusis
odynometer
odynophagia
odynophobia
oedipal
    conflict, o.
oedipism
Oedipus complex
Oehler's symptom
oestromania
OFD (oral-facial-digital)
    syndrome, O.
Ogilvie's syndrome
Oguchi's disease
Ohm's law
OI (osteogenesis imperfecta) types I-IV
oikofugic
oikomania
OKN (optokinetic nystagmus)
Oldberg dissector
Oldberg forceps
Oldberg retractor
olfactie
olfaction
olfactism
olfactometer
olfactory
    area, o.
    brain, o.
    bulb, o.
    esthesioneuroma, o.
    groove, o.

olfactory *(continued)*
  hallucinations, o.
  lobe, o.
  membrane, o.
  nerve (cranial nerve I), o.
  neuroblastoma, o.
  striae, o.
  sulcus, o.
  trigone, o.
olfactus
oligergasia
oligergastic
oligoastrocytoma
oligoclonal
  bands, o.
oligodendria
oligodendroblastoma
oligodendrocyte
oligodendroglia
oligodendroglioma
oligodipsia
oligoencephalon
oligoglia
oligophrenia
  moral o.
  phenylpyruvic o.
  polydystrophic o.
oligopnea
oligopsychia
oligoria
oligosynaptic
olisthetic
  vertebra, o.
olisthy
oliva
  cerebellaris, o.
olivary
  body, o.
olive
  cerebellar o.
  inferior o.
  spurge o.
  superior o.
Olivecrona clip
olivifugal
olivipetal

olivocerebellar
  atrophy, o.
  fibers, o.
olivopontocerebellar
  atrophy, o.
Ollier's disease
olophonia
omalgia
ombrophobia
omega sign
OMM (ophthalmomandibulomelic)
  syndrome, O.
Ommaya reservoir
Omnipaque
omnipotence of thought
omnipotent
omodynia
omohyoid
onanism
onanist
onchocerciasis
Ondine's curse
1-1/2 syndrome
oneiric
oneirism
oneiroanalysis
oneirodynia
oneirogenic
oneirogmus
oneiroid
oneirology
oneirophrenia
oneiroscopy
oniomania
onlay graft
on-off phenomenon
onomatomania
onomatophobia
onomatopoiesis
on-table x-ray
ontology
onychophagia
onychotillomania
oogenesis
OP (opening pressure)
opalgia

open-angle glaucoma
open spina bifida
opening pressure (OP)
operant conditioning
operating microscope
opercula (pl. of operculum)
opercular
operculum (pl. opercula)
   frontal o.
   frontoparietal o.
   insula, o. of
   occipital o.
   temporal o.
OPG (oculoplethysmography)
OPG/CPA (oculoplethysmography/ca-
   rotid phonoangiography)
OPG-Gee instrument
ophidiophobia
ophryon
ophryosis
ophthalmagra
ophthalmalgia
ophthalmencephalon
ophthalmia
ophthalmic
   zoster, o.
ophthalmodonesis
ophthalmodynamometry
ophthalmomandibulomelic (OMM)
ophthalmomyitis
ophthalmomyositis
ophthalmomyotomy
ophthalmoneuritis
ophthalmoneuromyelitis
ophthalmoplegia
   basal o.
   exophthalmic o.
   external o.
   fascicular o.
   internal o.
   internuclear o.
   nuclear o.
   orbital o.
   Parinaud's o.
   partial o.
   progressive external o.

ophthalmoplegia *(continued)*
   total o.
ophthalmoplegic
ophthalmoplegic-type progressive muscular dystrophy
ophthalmosonometry
ophthalmospasm
opiate
   abstinence syndrome, o.
   addiction, o.
   receptor, o.
   withdrawal, o.
opiatergic
opioid
   neuroadaptation, o.
   peptides, o.
opiomania
opiophagism
opisthenar
opisthencephalon
opisthiobasial
opisthion
opisthionasial
opisthocranion
opisthoporeia
opisthotonoid
opisthotonos
opium
opiumism
OPMI operating microscope
Oppenheim's disease
Oppenheim's gait
Oppenheim's sign
Oppenheim's syndrome
opponens
   splint, o.
oppositional
opprobrium
opsialgia
Op-Site
opsoclonia
opsoclonus
opsomania
Optacon (Optical Tactile Converter)
optesthesia
optic

optic *(continued)*
 chiasm, o.
 disk, o.
 foramen, o.
 glioma, o.
 nerve (cranial nerve II), o.
 neuritis, o.
 neuropathy, o.
 papilla, o.
 thalamus, o.
 tract, o.
opticochiasmatic
opticociliary
opticofacial winking
opticonasion
opticopupillary
optics
optochiasmic
optokinetic
 nystagmus (OKN), o.
optomeninx
optomyometer
optophone
optostriate
optotype
oral
 erotism, o.
 -facial-digital syndrome, o.
 gratification, o.
 sex, o.
orale
orality
orange reflex
Orbeli phenomenon
orbicularis
 oculi, o.
 oris, o.
orbicularis muscle
orbicularis sign
orbit
orbita (pl. orbitae)
orbitae (pl. of orbita)
orbital
 floor, o.
 gyrus, o.
 myositis, o.

orbital *(continued)*
 pneumotomography, o.
 rim, o.
 roof, o.
 sulcus, o.
orbivirus
orchioneuralgia
orexia
orexigenic
oreximania
organ of Corti
organic
 affective disorder, o.
 anxiety syndrome, o.
 brain syndrome (OBS), o.
 delusional syndrome, o.
 mental syndrome, o.
 mood syndrome, o.
 personality disorder, o.
 psychosis, o.
organoleptic
organs of special sense
orgasm
 expander, o.
orgasmic
orgone theory
orientation
oriented
 in all spheres, o.
 in three spheres, o.
 times three, o.
 times four, o.
 to person, place, and time, o.
orofaciodigital (OFD)
orofaciodigital syndrome
orolingual
oromeningitis
orrhomeningitis
orthergasia
orthesis
orthetic
orthetist
orthochorea
orthodromic
orthokinetic cuff
orthokinetics

orthomolecular
    psychiatry, o.
orthophony
orthophoria
orthophrenia
orthoplast jacket
orthopsychiatry
orthoptic
orthoptoscope
orthorrhachic
orthosis
orthostatic
    hypertension, o.
    hypotension, o.
orthosympathetic
orthotast
orthotherapy
orthotic
orthotist
orthotonos
Orthotron
orthropsia
Ortolani's sign
os (pl. ossa)
OSA (obstructive sleep apnea)
Osborne lesion
oscillating saw
oscillation
    bradykinetic o.
oscillopsia
Oseretsky test
Osler-Vasquez disease
osmatic
osmesthesia
osmodysphoria
osmolagnia
osmolar
osmometer
osmonosology
osmophobia
osmoreceptor
osmotherapy
osmotic disequilibrium syndrome
osphresiolagnia
osphresiology
osphresiometer

osphresis
osphretic
osphyomyelitis
ossa (pl. of os)
osseosonometry
Ossotome bur
osteoacusis
osteoanesthesia
osteoarthritic
    changes, o.
    lipping, o.
osteoarthritis
osteoarthropathy
osteocachexia
osteocampsia
osteochondral
osteochondritis
osteochondrodysplasia
osteochondrodystrophia
    deformans, o.
osteochondrodystrophy
osteochondrofibroma
osteochondrolysis
osteochondromatosis
osteochondromyxoma
osteochondropathia
    cretinoidea, o.
osteochondropathy
osteochondrophyte
osteochondrosarcoma
osteochondrosis
osteocomma
osteocope
osteodiastasis
osteodynia
osteodysplasty
    Melnick and Needles, o. of
osteodystrophia
osteodystrophy
osteoectasia
osteoenchondroma
osteofibrochondrosarcoma
osteofibromatosis
osteogenic
osteogenesis
    imperfecta cystica, o.

osteogenesis *(continued)*
  imperfecta (OI), types I through IV, o.
osteogenetic
osteogenic
osteogenous
osteogram
osteohalisteresis
osteoid
  osteoma, o.
osteolysis
osteolytic
osteoma
osteomalacia
osteomalacic
osteomatosis
osteomere
osteomiosis
osteomyelitic
osteomyelitis
osteomyelodysplasia
osteomyelography
osteomyxochondroma
osteonecrosis
osteoneuralgia
osteopathia
osteopathy
osteopenia
osteopetrosis
osteophagia
osteophony
osteophyte
  formation, o.
osteophytosis
osteoporosis
  circumscripta cranii, o.
  disuse, o. of
  postmenopausal o.
  post-traumatic o.
  senile o.
osteoporotic
osteopsathyrosis
osteosclerosis
osteosis
Osteo-Stim
osteosynovitis
osteosynthesis

osteotabes
osteotome
osteotomy
osteotympanic
osthexia
ostia (pl. of ostium)
ostial
ostium (pl. ostia)
ostomate
ostomy
  club, o.
ostosis
ostracosis
Ostrum-Furst syndrome
OT (occupational therapy)
otacoustic
otagra
otalgia
oticodinia
otitic
  hydrocephalus, o.
otitis
otocerebritis
otocleisis
otocranium
otodynia
otoencephalitis
otohemineurasthenia
otomastoiditis
otomyasthenia
otoneuralgia
otoneurasthenia
otoneurologic
otoneurology
otoplasty
otorrhea
otosclerosis
otosis
otospongiosis
otospongiosis/otosclerosis syndrome
Ototome drill
ototoxic
ototoxicity
out-of-body experience
outpouching
outrigging

ovariodysneuria
overaccepting
Overall and Gorham's Brief Psychiatric
   Rating Scale
overanxious
overcompensation
overcontrolled
overdetermination
overdose (OD)
overdosed (OD'd)
overdosing
overextension
overflow tears
overgeneralization
overgrowth
overhead trapeze
overhydration
overideational
overlap syndrome
overlay
   emotional o.
   psychogenic o.
overprotective
overpull
overreact
overreaction
overresponse
overriding
overshooting
overstrain
overstress
overt
overtoe
overtone
   psychic o.

overvalued idea
overventilation
overzealous
oxalic acid poisoning
oximeter
   ear o.
   pulse o.
oximetry
oxyachrestia
oxyblepsia
oxycephaly
oxycinesia
oxyecoia
oxyesthesia
oxygen (O2)
   catheter, o.
   cisternography, o.
   mask, o.
   myelography, o.
   tent, o.
oxygenation
oxygeusia
oxyhydrocephalus
oxylalia
oxynervon
oxyopia
oxyosmia
oxyosphresia
oxypathia
oxypathy
oxyphonia
oxyrhine
oxytocin

Additional entries

Additional entries

P

P300 test for dementia
Paas' disease
pacchionian
    bodies, p.
    depressions, p.
    granulations, p.
pachycephaly
pachydermatocele
pachydermoperiostosis
pachygyria
pachyleptomeningitis
pachymeninges
pachymeningitis
    cerebral p.
    circumscribed p.
    external p.
    hemorrhagic internal p.
    internal p.
    intralamellaris, p.
    purulent p.
    serous internal p.
    spinal p.
    syphilitic p.
pachymeningopathy
pachymeninx (pachymeninges)
Pacini's corpuscles
pacinian corpuscles
paganism
page turner
Paget's disease
Pagitane hydrochloride
pagophagia
pagoplexia
pain
    aching p.
    boring p.
    Brodie's p.
    burning p.
    central p.
    chronic intractable p.
    contralateral p.
    dull aching p.
    eccentric p.

pain *(continued)*
    fulgurant p.
    girdle p.
    growing p.
    head p.
    heteropic p.
    homotropic p.
    ideogenous p.
    imperative p.
    intractable p.
    jumping p.
    lancinating p.
    lightning p.
    mental p.
    migraine p.
    mind p.
    mobile p.
    movement p.
    neuralgic p.
    night p.
    noise p.
    objective p.
    osteoscopic p.
    parenchymatous p.
    paresthetic p.
    phantom limb p.
    pseudomyelic p.
    psychic p.
    psychogenic p.
    psychosomatic p.
    radicular p.
    referred p.
    remittent p.
    rest p.
    root p.
    shifting p.
    shooting p.
    spot p.
    starting p.
    terebrant p.
    terebrating p.
    theralgesic p.
    throbbing p.

pain *(continued)*
    wandering p.
pain complex
pain game
pain threshold
painful stimulus
painter's encephalopathy
Pal's modification of Wiegert's myelin
    sheath
palaeocerebellum
palaeocortex
palatal nystagmus
palatal reflex
palate
    artificial p.
palatognathous
palatopharyngoplasty
palatoplasty
palatoplegia
palatorrhaphy
palatoschisis
pale infarct
paleencephalon
paleocerebellar
paleocerebellum
paleocortex
paleoencephalon
paleokinetic
paleopallium
paleophrenia
paleosensation
paleostriatal
paleostriatum
paleothalamus
palikinesia
palilalia
palinal
palinesthesia
palingraphia
palinmnesis
palinopsia
palinphrasia
paliphrasia
palisade effect
pallanesthesia
pallesthesia

pallesthetic
pallhypesthesia
pallial
palliation
palliative
pallid
pallidal
pallidectomy
pallidoansection
pallidoansotomy
pallidofugal
pallidotomy
pallidum
pallium
pallor
palmanesthesia
palmar
    crease, p.
    cuff, p.
    flexion, p.
    grasp reflex, p.
palmaris
palmature
palm-chin reflex
palmesthesia
palmesthetic
palmomental
    reflex, p.
    reflex of Marinesco-Radovici, p.
palmoplantar
palmus
palpatometry
palpebral fissure
palpebrate
palpebration
palpitant
palsy
    backpack p.
    Bell's p.
    birth p.
    brachial p.
    bulbar p.
    cerebral p.
    crossed leg p.
    crutch p.
    diver's p.

palsy *(continued)*
    Erb's p.
    Erb-Duchenne p.
    facial p.
    hammer p.
    handlebar p.
    ischemic p.
    Klumpkie's p.
    Landry's p.
    lead p.
    night p.
    ocular muscle p.
    peroneal p.
    printer's p.
    progressive supranuclear p.
    pseudobulbar p.
    radial nerve p.
    Saturday night p.
    sciatic p.
    scrivener's p.
    shaking p.
    spastic bulbar p.
    supranuclear p.
    tardy median nerve p.
    tardy ulnar nerve p.
    Todd's p.
    transverse p.
    ulnar p.
    wasting p.
Pamelor
pampiniform plexus
pamplegia
PAN (periodic alternating nystagmus)
pananxiety
panasthenia
panatrophy
panautomonic
Pancoast syndrome
Pancoast tumor
Pancoast procedure
pancytopenia-dysmelia syndrome
pandiculation
Pandy's test
pandysautonomia
panencephalitis
    Pette-Doring p.

panencephalitis *(continued)*
    subacute sclerosing p.
panesthesia
pang
panglossia
panhypopituitarism
panic
    homosexual p.
panic attack
panic disorder
Panje voice button
panneuritis
panneurosis
panphobia
panophobia
panplegia
panpsychism
Pansch's fissure
pantalgia
pantamorphia
pantanencephaly
pantaphobia
pantatrophia
pantatrophy
pantheism
panthodic
pantomorphia
Pantopaque
pantophobia
pantothenic acid
pantothermia
papilla (pl. papillae)
papillae (pl. of papilla)
papillary muscle
papilledema
papilloma
    neuroticum, p.
papovavirus
para-analgesia
para-anesthesia
parablepsia
parables
parabulia
paracenesthesia
paracentral
    lobule, p.

paracephalus
paracerebellar
parachute reflex
paracinesia
paracinesis
paracoccidioidomycosis
paracoele
paracortex
paracoxalgia
paracusia
  acris, p.
  duplicata, p.
  loci, p.
  willisiana, p.
paracusis
  Willis, p. of
Paradione
paradipsia
paradox
paradoxic
  sleep, p.
paradoxical
  embolus, p.
  respiration, p.
paraepilepsy
paraequilibrium
parafalx
parafascicular (PF)
  nucleus, p.
  thalamotomy (PFT), p.
Parafon Forte
parafunctional
paragammacism
paraganglia (pl. of paraganglion)
paraganglioma
paraganglion (pl. paraganglia)
parageusia
paragonimiasis
paragrammatism
paragranuloma
paragraphia
parahypnosis
parahypophysis
parakinesia
parakinetic
paralalia

paralalia *(continued)*
  literalis, p.
paralepsy
paralambdacism
paralexia
paralgesia
paralgia
parallax
paralogia
  benign p.
  thematic p.
paralogism
paralogy
paralyses (pl. of paralysis)
paralysis (pl. paralyses)
  abducens p.
  abducens-facial p.
  accommodation, p. of
  acoustic p.
  acute ascending spinal p.
  acute atrophic p.
  acute bulbar p.
  acute infectious p.
  acute wasting p.
  agitans, p.
  alcoholic p.
  alternate p.
  alternating p.
  ambiguo-accessorius p.
  ambiguo-accessorius-hypoglossal p.
  ambiguospinothalamic p.
  anesthesia p.
  anterior spinal p.
  arsenical p.
  ascending p.
  association p.
  asthenic bulbar p.
  asthenobulbospinal p.
  atrophic spinal p.
  Avellis' p.
  Bell's p.
  bilateral p.
  birth p.
  brachial p.
  brachiofacial p.
  Brown-Sequard p.

paralysis (pl. paralyses) *(continued)*
    bulbar p.
    bulbospinal p.
    cage p.
    central p.
    centrocapsular p.
    cerebral p.
    cerebral spastic p.
    Chastek p.
    Chaves-Rapp p.
    circumflex p.
    complete p.
    compression p.
    congenital abducens-facial p.
    congenital oculofacial p.
    conjugate p.
    cortical p.
    crossed p.
    cruciate p.
    crural p.
    crutch p.
    Cruveilhier's p.
    decubitus p.
    Dejerine-Klumpke p.
    Dewar-Harris p.
    diaphragmatic p.
    Dickson p.
    diphtheric p.
    diphtheritic p.
    divers' p.
    Duchenne's p.
    Duchenne-Erh p
    epidemic infantile p.
    Erb's p.
    Erb-Duchenne p.
    essential p.
    exhaustion p.
    facial p.
    false p.
    familial periodic p.
    Felton's p.
    Fereol-Graux p.
    flaccid p.
    functional p.
    gaze, p. of
    general p. of the insane

paralysis (pl. paralyses) *(continued)*
    ginger p.
    glossolabial p.
    glossopharyngolabial p.
    Gubler's p.
    Hass p.
    Henry p.
    hereditary cerebrospinal p.
    histrionic p.
    hyperkalemic periodic p.
    hypoglossal p.
    hypokalemic periodic p.
    hysterical p.
    immune p.
    immunologic p.
    incomplete p.
    Indian bow p.
    infantile p.
    infantile cerebral ataxic p.
    infantile cerebrocerebellar diplegic p.
    infantile spastic p.
    infantile spinal p.
    infectious bulbar p.
    ischemic p.
    jake p.
    Jamaica ginger p.
    juvenile p.
    Klumpke's p.
    Klumpke-Dejerine p.
    Kussmaul's p.
    Kussmaul-Landry p.
    labial p.
    labioglossolaryngeal p.
    labioglossopharyngeal p.
    Landry's p.
    laryngeal p.
    lead p.
    lingual p.
    Lissauer's p.
    local p.
    masticatory p.
    medullary tegmental p.
    Millard-Gubler p.
    mimetic p.
    mixed p.
    motor p.

paralysis (pl. paralyses) *(continued)*
  muscular p.
  musculospiral p.
  myopathic p.
  narcosis p.
  normokalemic periodic p.
  notariorum, p.
  nuclear
  obstetric p.
  ocular p.
  oculofacial p.
  oculomotor p.
  organic p.
  parotitic p.
  periodic p.
  periodica paramyotonia, p.
  peripheral p.
  peroneal p.
  phonetic p.
  postdiphtheric p.
  posthemiplegic p.
  posticus p.
  Pott's p.
  pressure p.
  primary periodic p.
  progressive bulbar p.
  pseudobulbar p.
  pseudohypertrophic muscular p.
  radial p.
  Ramsay Hunt p.
  reflex p.
  Remak's p.
  rucksack p.
  Saturday night p.
  sensory p.
  serum p.
  sleep p.
  spastic p.
  spastic spinal p.
  spinal p.
  spinomuscular p.
  supranuclear p.
  tick-bite p.
  Todd's p.
  tourniquet p.
  trigeminal p.

paralysis (pl. paralyses) *(continued)*
  vacillans, p.
  vasomotor p.
  Vastamaki p.
  Volkmann's ischemic p.
  waking p.
  wasting p.
  Weber's p.
  Werdnig-Hoffman p.
  Whitman p.
  writers' p.
paralysor
paralyssa
paralytic
  bladder, p.
  dementia, p.
  ileus, p.
  squint, p.
paralytogenic
paralyzant
paralyze
paralyzer
paramania
paramedian
parameningeal
paramesial
paramimia
paramnesia
paramusia
paramyelin
paramyoclonus
  multiplex, p.
  simplex, p.
paramyosinogen
paramyotone
paramyotonia
  ataxia p.
  congenita, p.
  symptomatic p.
paramyotonus
paramyxovirus
paranalgesia
paraneoplastic
paranephroma
paranephros
paranesthesia

paraneural
paranoia
   hallucinatoria, p.
   heboid p.
   litigious p.
   originaria, p.
   querulous p.
   simplex, p.
paranoiac
paranoid
   delusions, p.
   ideation, p.
   personality, p.
   reaction type, p.
   schizophrenia, p.
paranoidism
paranomia
   myotactic p.
   visual p.
paranormal
paranosic
paranosis
paraosmia
paraparesis
paraparetic
parapathia
paraphasia
   central p.
   literal p.
   verbal p.
paraphasic
paraphasis
paraphemia
paraphia
paraphilia
paraphiliac
paraphobia
paraphonia
paraphora
paraphrasia
paraphrenia
   confabulans, p.
   expansiva, p.
   phantastica, p.
   systematica, p.
paraphrenic

paraphronia
paraplectic
paraplegia
   alcoholic p.
   ataxic p.
   cerebral p.
   congenital spastic p.
   dolorosa, p.
   Erb's spastic p.
   Erb's syphilitic spastic p.
   flaccid p.
   infantile spastic p.
   peripheral p.
   Pott's p.
   reflex p.
   senile p.
   spastic p.
   superior, p.
   syphilitic p.
   tetanoid p.
   toxic p.
paraplegic
paraplegiform
paraplexus
parapophysis
parapoplexy
parapraxia
parapraxis
parapsia
parapsis
parapsychology
parapsychosis
parapyknomorphous
paraqueduct
parareaction
parareflexia
pararhotacism
pararthria
parasacral
parasagittal
parasellar
parasexual
parasexuality
parasigmatism
parasinusoidal space
parasitophobia

parasitosis
parasomnia
paraspasm
paraspasmus
  faciale, p.
paraspinal
  musculature, p.
paraspinous
  muscle mass, p.
parasthenia
parasuicide
parasympathetic
  nervous system, p.
parasympathicotonia
parasympathin
parasympatholytic
parasympathomimetic
parataxic
  distortion, p.
paratereseomania
parathormone
parathymia
parathyroid
  tetany, p.
parathyropathy
parathyroprival
parathyrotropic
paratonia
paratrigeminal syndrome
paratrophy
paravertebral
  block, p.
  musculature, p.
  space, p.
  triangle, p.
paraxial
  hemimelia, p.
paraxon
parchment skin
parectropia
pareidolia
parelectronomy
parencephalia
parencephalocele
parencephalon
parencephalous

parenchymal
parenchymatous neurosyphilis
parent
  fixation, p.
parenting
  surrogate p.
parepithymia
paresis
paresthesia
  Berger's p.
  Bernhardt's p.
  visceral p.
paresthetic
  meralgia, p.
paretic
  neurosyphilis, p.
parietal
  bosses, p.
  gyrus, p.
  lobe, p.
  lobe tumor, p.
parietofrontal
parieto-occipital
  fissure, p.
  sulcus, p.
parietosphenoid
parietosplanchnic
parietosquamosal
parietotemporal
  projection, p.
Parinaud's syndrome
Parkinson's dementia
Parkinson's disease
Parkinson's facies
Parkinson's mask
Parkinson's sign
Parkinson's syndrome
parkinsonian
parkinsonism
  drug-induced p.
  postencephalitic p.
  primary p.
  secondary p.
  vascular p.
parkinsonism-plus
Parkside Behavior Rating Scale

Parlodel
paroccipital
parolivary
Parona's space
paroniria
  ambulans, p.
  salax, p.
parorexia
parosmia
parosphresia
parotid
parotitis
paroxysm
paroxysmal
  activity, p.
  burst, p.
  depolarization shift (PDS), p.
  discharge, p.
  dyskinesia, p.
  dystonia, p.
  kinesigenic choreoathetosis, p.
  labyrinthine vertigo, p.
  nocturnal hemoglobinuria, p.
  sleep, p.
  slowing, p.
Parrot's atrophy of the newborn
Parrot's disease
Parrot's pseudoparalysis
Parrot's sign
Parry-Romberg syndrome
pars (pl. partes)
  centralis ventriculi lateralis cerebri, p.
  cervicalis medullae spinalis, p.
  frontalis radiationes corporis callosi, p.
  inferior fossae rhomboideae, p.
  inferior gyri frontalis medii, p.
  intermedia fossae rhomboideae, p.
  lumbalis medullae spinalis, p.
  marginalis sulci cinguli, p.
  occipitalis radiationis corporis
    callosi, p.
  opercularis gyri frontalis inferioris, p.
  orbitalis gyri frontalis inferioris, p.
  parasympathica systematis nervois au-
    tonomici, p.
  parietalis operculi, p.

pars (pl. partes) *(continued)*
  parietalis radiationis corporis
    callosi, p.
  petrosa ossis temporalis, p.
  posterior commissurae anterioris
    cerebri, p.
  posterior rhinencephali, p.
  subfrontalis sulci cinguli, p.
  superior fossae rhomboideae, p.
  superior gryi frontalis medii, p.
  sympathica systematis nervosi au-
    tonomici, p.
partes (pl. of pars)
parthenophobia
partial thenar atrophy
partial weight-bearing
parturient
paralysis
parturiphobia
Pascal's law
PASG (pneumatic antishock garment)
passive
  -aggressive, p.
  -dependence reaction, p.
  -dependent, p.
  exercise, p.
  hyperventilation, p.
  motion, p.
  range of motion, p.
passivism
passivity
  feelings, p.
past-pointing
Patau's syndrome
patchy distribution
patella
patellar
  jerk, p.
  reflex, p.
patelloquadriceps tendon
Paterson clip
pathematology
pathergasia
pathetic
pathetism
pathodixia

pathoformic
pathogenesis
pathogenetic
pathognomonic
pathologic
    gambling, p.
    reflex, p.
pathological
pathological reaction to alcohol
pathomania
pathomimesis
pathomimia
pathomimicry
pathoneurosis
pathophilia
pathophobia
pathopsychology
pathopsychosis
pathway
    afferent p.
    dopaminergic nigrostriatal p.
    efferent p.
    final common p.
    internuncial p.
patient-controlled analgesic (PCA) system
Patil sterotactic system
patriarch
patriarchal
Patrick's sign
Patrick's test
pattern reversal stimuli
pattern shift style
patterned movement
patterning
paucisynaptic
paucity
    findings, p. of
    speech, p. of
Pavlik harness
pavlovian conditioning
pavlovian reflex
pavor
    diurnus, p.
    incubus, p.
    nocturnus, p.
Payr sign

PCA (patient-controlled analgesia or posterior communicating artery)
    system, P.
PCP (phencyclidine)
PDS (paroxysmal depolarization shift)
Peabody Individual Achievement Test
peace pill
peak-to-peak amplitude
peapod chisel
peccatiphobia
Pecquet's cistern
Pecquet's reservoir
pectoralgia
pederast
pederasty
pederosis
pedialgia
pedicle
    vertebral arch, p. of
pediculophobia
pedigree analysis
pedionalgia
pediophilic
pediophobia
pedomorphism
pedophile
pedophilia
pedophobia
peduncle
peduncular
    hallucinosis, p.
pedunculi (pl. of pedunculus)
pedunculotomy
pedunculus (pl. pedunculi)
peer
    pressure, p.
    relationship, p.
Peet splanchnic resection
PEG (pneumoencephalography)
Peganone
Pel's crisis
Pel-Ebstein disease
Pelizaeus-Merzbacher disease
Pelizaeus-Merzbacher sclerosis
pellagra
Pellizzi's syndrome

pellote
pelvic girdle
pelvospondylitis
PEMF (pulsating electromagnetic field)
pemoline
Pende's sign
Pendred's syndrome
pendular nystagmus
penectomy
penetrance
peniaphobia
penile implant
penile prosthesis
penile tumescence
penis envy
pension neurosis
pentobarbital
pentogram
Pentothal interview
peotillomania
Pepper's syndrome
peptidergic nervous system
perceive
percentile
perception
   constant-touch p.
   depth p.
   extrasensory p. (ESP)
   facial p.
   stereognostic p.
perceptivity
perceptorium
perceptual
percipient
percutaneous automated diskectomy
perencephaly
Perez's sign
perfectionism
perfectionist
perfectionistic
perforans
   manus, p.
pergolide mesylate
periaqueductal
   gray electrode, p.
periaxial

periaxonal
pericallosal
pericephalic
pericranial
pericranitis
pericranium
peridendritic
peridural
peridurogram
peridurography
periencephalitis
periencephalography
perifascicular
periganglionic
periglial
perimedullary
perimeningitis
perimolysis
perimyelitis
perimyelography
perimyositis
perimysia
perimysial
perimysiitis
perimysium (perimysia)
perineural
   channel, p.
   fibroblastoma, p.
perineurial
   cyst, p.
   neurorrhaphy, p.
perineuritic
perineuritis
perineurium
perineuronal satellite cell
periodic
   alternating nystagmus (PAN), p.
   lateralized epileptiform discharges
     (PLEDs), p.
   paralysis, p.
perioral cyanosis
periosteal
   elevator, p.
periosteum
peripachymeningitis
peripherad

peripheral
  anesthesia, p.
  cyanosis, p.
  effector neuron, p.
  facial paralysis, p.
  nerve, p.
  nerve block, p.
  nervous system (PNS), p.
  neuritis, p.
  neuropathy, p.
  venous stasis, p.
  vision, p.
peripheraphose
peripherocentral
peripheroceptor
peripheromittor
peripherophose
periphery
periphoria
periphrastic
periradicular
perispondylic
perispondylitis
perivascular
perivascularity
perivasculitis
periventricular
perivertebral
Perkins Brailler
PERLA (pupils equal and react to light
  and accommodation)
Perls theory
permanent and stationary
permanent disability
permanent section
pernicious anemia
peronarthrosis
peroneal
  muscular atrophy, p.
  nerve, p.
  sign, p.
peroneotibial
peronia
Perrin-Ferraton disease
PERRLA (pupils equal, round, and react
  to light and accommodation)

Perry-Robinson cervical technique
persecution
persecutory
perseverate
perseveration
perseverative chaining
persistent vegetative state (PVS)
person in need of supervision (PINS)
persona
personality
  affective p.
  alternating p.
  anancastic p.
  antisocial p.
  as-if p.
  asthenic p.
  avoidant p.
  borderline p.
  compulsive p.
  cycloid p.
  cyclothymic p.
  dependent p.
  disordered p.
  double p.
  dual p.
  dyssocial p.
  epileptoid p.
  explosive p.
  extroverted p.
  histrionic p.
  hypomanic p.
  hysterical p.
  inadequate p.
  multiple p.
  narcissistic p.
  neurotic p.
  obsessive p.
  obsessive-compulsive p.
  paranoid p.
  passive-aggressive p.
  passive-dependent p.
  phobic p.
  psychopathic p.
  sadistic p.
  schizoid p.
  schizotypal p.

personality *(continued)*
  seclusive p.
  self-defeating p.
  shut-in p.
  sociopathic p.
  split p.
  thymic p.
personality change
personality disorder
personality features
personality style
personality trait
personologic
personology
persuasion
persuasive
perturbation level lethality
pervasive
pervasiveness
perverse
  triangle, p.
perversion
pervert
  sexual p.
perverted
pervigilium
pessimism
  therapeutic p.
pessimist
pessimistic
pet therapy
PET (positron emission tomography)
  scan, P.
petit mal
  epilepsy, p.
  seizure, p.
  triad, p.
petit pas gait
petroclinoid
petro-occipital
petrosal
  nerve, p.
  sinus, p.
petroso-occipital synchondrosis
petrosphenoid
petrous

petrous *(continued)*
  pyramid, p.
  ridge, p.
Petruschky's spinalgia
PETT (positron emission transaxial tomography)
  scan, P.
Pett-Doring panencephalitis
Peyer's patches
peyote
peyotl
Peyronie's disease
Peyton brain spatula
PF (parafascicular)
  nucleus, P.
Pfeiffer's syndrome
Pfluger's law
PFT (parafascicular thalamotomy)
PGO spikes
phagocytosis
phagomania
phagophobia
Phalen's maneuver
Phalen's sign
phallic
  symbol, p.
  -narcissistic character, p.
phallus
phaneromania
phantasia
phantasm
phantasmatomoria
phantasmology
phantasmoscopia
phantasy
phantogeusia
phantom
  limb, p.
  pain, p.
  spike and wave, p.
  vision, p.
phantosmia
pharmacomania
pharmacophilia
pharmacophobia
pharmacopsychosis

pharmacotherapy
pharyngeal reflex
pharyngismus
pharyngoparalysis
pharyngoplegia
pharyngospasm
phase
  bed p.
  cane-walking p.
  stair-climbing p.
  standing p.
phase advance syndrome
phase delay syndrome
phase of life problem
phase reversal
phasic activity
phasmophobia
phenacemide
phencyclidine hydrochloride (PCP)
phenelzine sulfate
phengophobia
phenobarbital
phenomenologic
phenomenology
phenomomen
  arm p.
  Aubert's p.
  autokinetic visible light p.
  Babinski's p.
  Becker's p.
  Bell's p.
  brake p.
  break-off p.
  cheek p.
  cogwheel p.
  Cushing's p.
  doll's p.
  head p.
  Duckworth's p.
  Erb's p.
  face p.
  facialis p.
  finger p.
  flicker p.
  Galassi's pupillary p.
  Gowers' p.

phenomomen *(continued)*
  Grasset's p.
  Grasset-Gaussel p.
  Gunn's p.
  Gunn's pupillary p.
  Hammerschlag's p.
  Hertwig-Magendie p.
  hip-flexion p.
  Hochsinger's p.
  Hoffmann's p.
  Holmes' p.
  Holmes-Stewart p.
  Hunt's paradoxical p.
  jaw-winking p.
  Kuhne's muscular p.
  LeGrand-Geblewics p.
  Leichtenstern's p.
  Lust's p.
  Marcus Gunn p.
  Marcus Gunn pupillary p.
  muscle p.
  Negro's p.
  Orbeli p.
  orbicularis p.
  paradoxical p. of dystonia
  paradoxical pupillary p.
  peroneal nerve p.
  phi p.
  Piltz-Westphal p.
  Pool's p.
  Porret's p.
  psi p.
  Purkinje's p.
  Queckenstedt's p.
  radial p.
  Raynaud's p.
  rebound p.
  release p.
  Rieger's p.
  Ritter-Rollet p.
  Rust's p.
  Schramm's p.
  Schuller's p.
  Sherrington p.
  Sinkler's p.
  Souques' p.

phenomomen *(continued)*
  springlike p.
  staircase p.
  Strumpell p.
  toe p.
  tongue p.
  Trousseau's p.
  Wedensky's p.
  Westphal's p.
  Westphal-Piltz p.
phenothiazine
Phenurone
phenylalanine
phenylalaninemia
pheynlketonuria (PKU)
phenylpyruvic
  acid, p.
  amentia, p.
  idiocy, p.
  oligophrenia, p.
pheochrome bodies
pheochromocytoma
pheromone
phi phenomenon
Philippe-Gombault tract
Philippson's reflex
philoneism
philosophical
philosophy
philter
phlebalgia
phlegmatic
PHN (postherpetic neuralgia)
phobanthropy
phobia
phobic
  desensitization, p.
  neurosis, p.
  personality, p.
  psychoneurosis p.
phobophobia
phonasthenia
phonation
phonautograph
phoneme
phonetics

phoniatrician
phoniatrics
phonic
phonism
phonology
phonomania
phonomyoclonus
phonomyogram
phonomyography
phonopathy
phonophobia
phonophotography
phonopsia
phoria
phose
phosis
phosphene
phosphocreatine
phosphoproteins
phosphor bronze wire
photalgia
photaugiaphobia
photesthesis
photic
  driving, p.
  epilepsy, p.
  sneezing, p.
  stimulation, p.
photism
photoconvulsive
photodynia
photodysphoria
photogene
photogenic epilepsy
photomania
photometer
photomotogram
photomotor
photomyoclonic
photomyogenic
photon densitometry
photoparoxysmal
photopathy
photoperceptive
photoperiodism
photophilic

photophobia
photophthalmia
photopia
photoplethysmography
photopsia
phren
phrenalgia
phrenemphraxis
phrenetic
phrenic
   nerve, p.
phrenicectomize
phrenicectomy
phrenicoexeresis
phreniconeurectomy
phrenicotomy
phrenicotripsy
phrenocardia
phrenopathy
phrenoplegia
phrenospasm
phrenotropic
phrictopathic
phronema
phthiriophobia
phthisiomania
phthisiophobia
Phynox cobalt alloy clip
physical therapy (PT)
physiologic
   reflexes, p.
   zero, p.
physiopathic
physiopsychic
physiotherapy
physocephaly
physostigmine
pia
   -arachnitis, p.
   -arachnoid, p.
   -glia, p.
pia mater
   encephali, p.m.
   spinalis, p.m.
pial
   funnel, p.

pial *(continued)*
   sheath, p.
piamatral
pianists' cramp
piarachnitis
piarachnoid
piblokto
pica
PICA (posterior inferior cerebellar or
   communicating artery)
Pick's bodies
Pick's convolutional atrophy
Pick's dementia
Pick's disease
Pick's syndrome
pickup walker
pickwickian syndrome
picornavirus
picrogeusia
pictograph
piecemeal
Pierre-Robin syndrome
piesesthesia
piesimeter
pigmented xerodermoid
piitis
pileus
pill-rolling tremor
Pillet hand prosthesis
pillion
piloerection
pilomotor
   nerve, p.
   reflex, p.
pilot's vertigo
Piltz's reflex
Piltz's sign
Piltz-Westphal phenomenon
pin
   fixation headholder, p.
   headrest, p.
   sensation, p.
pinch and grip
pinch meter
pineal
   body, p.

pinealectomy
pinealism
pinealoblastoma
pinealoma
Pinel's system
ping-pong fracture
ping-pong gaze
pinhole pupil
pinion headrest
pink disease
pinpoint pupil
pinprick sensation
PINS (person in need of supervision)
pins and needles sensation
pinus
pinwheel hypesthesia
pinwheel test
Piotrowski's sign
pipecolatemia
piriform
Pisces spinal cord stimulation system
pith
pithiatism
pithing
Pitre's sections
Pitt talking tracheostomy tube
Pittsburgh triangular frame
pituicyte
pituitarigenic
pituitarism
pituitary
    adenoma, p.
    apoplexy, p.
    cachexia, p.
    grasper, p.
    rongeur, p.
pituitectomy
PKU (phenylketonuria)
placebo
    effect, p.
placing reflex
placing response
plagiocephalic
plagiocephaly
plain film
plana (pl. of planum)

plane
    Aeby's p.
    axial p.
    Baer's p.
    coronal p.
    datum p.
    Daubenton's p.
    Frankfort horizontal p.
    Morton's p.
    sagittal p.
planotopokinesia
plantalgia
plantar
    flexion, p.
    flexors, p.
    grasp reflex, p.
    nerve, p.
    reflex, p.
    response, p.
planum (pl. plana)
plaque
    argyrophil p.
    attachment p.
    fibromyelinic p.
    Hollenhorst p.
    Lichtheim p.
    Redlich-Fisher miliary p.
    senile p.
plaquing
plasmapheresis
plastic rigidity
Plastizote cervical collar
Plasti-Pore
plate
    Hoen's skull p.
    tantalum p.
plateau
plateauing
platybasia
platycrania
platysma
platysmal
    reflex, p.
platyspondylia
platyspondylisis
pleasure principle

pleasure-pain principle
PLEDs (periodic lateralized epileptiform
   discharges)
pledget
pleocytosis
pleonexia
pleurodynia
pleurothotonos
plexal
plexectomy
plexiform
   neurofibroma, p.
   neuroma p.
plexitis
plexogenic
plexopathy
   lumbar p.
plexus
   autonomic p.
   brachial p.
   carotid p.
   cervical p.
   choroid p.
   lumbosacral p.
   nerve p.
   prevertebral p.
   vertebral p.
PLIF (posterior lumbar interbody fusion)
plug
Plummer's sign
Plutchik Geriatric Rating Scale
plutomania
PMMA (antibiotic-impregnated polymethyl methacrylate)
PMS (premenstrual syndrome)
PMT (premenstrual tension)
pneopneic reflex
pneumatic sign
pneumatocele
   extracranial p.
   intracranial p.
pneumatocephalus
pneumatology
pneumatophobia
pneumatorrhachis
pneumencephalogram

pneumencephalography
pneumencephalon
   artificiale, p.
pneumocephalus
pneumocisternogram
pneumocisternography
pneumocrania
pneumocranium
Pneumocystis carinii
pneumoencephalitis
pneumoencephalogram
pneumoencephalography (PEG)
pneumoencephalomyelogram
pneumoencephalomyelography
pneumoencephalos
pneumoencephalus
pneumogastric nerve
pneumography
pneumomyelography
pneumophonia
pneumorachicentesis
pneumorachis
pneumoroentgenography
pneumotomography
pneumoventiculogram
pneumoventricle
pneumoventriculography
PNI (psychoneuroimmunology)
pnigophobia
PNS (partial nonprogressing stroke or peripheral nervous system)
podencephalus
pododynamometer
pododynia
POEMS (polyneuropathy, organomegaly,
   endocrinopathy, monoclonal protein,
   skin change)
   syndrome, P.
poikilothermia
point
   Ar, p.
   B, p.
   Bo, p.
   craniometric p.
   deaf p. of ear
   Erb's p.

point *(continued)*
   Gueneau de Mussy's p.
   hot p.
   hysterogenic p.
   motor p.
   painful p.
   Po, p.
   pressure p.
   R, p.
   SE, p.
   SO, p.
   supra-auricular p.
   supranasal p.
   supraorbital p.
   trigger p.
   Trousseau's apophysiary p.
   Valleix's p.
   vital p.
   Z, p.
point tenderness
poker back
poker facies
poker spine
pokeroot poisoning
Poland's syndrome
polarity
polarization
polarize
poli (pl. of polus)
polio
poliocidal
polioclastic
poliodystrophia
poliodystrophy
polioencephalitis
   acute superior hemorrhagic p.
   acuta infantum, p.
   acute bulbar p.
   inferior p.
   posterior p.
   superior hemorrhagic p.
polioencephalomeningomyelitis
polioencephalomyelitis
polioencephalopathy
polioencephalotropic
poliomyelencephalitis

poliomyeliticidal
poliomyelitis
   acute anterior p.
   acute lateral p.
   anterior p.
   ascending p.
   bulbar p.
   cerebral p.
   endemic p.
   epidemic p.
   postinoculation p.
   post-tonsillectomy p.
   postvaccinal p.
   spinal paralytic p.
poliomyeloencephalitis
poliomyelopathy
polioneuromere
poliovirus
   vaccine, p.
pollakidipsia
Polli surgical garment
poltergeist
polus (pl. poli)
polyalcoholism
polyalgesia
polyarteritis
   nodosa, p.
polyaxon
polyclonal bands
polyclonia
polycystic kidneys
polycythemia
   vera, p.
polydipsia
polydrug
polydysplasia
polydysspondylism
polydystrophic
polydystrophy
   pseudo-Hurler p.
polyendocrinopathy
polyesthesia
polyesthetic
polygraph
polygyria
polymerization

polymethyl methacrylate, antibiotic-impregnated (PMMA)
polymicrogyria
polymodal
nociceptor, p.
polymorphic
delta activity, p.
slowing p.
wave, p.
polymorphism
polymyalgia
arteritica, p.
rheumatica p.
polymyoclonus
polymyositis
polyneural
polyneuralgia
polyneuritic
polyneuritis
acute febrile p.
acute idiopathic p.
acute infective p.
acute postinfectious p.
anemic p.
cerebralis menieriformis, p.
endemic p.
Guillain-Barre p.
Jamaica ginger p.
postinfectious p.
potatorum, p. p.
polyneuromyositis
polyneuropathy
acute postinfectious p.
amyloid p.
buckthorn p.
erythredema p.
porphyric p.
progressive hypertrophic p.
symmetrical p.
uremic p.
polyneuroradiculitis
polynuclear
polyopia
polyparesis
polypeptide
polypeptidorrhachia

polyperiostitis
hyperesthetica, p.
polyphagia
polypharmacy
polyphobia
polyphrasia
polyplegia
polyposia
polypragmasy
polyradiculitis
polyradiculoneuritis
polyradiculoneuropathy
polyradiculopathy
polysensitivity
polysensory
polysomnogram
polysomnography
polysubstance
abuse, p.
dependence, p.
polysurgery
polysurgical addiction
polysynaptic
polytef
polytheist
polytomography
polyurethane foam embolus
polyvinyl
Pompe's disease
pond fracture
ponesiatrics
ponograph
ponophobia
pons (pl. pontes)
cerebelli, p.
tarini, p.
varolii, p.
pons-oblongata
pontes (pl. of pons)
pontibrachium
ponticulus
pontile
hemiplegia, p.
nuclei, p.
pontine
angle, p.

pontine *(continued)*
   fissure, p.
pontobulbar
pontobulbia
pontocerebellar
pontogeniculo-occipital spike
pontomedullary
pontomesencephalic
pontopeduncular
Pool's phenomenon
Pool-Schlesinger sign
Poppen forceps
porencephalia
porencephalic
porencephaly
poriomania
porion
Porites coral
pornographic
pornographomania
pornography
pornolagnia
Porocoat
porosis
porotic
porphyria
porphyrism
porphyrismus
Porret's phenomenon
Port-A-Cath
port-wine nevus
Porteus Maze Test
portio (pl. portiones)
portiones (pl. of portio)
Portnoy ventricular cannula
portosystemic encephalopathy
porus
acousticus
Posey belt
Posey restraint
Posey vest
posey'd
position sense
positive
   attitude, p.
   behavior, p.

positive *(continued)*
   reinforcement, p.
positrocephalogram
positrocephalography
positron
   emission tomography (PET), p.
   emission transaxial tomography
     (PETT), p.
   scan, p.
possessed
possession
   demoniacal p.
Possum (Patient-Operated Selector Mechanism)
postanoxic
   encephalopathy, p.
postaxial polydactyly
postbasic stare
postbulbar
postcentral
   fissure, p.
   gyrus, p.
   sulcus, p.
postcentralis
postcisterna
postcoital cephalalgia
postcondylare
postcontrast
postconvulsive
postcornu
postcranial
postdormital
   hallucinations, p.
postdormitum
postencephalitic
postepileptic
posterior
   central gyrus, p.
   column, p.
   commissure, p.
   communicating artery (PCA), p.
   gray column, p.
   horn, p.
   inferior cerebellar artery (PICA), p.
   inferior communicating artery
     (PICA), p.

posterior *(continued)*
   lumbar interbody fusion (PLIF), p.
posterolateral
   sclerosis, p.
posteromedian
posteroparietal
posterotemporal
postganglionic
   fiber, p.
   neuron, p.
postglenoid
posthemiplegic
   paralysis, p.
postherpetic
   neuralgia (PHN), p.
posthypnotic
   suggestion, p.
posthypophysis
posthypoxic
postictal
   confusion, p.
   state, p.
postinfectious encephalomyelitis
postneuritic
postocular neuritis
postoperative psychosis
postparalytic
postpartum
   blues, p.
   depression, p.
   psychosis, p.
postpituitary
postpoliomyelitis muscular atrophy
   (PPMA)
postpontile
postpuberty
postpubescent
postpump psychosis
postpyramidal
postrolandic
postsacral
postsphenoid
poststroke
   parkinsonism, p.
postsylvian
postsynaptic

post-tap headache
post-transfusion psychosis
post-traumatic
   amnesia, p.
   cerebral syndrome, p.
   encephalopathy, p.
   stress syndrome, p.
postural
   changes, p.
   claudication, p.
   hypertension, p.
   hypotension, p.
   tremor, p.
posture
posturing
postvaccinal
post-Vietnam syndrome
postviral fatigue syndrome
pot (marijuana)
potamophobia
potential
   action p.
   brain stem auditory evoked p.
   demarcation p.
   injury p.
   somatosensory evoked p.
   visual evoked p.
potentiate
potentiation
potomania
Pott's disease
Pott's paralysis
Pott's puffy tumor
Potts' abscess
Potts' curvature
Potts' disease
Potts' paraplegia
Pottenger's sign
Potter facies
Potter's syndrome
pouch
pouching
poverty of movement
poverty of thought
Powassan encephalitis
Powassan virus

PPMA (postpoliomyelitis muscular atrophy)
Prader-Willi syndrome
pragmatagnosia
pragmatamnesia
    visual p.
pragmatic
pragmatism
pragmatist
Pratt curette
praxiology
praxis
prazepam
PRE (progressive resistive exercises)
preataxic
precentral
    convolution, p.
    fissure, p.
    gyrus, p.
    sulcus, p.
Prechtl's movements
precocious
    adrenarche, p.
    pseudopuberty, p.
    puberty, p.
precocity
precognition
precoma
preconscious
preconvulsant
preconvulsive
preoulmonate fissure
precuneus
predictor
predilection
predisposed
predisposition
predormital
    hallucinations, p.
predormition
predormitum
preeclampsia
prefrontal
    lobotomy, p.
preganglionic
    fiber, p.

preganglionic *(continued)*
    neuron, p.
pregenital
prehemiplegic
prehypophyseal
prehypophysis
preictal
preiotation
prelimbic
prelocomotion
Premack's principle
premature ejaculation
premenstrual
    syndrome (PMS), p.
    tension (PMT), p.
premonition
premonitory
premorbid
premotor cortex
preoblongata
preoccipital notch
preoptic
preparalytic
preperception
prepubescent
prepyramidal fissure
preretinal hemorrhage
prerolandic gyrus
presacral
    neurectomy, p.
presbyope
presbyophrenia
presbyopia
presenile
    dementia, p.
presenility
presenium
prespinal
prespondylolisthesis
pressor
    nerves, p.
    reflex, p.
pressoreceptive
pressoreceptor
pressure
    palsy, p.

pressure *(continued)*
   paralysis, p.
   phenomenon, p.
   point, p.
   sore, p.
pressured speech
PressureSense Monitor
Preston ligamentum flavum forceps
Preston pinch gauge
presylvian fissure
presynaptic
presyncopal spell
presyncope
pretectal
preternaturalism
pretraumatic
   amnesia, p.
prevertebral
   fascia, p.
   ganglia, p.
   space, p.
prevocational evaluation
Prevost's law
Prevost's sign
Preyer's reflex
prezygapophysis
priapism
   stuttering p.
prickling sensation
primal
   scene, p.
   scream, p.
   therapy, p.
primary
   affective witzelsucht, p.
   aldosteronism, p.
   epilepsy, p.
   gaze, p.
   mover, p.
primitive
   instinct, p.
   reflex, p.
prion
prism test
prison neurosis
prison psychosis

privileged communication
proactive
proatlas
proband
problematic
procephalic
process
processus
procoelia
procrastinate
procrastination
proctoplegia
procursive
procurvation
prodromal
prodrome
proencephalus
progeria
progression
   backward p.
   cross-legged p.
   metadromic p.
progressive
   bulbar palsy, p.
   cerebellar dyssynergia, p.
   hearing loss, p.
   multifocal leukoencephalopathy, p.
   muscular atrophy, p.
   muscular dystrophy, p.
   ossifying myositis, p.
   resistive exercise (PRE), p.
   spinal muscular atrophy, p.
   supranuclear palsy, p.
projection
   eccentric p.
   erroneous p.
   thalamocortical p.
projective
   identification, p.
   test, p.
prolactinoma
prolepsia
prolepsis
promontory
pronate
pronation

pronation *(continued)*
   sign, p.
   supination, p. and
pronatoflexor
pronator
   drift, p.
   syndrome, p.
prone
proneness
pronometer
propanolol
propel
proper fasciculus
Proplast
proprioception
proprioceptive
   impulses, p.
   sense, p.
proprioceptor
propriospinal
propulsion
prosencephalon
prosocoele
prosody
prosopagnosia
prosopalgia
prosophenosia
prosopoanoschisis
prosopodiplegia
prosopodysmorphia
prosopodynia
prosoponeuralgia
prosopoplegia
prosoposchisis
prosopospasm
prosopus varus
prostatic syncope
prosthesis
prosthetic
prosthetist
Prostigmin test
prostitute
prostitution
prostrate
prostration
   heat p.

prostration *(continued)*
   nervous p.
protective custody
proteinphobia
proton beam
protoneuron
protopathic
   pain, p.
   sensibility, p.
Protoplast
protospasm
Protouch padding
protovertebra
protriptyline hydrochloride
protruding disk
protrusion
protuberance
protuberant
proverbs
proxemics
proximoataxia
psalis
psalterium
psammoma
   body, p.
pselaphesia
psellism
pseudacousis
pseudacousma
pseudagraphia
pseudaphia
pseudarthrosis
pseudencephalus
pseudesthesia
pseudoagraphia
pseudoanaphylaxis
pseudoaneurysm
pseudoangina
pseudankylosis
pseudoantagonist
pseudoapoplexy
pseudoathetosis
pseudo-Babinski sign
pseudobulbar
   -type palsy, p.
pseudocele

pseudocephalocele
pseudochorea
pseudochromesthesia
pseudoclaudication
pseudoclonus
pseudocoele
pseudocoma
pseudocoxalgia
pseudocyesis
pseudocyst
pseudodelirium
pseudodementia
pseudoencapsulated
pseudoencephalomalacia
pseudoesthesia
pseudofracture
pseudoganglion
pseudogeusesthesia
pseudogeusia
pseudoglioma
pseudo-Graefe sign
pseudographia
pseudohallucination
pseudohermaphrodite
pseudohermaphroditism
   female p.
   male p.
pseudoheterotopia
pseudohydrocephalus
pseudohypertrophic
pseudohypertrophy
pseudohypoparathyroidism
pseudohypophosphatasia
pseudohypothyroidism
pseudoincontinence
pseudoinsomnia
pseudolaminar
pseudologia
   fantastica, p.
pseudoluxation
pseudomania
pseudomasturbation
pseudomelia
   paraesthetica, p.
pseudomeningitis
pseudomicrocephalus

pseudomnesia
pseudomotor
   cerebri, p.
pseudomyopia
pseudonarcotic
pseudonarcotism
pseudoneuritis
pseudoneurological
pseudoneuroma
pseudoneuronophagia
pseudoneurotic
pseudonystagmus
pseudopapilledema
pseudoparalysis
   agitans, p.
   arthritic general p.
   congenital atonic p.
   Parrot's p.
   syphilitic p.
pseudoparaphrasia
pseudoparaplegia
pseudoparesis
pseudoparkinsonism
pseudophotesthesia
pseudoplegia
pseudopoliomyelitis
pseudopolymelia
   paraesthetica, p.
pseudopregnancy
pseudopseudohypoparathyroidism
pseudopsia
pseudopsychopathic
pseudopsychosis
pseudoptosis
pseudopuberty
pseudorosette
pseudosclerosis
   spastica, p.
   Westfall-Strumpell p.
pseudoseizure
pseudosmia
pseudosteppage gait
pseudosyncope
pseudotabes
pseudotetanus
pseudotrismus

pseudotumor
   cerebri, p.
pseudouremia
pseudovoice
psi phenomenon
psilocin
psilocybin
psoas
   abscess, p.
   muscle, p.
   shadow, p.
   sign, p.
psoitis
psomophagia
psychagogy
psychalgia
psychanalysis
psychanopsia
psychasthene
psychasthenia
   reaction, p.
psychataxia
psychauditory
psyche
psycheclampsia
psychedelic
psychiater
psychiatric
psychiatrist
psychiatry
   biological p.
   community p.
   cross-cultural p.
   descriptive p.
   dynamic p.
   existential p.
   forensic p.
   industrial p.
   occupational p.
   organic p.
   orthomolecular p.
   preventive p.
   social p.
   transcultural p.
psychic
   blindness, p.

psychic *(continued)*
   contagion, p.
   deafness, p.
   determinism, p.
   energizer, p.
   energy, p.
   equivalent, p.
   force, p.
   healing, p.
   numbness, p.
   overlay, p.
   overtone, p.
   phenomenon, p.
   suicide, p.
   surgery, p.
   trauma, p.
psychical
   research, p.
psychicism
psychinosis
psychism
psychlampsia
psychoactive
psychoalgalia
psychoallergy
psychoanaleptic
psychoanalysis
psychoanalyst
psychoanalytic
psychoanalyze
psychoasthenics
psychoauditory
psychobacillosis
psychobiological
psychobiology
psychocatharsis
psychocentric
psychochemistry
psychochrome
psychochromesthesia
psychocoma
psychocortical
psychocutaneous
psychodiagnosis
psychodiagnostics
psychodometer

psychodometry
psychodrama
psychodynamics
psychodysleptic
psychoendocrinology
psychoepilepsy
psychoevolutionary
psychoextended hand
psychoflexed hand
psychogalvanic response
psychogalvanometer
psychogenesis
psychogenetics
psychogenia
psychogenic
   amenorrhea, p.
   amnesia, p.
   feud, p.
   fugue, p.
   overlay, p.
   pain, p.
   palpitations, p.
psychogenous
psychogeriatrics
psychogeusic
psychognosis
psychognostic
psychogogic
psychogram
psychograph
psychography
psychokinesis
psychokym
psycholagny
psycholepsy
psycholeptic
psycholinguistics
psychologic
psychological
   moment, p.
   overlay, p.
   overtones, p.
   sex, p.
   warfare, p.
psychologist
psychologue

psychology
   abnormal p.
   analytic p.
   analytical p.
   applied p.
   behavioristic p.
   child p.
   clinical p.
   cognitive p.
   community p.
   comparative p.
   criminal p.
   depth p.
   developmental p.
   dynamic p.
   environmental p.
   experimental p.
   genetic p.
   gestalt p.
   individual p.
   industrial p.
   physiological p.
   social p.
   sports p.
psychomathematics
psychometer
psychometrician
psychometrics
psychometry
psychomotor
   activity, p.
   agitation, p.
   epilepsy, p.
   retardation, p.
   seizure, p.
   variant, p.
psychoneural
psychoneuroendocrinology
psychoneuroimmunology
psychoneurology
psychoneuroses (pl. of psychoneurosis)
psychoneurosis (pl. psychoneuroses)
   anxiety p.
   anxiety reaction p.
   converse reaction p.
   defense p.

psychoneurosis (pl. psychoneuroses)
  (continued)
    depressive reaction p.
    dissociated reaction p.
    maidica, p.
    obsessive-compulsive p.
    paranoid p.
    phobic reaction p.
psychoneurotic
psychonomy
psychonosema
psychonosis
psychoparesis
psychopath
psychopathia
    martialis, p.
    sexualis, p.
psychopathic
    inferiority, p.
    personality, p.
psychopathist
psychopathology
psychopathosis
psychopathy
psychopharmacology
psychophonasthenia
psychophylaxis
psychophysical
psychophysics
psychophysiologic
psychophysiology
psychoplegia
psychoplegic
psychopneumatology
psychoprophylactic
    preparation for childbirth, p.
psychoprophylaxis
psychoreaction
psychorhythmia
psychorrhagia
psychorrhagy
psychorrhea
psychorrhexis
psychosedation
psychosedative
psychosensorial

psychosensory
psychoses (pl. of psychosis)
psychosexual
    development, p.
    disorder, p.
    dysfunction, p.
psychosine
psychosis (pl. psychoses)
    affective p.
    alcoholic p.
    bipolar p.
    brief reactive p.
    Cheyne-Stokes p.
    circular p.
    depressive p.
    drug p.
    exhaustion p.
    functional p.
    gestational p.
    hysterical p.
    idiophrenic p.
    involutional p.
    Korsakoff's p.
    manic p.
    manic-depressive p.
    organic p.
    paranoiac p.
    paranoid p.
    polyneuritic p.
    polyneuritica, p.
    postinfectious p.
    postpartum p.
    postpump p.
    posttransfusion p.
    prison p.
    puerperal p.
    schizoaffective p.
    schizophrenic p.
    senile p.
    situational p.
    symbiotic p.
    symbiotic infantile p.
    toxic p.
    traumatic p.
    unipolar p.
    zoophil p.

psychosocial
   dwarfism, p.
psychosociology
psychosolytic
psychosomatic
   medicine, p.
psychosomaticist
psychosomimetic
psychosophy
psychostimulant
psychosurgery
psychosynthesis
psychotaxis
psychotechnics
psychotechnology
psychotherapeutic
psychotherapist
psychotherapy
   brief p.
   existential p.
   group p.
   personologic p.
   supportive p.
psychotic
   features, p.
   indices, p.
   resolution, p.
psychotogenic
psychotomimetic
psychotonic
psychotropic drugs
psychroalgia
psychroesthesia
psychrophobia
PT (physical therapy)
ptarmic
ptarmus
pterion
pterygoid process
pterygopalatine
ptosis
   abdominal p.
   morning p.
   waking p.
ptotic
puber

puberal
pubertal
pubertas
   praecox, p.
puberty
   precocious p.
pubescence
pubescent
Pudenz reservoir
Pudenz shunt
Pudenz valve
Pudenz-Heyer shunt
Pudenz-Heyer-Schulte valve
puerile
puerilism
puerperal
   convulsion, p.
   psychosis, p.
puerperalism
puffing of cheeks
puka chisel
puka technique
Pulfrich's phenomenon
pulley
pulpified
pulsating electromagnetic field (PEMF)
Pulsavac lavage debridement system
pulse oximetry
pulseless disease
PULSES profile (physical condition,
   upper extremity function, lower
   extremity function, sensory and communication abilities, excretory
   control, social support)
pulsing current
pulvinar
punchdrunk encephalitis
puncture
   Bernard's p.
   cisternal p.
   Corning p.
   cranial p.
   diabetic p.
   intracisternal p.
   Kronecker's p.
   lumbar p.

puncture *(continued)*
   Quincke's p.
   spinal p.
   suboccipital p.
   thecal p.
   transethmoidal p.
   ventricular p.
punitive
pupil size
pupillary reflex
pupillomotor reflex
pupilloplegia
pure tone audiometry
Purkinje cells
Purkinje fibers
Purkinje phenomenon
purposeful movements
purposeless movements
purpura
   thrombocytopenic p.
purpuric
pursuit
   mechanism, p.
   movements, p.
   system, p.
putamen
Putnam type
Putnam-Dana syndrome
Puusepp's operation

Puusepp's reflex
PVS (persistent vegetative state)
pyencephalus
pygmalionism
pyknic
pyknodysostosis
pyknoepilepsy
pyknolepsy
pyknomorphous
pyknophrasia
Pyle's disease
pyocephalus
pyomyositis
pyramid
pyramidal
   cell, p.
   signs, p.
   tract, p.
pyramides (pl. of pyramis)
pyramidotomy
pyramis (pl. pyramides)
pyridoxine
pyrolagnia
pyromania
   erotic p.
pyrophobia
pyruvate carboxylase deficiency
pyruvate dehydrogenase complex deficiency

Additional entries

_____

_____

_____

_____

_____

_____

_____

_____

_____

Additional entries

Q

Q angle
Q disk
QCT (quantitative computed tomography)
Quaalude
quad (quadriceps or quadripod)
   cane, q.
   -setting exercises, q.
quadrangular
   lobe, q.
quadrantanopia
quadrantanopsia
quadrate
   lobule, q.
quadratipronator
quadratus
   femoris muscle, q.
   lumborum muscle, q.
quadriceps
   apron, q.
   femoris muscle, q.
   jerk, q.
   muscle, q.
   reflex, q.
   tendon, q.
   wasting, q.
quadricepsplasty
quadrigeminal
quadrilateral
quadriparesis
quadriparetic
quadriplegia
quadriplegic
   standing frame, q.
quadripod cane

quadruped
quadrupedal extensor
   reflex, q.
qualitative
quality of life
Quant's sign
quantal
quantitated computed tomography (QCT)
quantitative
   neurochemical analysis, q.
quasipurposeful
Quatrefages' angle
Queckenstedt maneuver
Queckenstedt phenomenon
Queckenstedt sign
Queckenstedt test
querulent
querulous
Quervain's disease
Quide
Quincke's disease
Quincke's meningitis
Quincke's puncture
Quine
Quinidex
quinine sulfate
Quinquaud's sign
quotient
   achievement q.
   Ayala's q.
   conceptual q.
   intelligence q.
   rachidian q.
   spinal q.

Additional entries

R

RAB (remote afterloading brachytherapy)
rabbetting
rabbit syndrome
rabid
rabies
   dumb r.
   furious r.
   paralytic r.
raccoon eyes
rachialbuminimeter
rachialbuminimetry
rachialgia
rachianalgesia
rachianesthesia
rachicele
rachicentesis
rachidial
rachidian
rachigraph
rachilysis
rachiocampsis
rachiocentesis
rachiochysis
rachiocyphosis
rachiodynia
rachiokyphosis
rachiometer
rachiomyelitis
rachioparalysis
rachiopathy
rachioplegia
rachioscoliosis
rachiotome
rachiotomy
rachiresistance
rachiresistant
rachis
rachisagra
rachischisis
   paralyticus, r.
   posterior, r.
   totalis, r.
rachisensibility

rachisensible
rachitic
   rosary sign, r.
rachitis
rachitism
rachitogenic
rachitome
rachitomy
racial unconscious
racing heart
racing thoughts
rad (radiation absorbed dose)
radiad
radial
   drift, r.
   nerve, r.
   notch, r.
   palsy, r.
   reflex, r.
radialis
radian
radiathermy
radiatio (pl. radiationes)
radiation
   myelopathy, r.
   therapy, r.
radiationes (pl. of radiatio)
radices (pl. of radix)
radicle
radicotomy
radiculalgia
radicular
   pain, r.
radiculectomy
radiculitis
radiculoganglionitis
radiculomedullary
radiculomeningomyelitis
radiculomyelopathy
radiculoneuritis
radiculoneuropathy
radiculopathy
   cervical r.

radiculopathy *(continued)*
  lumbar r.
  spondylitic caudal r.
radiectomy
radioactive
  brain scan, r.
  iodine (RAI), r.
  iodine scan, r.
  iodine uptake, r.
  tracer, r.
radioactivity
radiocarcinogenesis
radiodense
radiodensity
radioencephalogram (REG)
radioencephalography
radiofrequency
  electrophrenic respiration, r.
  neurotomy, r.
radiogenic
radiogram
radiograph
radiography
radioiodinated seruim albumin (RISA)
radioiodine
radioisotope
  scanning, r.
radiolesion
radiolucency
radiolucent
  density, r.
radiomuscular
radioneuritis
radionuclide
  brain scan, r.
  cisternography, r.
radiopacity
radiopaque
  density, r.
radioparency
radioparent
radiophobia
radiophosphorus
radioprotective
radioresponsive
radiosensitive

radiosurgery
radium
  needle, r.
radix (pl. radices)
Rado theory
Radovici's sign
Raeder's syndrome
rage
raging
ragged red fibers
RAI (radioactive iodine)
  scan, R.
  uptake, R.
railroad nystagmus
railway sickness
railway spine
Raimiste's leg sign
Raimondi scalp hemostatic forceps
Raimondi ventricular catheter
rainbow coverage
RAM (rapid alternating movements)
rami (pl. of ramus)
ramicotomy
Ramirez's shunt
ramisection
ramisectomy
ramitis
ramollissement
ramose
Ramsay Hunt disease
Ramsay Hunt paralysis
Ramsay Hunt syndrome
ramuli (pl. of ramulus)
ramulus (pl. ramuli)
ramus (pl. rami)
random blood sugar
random waves
Raney clip
Raney curette
Raney drill
Raney-Crutchfield tongs
Raney Gigli saw guide
range of motion (ROM)
Rank theory
Ranke's angle
Ranson's pyridine silver stain

Ranvier's crosses
Ranvier's segments
Ranvier's tactile disks
rape
    date r,
    marital r.
    prison r.
    statutory r.
rape counseling
rape-trauma syndrome
raphe
rapid
    alternating movements (RAM), r.
    cycling, r.
    eye movement (REM), r.
rapport
raptus
Rasin's sign
Raskin Depression Scale
raspatory
Rathke's pouch
Rathke's trabeculae
Rathke's tumor
rational
    -emotive therapy, r.
rationale
rationalization
rationalize
rat-tooth forceps
rauwolfia
rave
Raven's Progressive Matrices
raving
Ray's mania
Rayleigh scattering law
Raymond's apoplexy
Raymond-Cestan syndrome
Raynaud's disease
Raynaud's phenomenon
Raynaud's sign
rCBF (regional cerebral blood flow)
rCBV (regional cerebral blood volume)
rCPP (regional cerebral perfusion pressure)
RDI (respiratory disturbance index)
reacher

react
reacting
reaction
    acute situational r.
    acute stress r.
    adjustment r.
    alarm r.
    anamnestic r.
    anaphylactoid r.
    anxiety r.
    associative r.
    Bekhterev's r.
    cadaveric r.
    consensual r.
    conversion r.
    Cushing's r.
    defense r.
    degeneration, r. of
    delayed hypersensitivity r.
    depressive r.
    dissociative r.
    dysergastic r.
    electric r.
    false-negative r.
    false-positive r.
    fight-or-flight r.
    Ghilarducci's r.
    gross stress r.
    hemianopic pupillary r.
    hyperkinetic r. of childhood
    hypersensitivity r.
    involutional psychotic r.
    Jarisch-Herxheimer r.
    Jolly's r.
    lengthening r.
    manic-depressive r.
    Marchi's r.
    myasthenic r.
    myotonic r.
    near-point r.
    Neisser's r.
    neurotonic r.
    Nonne-Apelt r.
    obsessive-compulsive r.
    phobic r.
    psychotic depressive r.

reaction *(continued)*
    reversal r.
    schizophrenic r.
    shortening r.
    startle r.
    stress r.
    sympathetic r.
    stress r.
    tendon r.
    upgrading r.
    Weichbrodt's r.
    Wernicke's r.
reaction-formation
reaction time
reactive
    attachment disorder of infancy, r.
    depression, r.
reactivity
reactology
reading
    lip r.
    speech r.
reading disorders
real-time ultrasonography
reality
    principle, r.
    testing, r.
    therapy, r.
reamer
reaming
rebel
rebellion
rebellious
rebound
    headache, r.
    phenomenon, r.
    phenomenom of Holmes, r.
recall
recent memory
recent recall
receptaculi (pl. of receptaculum)
receptaculum (pl. receptaculi)
receptive
    aphasia, r.
    dysphasia, r.
receptor

recess
recessive
    gene, r.
    trait, r.
recessus
    infundibuli, r.
    lateralis fossae rhomboidei, r.
    lateralis ventriculi quarti, r.
    pinealis, r.
    suprapinealis, r.
    trangularis, r.
recidivation
recidivism
recidivist
recipiomotor
reciprocal inhibition
reciprocal innervation
reciprocation
Recklinghausen's disease
recreational drugs
recreational sex
recruitment
    end organs, r. of
    test, r.
rectal
    alimentation, r.
    anesthesia, r.
    crisis, r.
recti
rectophobia
rectus (recti)
recurrent artery of Heubner
recurrent laryngeal nerve
recurvation
red
    blindness, r.
    infarct, r.
    nucleus, r.
    -out, r.
    reflex, r.
    softening, r.
Redi head halter
redintegration
Redlich-Fisher miliary plaques
red Robinson catheter
Reed-Hodgkin disease

re-education
reel foot
reeling gait
Reese stimulator
referred pain
reflex
   abdominal r.
   abdominocardiac r.
   Achilles tendon r.
   accommodation r.
   acoustic r.
   adductor r.
   after-discharge of r.
   allied r.
   anal r.
   ankle jerk r.
   antagonistic r.
   Aschner's r.
   attention r. of pupil
   attitudinal r.
   audito-oculogyric r.
   auditory r.
   aural r.
   auricle r.
   auriculocervical nerve r.
   autonomic r.
   axon r.
   Babinski's r.
   Babkin r.
   Bekhterev's r.
   Bekhterev-Mendel r.
   biceps r.
   bladder r.
   blink r.
   blink reflex of Descartes r.
   Brain's r.
   brachioradialis r.
   bregmocardiac r.
   Brissaud's r.
   bulbomimic r.
   carotid sinus r.
   cerebral cortex r.
   cat's eye r.
   cerebral cortex r.
   Chaddock's r.
   chain r.

reflex *(continued)*
   chin r.
   chocked r.
   ciliary r.
   ciliospinal r.
   clasp-knife r.
   cochleo-orbicular r.
   cochleopalpebral r.
   cochleopupillary r,
   cochleostapedial r.
   concealed r.
   conditioned r.
   consensual r.
   consensual light r.
   convulsive r.
   coordinated r.
   corneal r.
   corneomandibular r.
   corneopterygoid r.
   corneomental r.
   cough r.
   cranial r.
   cremasteric r.
   crossed r.
   crossed extension r.
   cuboidodigital r.
   cutaneous pupillary r.
   dazzle r.
   deep r.
   deep tendon r.
   defense r.
   delayed r.
   depressor r.
   digital r.
   direct r.
   direct light r.
   diving r.
   doll's eye r.
   dorsal r.
   dorsocuboidal r.
   elbow r.
   elementary r.
   embrace r.
   emergency light r.
   Erben's r.
   erector spinae r.

reflex *(continued)*
- extensor plantar r.
- extensor thrust r.
- eyeball compression r.
- eyelid closure r.
- facial r.
- femoral r.
- finger-thumb r.
- flexion r.
- flexor r.
- flexor plantar r.
- flexor withdrawal r.
- fontanelle r.
- front-tap r.
- fundus r.
- gag r.
- gastrocnemius r.
- Gault's cochleopalpebral r.
- Gifford's r.
- Gifford-Galassi r.
- glabella r.
- gluteal r.
- Gonda r.
- Gordon's r.
- grasp r.
- grasping r.
- Grunfelder's r.
- gustolacrimal r.
- H r.
- Haab's r.
- head retraction r.
- heel-tap r.
- Hering-Breuer r.
- Hirschberg's r.
- Hoffman's r.
- hung-up r.
- inborn r.
- indirect r.
- infraspinatus r.
- inhibition of r.
- interscapular r.
- intersegmental r.
- intrasegmental r.
- inverted radial r.
- iris contraction r.
- ischemic r.

reflex *(continued)*
- jaw r.
- jaw jerk r.
- Joffroy's r.
- Juster r.
- kinetic r.
- knee jerk r.
- Kocher's r.
- labyrinthine r.
- Landau r.
- lid r.
- Liddell and Sherrington r.
- light r.
- lip r.
- local r.
- long r.
- Loven r.
- lumbar r.
- Lust's r.
- Magnus and de Kleijn neck r.
- mandibular r.
- Marinesco-Radovici r.
- mass r.
- Mayer's r.
- maxillary r.
- McCarthy's r.
- McCormac's r.
- Mendel's r.
- Mendel-Bekhterev r.
- monosynaptic r.
- Morley's peritoneocutaneous r.
- Moro r.
- Moro embrace r.
- motor r.
- muscle stretch r.
- muscular r.
- myenteric r.
- myopic r.
- myotatic r.
- nasal r.
- nasolabial r.
- nasomental r.
- near r.
- neck-righting r.
- nociceptive r.
- oculocardiac r.

reflex *(continued)*
  oculocephalogyric r.
  oculopharyngeal r.
  oculopupillary r.
  oculosensory cell r.
  optical righting r.
  opticofacial winking r.
  orbicularis r.
  orbicularis oculi r.
  orbicularis pupillary r.
  palatal r.
  palmar grasp r.
  palm-chin r.
  palmomental r.
  parachute r.
  paradoxical pupillary r.
  patellar r.
  patellar tendon r.
  patelloadductor r.
  pathologic r.
  pectoral r.
  periosteoradial r.
  periosteo-ulnar r.
  pharyngeal r.
  phasic r.
  Philippson's r.
  pilomotor r.
  Piltz's r.
  placing r.
  plantar r.
  plantar grasp r.
  polysynaptic r.
  postural r.
  pressor r.
  Preyer's r.
  proprioceptive r.
  psychic r.
  psychocardiac r.
  psychogalvanic r.
  pulmonocoronary r.
  pupillary r.
  Puusepp's r.
  quadriceps r.
  quadrupedal extensor r.
  radial r.
  red r.

reflex *(continued)*
  regional r.
  Remak's r.
  resistance r.
  retrobulbar pupillary r.
  reversed pupillary r.
  Riddoch's mass r.
  righting r.
  rooting r.
  Rossolimo's r.
  Ruggeri's r.
  Schaffer's r.
  segmental r.
  sexual r.
  short r.
  simple r.
  skin pupillary r.
  sneeze r.
  Snellen's r.
  snout r.
  sole r.
  somatic r.
  spinal r.
  stapedial r.
  startle r.
  static r.
  statokinetic r.
  statotomic r.
  stepping r.
  Stookey r.
  Stransky r.
  stretch r.
  Strumpell's r.
  sucking r.
  superficial r.
  supinator longus r.
  supraorbital r.
  suprapatellar r.
  swallowing r.
  tapetal light r.
  tarsophalangeal r.
  tendon r.
  tendon jerk r.
  threat r.
  Throckmorton's r.
  tibioadductor r.

reflex *(continued)*
  toe r.
  tonic r.
  tonic neck r.
  trained r.
  triceps r.
  triceps surae r.
  trigeminus r.
  ulnar r.
  unconditioned r.
  urinary r.
  uvular r.
  vagus r.
  vasomotor r.
  vasopressor r.
  vertebra prominens r.
  vesicle r.
  vestibular r.
  vestibulo-ocular r.
  visceral r.
  viscerocardiac r.
  visceromotor r.
  viscerosensory r.
  Weiss' r.
  Westphal's pupillary r.
  Westphal-Piltz r.
  withdrawal r.
  wrist clonus r.
  zygomatic r.
reflex act
reflex action
reflex akinesia
reflex arc
reflex center
reflex epilepsy
reflex incontinence
reflex irritability
reflex orgasm
reflex response
reflex therapy
reflexes equal and active
reflexogenic
reflexogenous
reflexograph
reflexology
reflexometer

reflexophil
reflexotherapy
refractory
refractory period
Refsum disease
REG (radioencephalogram)
Regen flexion exercises
regeneration
regional
  cerebral blood flow (rCBF), r.
  cerebral blood volume (rCBV), r.
  cerebral perfusion pressure (rCPP), r.
  reflex, r.
Reglan
regress
regression
  age r.
  atavistic r.
regression neurosis
regression therapy
regressive
  resistive exercise, r.
rehab (rehabilitation)
rehabilitate
rehabilitation
rehabilitee
Reichert/Mundinger (RM) stereotactic
  system
reichian psychology
Reid's base line
Reil's base line
Reil's island
Reil's ribbon
Reil's trigone
reinactment
reinforcement
  reflex, r. of
reinforcer
reinnervation
reintegration
Reitan battery
Reitan Trail Making Test
Reitan-Indiana aphasic screening test
Reitan-Klove Auditory-Perceptual Test
Reitan-Klove Lateral Dominance Test
rejection

relate to
related paraphasia
relaxant
relaxation
  general r.
  isometric r.
  local r.
relaxation response
relaxed movement
release phenomenon
REM (rapid eye movement)
  density, R.
  latency, R.
  rebound, R.
  sleep, R.
Remak's axis cylinder
Remak's band
Remak's fibers
Remak's axis cylinder
Remak's band
Remak's fibers
Remak's ganglion
Remak's paralysis
Remak's reflex
Remak's sign
Remak's symptom
Remak's type
remodeling
remote
  afterloading brachytherapy (RAB), r.
  memory, r.
  recall, r.
remotivate
remotivation
Renaut's bodies
Rendu's tremor
Rendu-Osler-Weber disease
renifleur
reovirus
repertoire
repetition of digits
Repoise
repressed
repression
repressive
Repro head halter

reserpine
reservoir
  Ommaya r.
  Pecquet r.
  Pudenz r.
  Rickham r.
  Rickham-Salmon r.
residua
residual
  hemiparesis, r.
  schizophrenia, r.
resistance
  reflex, r.
resistive
  exercises, r.
resolution
respiratory
  arrest, r.
  center, r.
  disturbance index (RDI), r.
  embarrassment, r.
  myoclonus, r.
response
rest cure
restibrachium
restiform
  body, r.
resting
  membrane potential, r.
  hand splint, r.
  pan splint, r.
  size of pupils, r.
  tremor, r.
restitution
restless legs syndrome
restlessness
Restoril
restrained
restraint
retardate
retardation
  growth r.
  mental r.
  psychomotor r.
retarded
rete

rete *(continued)*
   canalis hypoglossi, r.
retention sutures
reticular
   activating system, r.
   formation, r.
reticulate substance
reticulation
reticuloendothelial
   system, r.
reticulospinal
reticulovestibular
   pathway, r.
reticulum cell sarcoma
retiform
retina
retinal commotio
retinal correspondence
retinitis
   pigmentosa, r.
retinoblastoma-mental retardation syndrome
retinopathy
retinoschisis
retinotopic
retreat
retrieval
retrobulbar
   neuritis, r.
retrocochlear
retrocollic
retrocollis
retrocrural
retrocursive
retrodeviation
retroflex
retroflexed
retrogasserian
   neurotomy, r.
retrograde
   amnesia, r.
retrography
retrogress
retrogression
retrolisthesis
retropulsion

retrospect
retrospective
   falsification, r.
retrospondylolisthesis
Rett syndrome
Retzius' foramen
reversal
   digits, r. of
   lumbar curve, r. of
   sex, r. of
   reaction, r.
reverse angle Epstein curette
reversible ischemic neurologic deficit
   (RIND)
Revilliod's sign
revulsion
Rexed's laminae
Rey Auditory Verbal Learning Test
Rey and Taylor Complex Figure Test
Reye's syndrome
rhabdium
rhabdomyoblastoma
rhabdomyochondroma
rhabdomyolysis
   exertional r.
rhabdomyoma
rhabdomyomyxoma
rhabdomyosarcoma
rhabdophobia
rhabdosarcoma
rhabdovirus
rhachialgia
rhachioplegia
rhachioscoliosis
rhachischisis
rhachitis
rhachotomy
rhaebocrania
rhaeboscelia
rhaebosis
rheobase
rheobasic
rheonome
rheotachygraphy
rheumatalgia
rheumatic

rheumatic *(continued)*
   fever, r.
   heart disease, r.
rheumatism
rheumatoid
   arthritis, r.
   factor, r.
rheumatologist
rheumatology
rhexis
rhigosis
rhinalgia
rhinencephalon
rhinesthesia
rhinion
rhinodynia
rhinolalia
rhinorrhea
   cerebrospinal r.
rhizolysis
rhizomelic
   spondylitis, r.
   spondylosis, r.
rhizomeningomyelitis
rhizoneure
rhizotomy
   anterior r.
   dorsal r.
   posterior r.
   retrogasserian r.
rhombencephalography
rhombocoele
rhomboid
   Michaelis' r.
rhomboid fossa
rhomboid muscle
rhomboideus
rhombomere
rhotacism
Rhoton punch
Rhoton titanium microsurgical forceps
rhypophobia
rhythm
   alpha r.
   Berger r.
   beta r.

rhythm *(continued)*
   biological r.
   circadian r.
   circus r.
   delta r.
   diurnal r.
   gamma r.
   infradian r.
   nyctohemeral r.
   theta r.
   ultradian r.
rhythmical
rhythmicity
ribbon muscle
Ribes' ganglion
ribonucleic acid (RNA)
Richards-Rundle syndrome
richitism
Richmond bolt
rickets
rickettsial
rickettsialpox
Rickham intraventricular reservoir system
Rickham-Salmon reservoir
riders' bone
riders' sprain
Riddoch's mass reflex
ridge
riding the ventilator
Rieger's phenomenon
Rieger's syndrome
right-handed
right-handedness
right-left confusion
righting reflex
rigid
rigidity
   cerebellar r.
   clasp-knife r.
   cogwheel r.
   decerebrate r.
   hemiplegic r.
   lead-pipe r.
   mydriatic r.
   nuchal r.
   paratonic r.

rigidity *(continued)*
    spastic r.
rigor
    heat r.
    nervorum, r.
    tremens, r.
    water r.
Riley-Day syndrome
Riley-Smith syndrome
Rimbaud-Passouant-Vallat syndrome
rimula
RIND (reversible ischemic neurologic
    deficit)
ring-enhancing lesion
ring fracture
Ringer's lactate
Rinne test
Riolan's bouquet
Riolan's nosegay
ripa
Ripault's sign
RISA (radio-iodinated serum albumin)
risk behavior
risk factor
risky sex
Risser jacket
Risser localizer cast
risus
    caninus, r.
    sardonicus, r.
Ritalin
Ritter-Rollet phenomenon
Ritter-Rollet sign
Ritter-Valli law
ritual
    abuse, r.
    act, r.
    behavior, r.
    sacrifice, r.
ritualistic
    surgery, r.
rivalry strife
river blindness
Riviere's sign
RM (Reichert/Mundinger) stereotactic
    system

RNA (ribonucleic acid)
Robertson's pupil
Robertson's sign
Robertson's technique
Robin's syndrome
Robin's anomalad
Robinow's syndrome
Robinson cervical spine fusion
Robinson-Keppler test
Robinson-Riley cervical arthrodesis
Robinul
Robotrac passive retraction system
Rochester connector
Rochester elevator
rocker knife
rocking
Rocky Mountain spotted fever
rod
    cells, r.
    fixation, r.
rodding
Roger's symptom
Rogers cervical fusion
Rogers theory
Rokitansky-Cushing ulcers
rolandic
    epilepsy, r.
    fissure, r.
    vein syndrome, r.
Rolando's angle
Rolando's area
Rolando's cells
Rolando's gelatinous substance
Rolando's line
Rolando's zone
rolandometer
role
    model, r.
    playing, r.
    reversal, r.
rolfing
ROM (range of motion)
Romana's sign
Romano-Ward syndrome
Romberg's disease
Romberg's position

Romberg's sign
Romberg's spasm
Romberg's station
Romberg's test
rombergism
Rommelaere's sign
rongeur
rongeured
roof
    disk, r.
    nucleus, r.
    skull, r. of
    plate, r.
Roos procedure
root
    anterior r.
    dorsal r.
    motor r.
    nerve r.
    posterior r.
    sensory r.
    spinal r.
    ventral r.
root canal
root compression
root compression sign
root field
root pain
root signs
root sleeve
root zone
rooting reflex
rootlet
rope sign
Rorschach test
rosary
rachitic
Rose position
Rose's tetanus
Rosenbach's sign
Rosenthal's canal
Rosenthal's fibers
Rosenthal's vein
Roser's sign
Roser-Braun sign
rosette

Rosomoff cordotomy
Rossolimo's reflex
Rossolimo's sign
rostra (pl. of rostrum)
rostrad
rostral
    displacement, r.
    lamina, r.
rostralis
rostrally
rostrum (pl. rostra)
    corpus callosum, r. of
rosulate
rotary nystagmus
rotating tourniquet
rotatory
    spasm, r.
rotexed
rotexion
Rot's disease
Rot's syndrome
Rot-Bernhardt disease
Rot-Bernhardt syndrome
Roth's disease
Roth's spots
Roth's syndrome
Roth-Bernhardt disease
Roth-Bernhardt syndrome
Rothmund-Thomson syndrome
Roto-Kinetic bed
Roto-Rest bed
Rotter's Incomplete Sentence Test
Roussy-Cornil syndrome
Roussy-Dejerine syndrome
Roussy-Levy syndrome
Roven's IMDC (intramedullary metatar-
    sal decompression)
Roxanol
Royal Free disease
Royalite body jacket
rubella
Rubinstein's syndrome
Rubinstein-Taybi syndrome
rubor
rubrospinal
rubrothalamic

rucksack paralysis
Rud's syndrome
Ruffini's brushes
Ruffini's corpuscles
Ruggeri's reflex
rugine
rule
    dermatomal r.
    Jackson's r.
    nines, r. of
    Pitres, r. of
rum fits
ruminate
rumination
ruminative
Rumpf's sign

runner's high
running fit
running taxon
rupophobia
ruptured disk
rush
Rush driver-bender-extractor
Rush rod
Ruskin forceps
Russell dwarf
Russell's syndrome
Rust's disease
Rust's phenomenon
Rust's syndrome
rut-formation
Rye histopathologic classification

Additional entries

_____

_____

_____

_____

_____

_____

_____

_____

_____

_____

_____

_____

_____

_____

_____

_____

_____

S

Sabbat
Sabin vaccine
Sabin-Feldman syndrome
Sabolich foot
Sabouraud
    agar
saccade
saccadic
    following movements, s.
    pursuit, s.
    slowing, s.
saccaropinuria
saccular aneurysm
SACH heel
Sachs disease
Sachs exploring cannula
Sachs guard
Sachs needle
Sachs nerve separator
Sachs nerve spatula
Sachs tissue forceps
Sachs vein retractor
sacra
sacrad
sacral
    agenesis, s.
    anesthesia, s.
    block, s.
    bone, s.
    canal, s.
    dimple, s.
    edema, s.
    flexure, s.
    index, s.
    myotome, s.
    nerve, s.
    plexus, s.
    prominence, s.
    sparing, s.
    spinal cord, s.
    spine, s.
    vertebra, s.
sacralgia

sacralization
sacralize
sacralized transverse process
sacrarthrogenic
sacrectomy
sacroanterior
sacrococcygeal
sacrococcyx
sacrocoxalgia
sacrocoxitis
sacrodynia
Sacro-Eze lumbar support
sacroiliac (SI)
    joint (SIJ), s.
    notch, s.
    strain, s.
sacroiliitis
sacrolisthesis
sacrolithesis
sacrolumbar
    angle, s.
sacroposterior
sacropromontory
sacrosciatic
sacrospinal
sacrospinalis
sacrospinous
sacrotomy
sacrotransverse
sacrovertebral
    angle, s.
sacrum
    assimilation s.
    tilted s.
SAD (seasonal affective disorder)
sad
saddle anesthesia
saddle area
saddle back
saddle block
sadism
    anal s.
    oral s.

sadist
sadistic
sadness
sadomasochism
sadomasochist
sadomasochistic
SAE (subcortical atherosclerotic encephalopathy)
Saenger's sign
Saethre-Chotzen syndrome
safe sex
sagittal
  fontanelle, s.
  plane, s.
  roll spondylolisthesis, s.
  sinus, s.
  suture, s.
  synostosis, s.
sagittalis
SAH (subarachnoid hemorrhage)
Saint Vitus' dance
Sakati-Nyhan syndrome
salaam
  activity, s.
  convulsions, s.
  spasm, s.
salacious
Salibi clamp
salivate
salivation
Salk vaccine
salt-losing syndrome
saltation
saltatorial
saltatory
  conduction, s.
  spasm, s.
sand
  bodies, s.
  tray therapy, s.
sandbag
sandbagging
Sandhoff's disease
sane
Sanfillipo's syndrome
Sanger-Brown ataxia

sanity
Sansert
Sanson's images
Santavuori's disease
sapphism
Sarbo's sign
sarcoglia
sarcoid
sarcoidosis
sarcolemma
sarcoma
sarcoplasm
sarcoplast
sarcopoietic
sarcosinemia
sarcostyle
sardonic
  laugh, s.
  smile, s.
sartorius muscle
SAS (sleep apnea syndrome)
satanic cult
satanism
satanist
satellite lesion
satellitosis
Sattler veil
Saturday night arm
Saturday night palsy
Saturday night paralysis
saturnine gout
satyr
satyriasis
satyromania
saucer
saucerization
Saunders' sign
saw
sawtooth wave
Sayre's jacket
SBE (subacute bacterial endocarditis)
SBO (spina bifida occulta)
SBRN (sensory branch of radial nerve)
scabiphobia
scaleniotomy
scalenotomy

scalenus anticus syndrome
scalloping of vertebrae
scalp
  clip, s.
  electrode, s.
  flap, s.
  -recorded somatosensory evoked po-
    tential, s.
  retractor, s.
  tourniquet, s.
scamping speech
scan
scanning
  radioisotope s.
scanning speech
scanogram
scanography
scapegoating
scaphion
scaphocephaly
scaphohydrocephalus
scapula
  alar s.
  elevated s.
  Graves' s.
  scaphoid s.
  winged s.
scapular
  reflex, s.
scapulohumcral
  reflex, s.
scapuloperoneal syndrome
scapulovertebral
scar
  formation, s.
  revision, s.
  tissue, s.
Scarpa's nerve
Scarpa's triangle
scarred
  down, s.
  over, s.
scarring
scatology
SCD (subacute combined degeneration of
  spinal cord)

scelalgia
scelotyrbe
Schacher's ganglion
Schaefer's sign
Schafer's syndrome
Schaffer's reflex
Schanz collar
Schanz's syndrome
Schedule for Affective Disorders and
  Schizophrenia
Scheibe's deafness
Scheie's syndrome
Schepelmann's sign
Scheuermann's disease
Scheuermann's juvenile kyphosis
Schiefferdecker's disk
Schilder's disease
Schilder's encephalitis
Schilling test
schistasis
schistocephalus
schistoprosopia
schistorachia
schizaxon
schizencephalic
schizencephaly
schizoaffective
  schizophrenia, s.
schizogyria
schizoid
  personality disorder, s.
schizoidism
schizokinesis
schizophasia
schizophrenia
  acute s.
  ambulatory s.
  borderline s.
  catatonic s.
  childhood s.
  disorganized s.
  hebephrenic s.
  latent s.
  nuclear s.
  paranoid s.
  paraphrenic s.

schizophrenia *(continued)*
  prepsychotic s.
  process s.
  pseudoneurotic s.
  pseudopsychopathic s.
  reactive s.
  residual s.
  schizoaffective s.
  simple s.
  undifferentiated s.
schizophreniac
schizophrenic
schizophreniform
schizophrenosis
schizoprosopia
schizothymia
schizotonia
schizotrypanosomiasis
schizotypal
Schlesinger cervical rongeur
Schlesinger forceps
Schlesinger sign
Schlesinger's solution
Schlosser's treatment
Schmidt's syndrome
Schmidt-Lanterman incisures
Schmidt-Lanterman segment
Schmorl's body
Schmorl's disease
Schmorl's nodule
schnauzkrampf
Schober test
Scholz's disease
Schon's theory
Schonlein's purpura
school phobia
Schoser's treatment
Schramm's phenomenon
Schreiber's maneuver
Schroeder van der Kolk's law
Schrotter's chorea
Schuller's disease
Schuller's phenomenon
Schuller's syndrome
Schuller-Christian disease
Schuller-Christian syndrome

Schultze's acroparesthesia
Schultze's bundle
Schultze's sign
Schultze's tract
Schultze's type
Schultze-Chvostek sign
Schutz clip
Schutz forceps
Schwabach test
Schwalbe's corpuscles
Schwalbe's fissure
Schwalbe's foramen
Schwalbe's nucleus
Schwalbe's space
Schwann cell
Schwann membrane
Schwann nucleus
Schwann's substance
Schwann tumor
schwannitis
schwannoglioma
schwannoma
schwannosis
Schwartz clip
Schwartz-Jampel syndrome
sciatic
  hernia, s.
  nerve, s.
  notch, s.
  scoliosis, s.
  spine, s.
  stretch, s.
sciatica
scintigraphy
scintillating
scotoma
scintillation
scintiphotograph
scintiphotography
scintiscan
scissor leg
scissoring gait
scissors gait
scissors walking
sclerencephaly
scleroderma

sclerodermatomyositis
scleromeninx
scleromere
sclerosis
    Alzheimer's s.
    amyotrophic lateral s.
    annular s.
    anterolateral s.
    arterial s.
    arteriolar s.
    arteriopapillary s.
    benign s.
    bone s.
    bulbar s.
    cerebellar s.
    cerebral s.
    cerebrospinal s.
    cervical s.
    circumscripta pericardii, s.
    combined s.
    diffuse s.
    disseminated s.
    Erb's s.
    familial centrolobar s.
    focal s.
    hyperplastic s.
    insular s.
    Krabbe's s.
    lateral s.
    lobar s.
    Marie's s.
    mesial temporal s.
    miliary s.
    Monckeberg's s.
    multiple s.
    nodular s.
    Pelizaeus-Merzbacher s.
    posterior spinal s.
    posterolateral s.
    presenile s.
    primary lateral s.
    progressive systemic s.
    redux, s.
    renal arteriolar s.
    systemic s.
    transitional s.

sclerosis *(continued)*
    tuberosa, s.
    tuberous s.
    unicellular s.
    vascular s.
    ventrolateral s.
scleroskeleton
sclerostenosis
sclerotic
sclerotome
scoliokyphosis
scoliorachitic
scoliosis
    Brissaud's s.
    cicatricial s.
    congenital s.
    coxitic s.
    empyematic s.
    habit s.
    inflammatory s.
    ischiatic s.
    myopathic s.
    ocular s.
    ophthalmic s.
    osteopathic s.
    paralytic s.
    rachitic s.
    rheumatic s.
    sciatic s.
    static s.
scoliosis operating frame
scoliosometer
scoliosometry
scoliotic
scoliotone
scolopsia
scombroid poisoning
scopolagnia
scopolamine
scopophilia
scopophobia
scopophobiac
scordinema
scotodinia
scotoma (pl. scotomata)
    absolute s.

scotoma (pl. scotomata) *(continued)*
   annular s.
   arcuate s.
   aural s.
   Bjerrum's s.
   cecocentral s.
   central s.
   centrocecal s.
   color s.
   eclipse s.
   flittering s.
   hemianopic s.
   mental s.
   motile s.
   negative s.
   paracentral s.
   peripapillary s.
   peripheral s.
   physiologic s.
   positive s.
   relative s.
   ring s.
   scintillating s.
   Seidel's s.
scotomagraph
scotomata (pl. of scotoma)
scotomatous
scotometer
scotometry
scotomization
scotophilia
scotophobia
scotopia
scotopic vision
Scott cannula
scout film
scout view
Scoville clip
Scoville forceps
Scoville hemilaminectomy retractor
Scoville self-retaining retractor
Scoville-Lewis clip
scrapie
scraping toe
scream therapy
screatus

scribomania
scrim (speech/auditory discrimination)
scrotal reflex
scrub typhus
scruple
scrupulosity
scrupulous
scythropasmus
SDL (skills of daily living)
SE (spin echo)
sea blue histiocyte syndrome
sea fronds
Seabright bantam syndrome
seance
searching gaze
Seashore's Test
seasonal affective disorder (SAD)
seasonal depression
Seattle foot
sebastomania
Sechenoff's center
Sechenow's center
Seckel dwarf
Seckel syndrome
seclusion
secobarbital
second cranial nerve
second sight
second-person hallucinations
secretomotor
sectio (pl. sectiones)
sectiones (pl. of sectio)
sed (sedimentation) rate
sedate
sedated
sedation
sedative
sedentary
   lifestyle, s.
seeding
seeing double
seeing-eye dog
Seeligmuller's sign
Seessel's pouch
see-saw nystagmus
SEG (sonoencephalogram)

Seglas type
segment
segmenta (pl. of segmentum)
segmental
   reflex, s.
   static reaction, s.
segmentary syndrome
segmentation
segmentum (pl. segmenta)
Seguin's sign
Seguin's signal symptom
Seidel's scotoma
Seidel's sign
seisesthesia
seismesthesia
Seitelberger's disease
seize
seizure
   absence s.
   akinetic s.
   atonic s.
   audiogenic s.
   cerebral s.
   clonic s.
   febrile s.
   grand mal s.
   jackknife s.
   myoclonic s.
   neonatal s.
   partial s.
   petit mal s.
   photogenic s.
   psychic s.
   psychomotor s.
   tonic s.
   tonic/clonic s.
   tonoclonic s.
   uncinate s.
seizure activity
seizure precautions
sejunction
selective attention effect
selegine hydrochloride
selenoplegia
selenoplexia
Seletz ventricular cannula

self
   -abuse, s.
   -acceptance, s.
   -actualization, s.
   -affirmation, s.
   -alienated, s.
   -awareness, s.
   -centered, s.
   -confidence, s.
   -conscious, s.
   -criticism, s.
   -defeating, s.
   -deprecation, s.
   -destruction, s.
   -destructive, s.
   -determination, s.
   -directedness, s.
   -dramatization, s.
   -effacing, s.
   -esteem, s.
   -expression, s.
   -fulfillment, s.
   -hatred, s.
   -hypnosis, s.
   -identity, s.
   -image, s.
   -inventory, s.
   -medication, s.
   -mutilation, s.
   -realization, s.
   -reproach, s.
   -suggestion, s.
   -suspension, s.
   -transcendence, s.
selfish
selfishness
sella (pl. sellae)
   turcica, s.
sellae (pl. of sella)
sellar
Seller's stain
Sellick maneuver
Selter's disease
Selverstone clamp
Selye syndrome
semicoma

semicomatose
semicretinism
semidecussation
semiflexion
semilunar lobe
semiluxation
seminarcosis
seminoma
semiotic function
semiplegia
semipronation
semiprone
semirecumbent
semisideratio
semisomnus
semisopor
semispinalis muscle
semisupination
semisupine
semitendinosus
Semliki Forest encephalitis
Semon's law
Semon-Rosenbach law
senescence
senescent
senile
    chorea, s.
    dementia, s.
    gait, s.
    plaques, s.
    tremor, s.
senilism
senility
    premature s.
    psychosis of s.
senium
Senn operation
Senn retractor
Senn small rake retractor
Senn-Dingman retractor
sensate focus exercises
sensation
    altered s.
    burning s.
    catching s.
    cincture s.

sensation *(continued)*
    common s.
    concomitant s.
    cutaneous s.
    delayed s.
    dermal s.
    diminished s.
    epigastric s.
    external s.
    general s.
    girdle s.
    gnostic s.
    internal s.
    light touch s.
    negative s.
    new s.
    objective s.
    palmesthetic s.
    phantom s.
    pinprick s.
    prickling s.
    primary s.
    proprioceptive s.
    referred s.
    reflex s.
    skin s.
    somesthetic s.
    strain s.
    subjective s.
    tactile s.
    tingling s.
    touch s.
    transferred s.
    vibration s.
    warmth, s. of
sensation level
sense
    color s.
    equilibrium s.
    internal s.
    kinesthetic s.
    labyrinthine s.
    light s.
    muscle s.
    posture s.
    pressure s.

sense *(continued)*
   proprioception s.
   proprioceptive s.
   seventh s.
   sixth s.
   space s.
   special s.
   static s.
   stereognostic s.
   temperature s.
   time s.
   tone s.
   visceral s.
sensibility
   bone s.
   common s.
   cortical s.
   deep s.
   electromuscular s.
   epicritic s.
   joint s.
   mesoblastic s.
   pallesthetic s.
   palmesthetic s.
   proprioceptive s.
   protopathic s.
   recurrent s.
   somesthetic s.
   splanchnesthetic s.
   vibratory s.
sensibilization
sensible
sensiferous
sensigenous
sensimeter
sensitive
sensitivity
   training, s.
sensomobile
sensomobility
sensor
   deprivation syndrome, s.
sensorial
sensoriglandular
sensorimetabolism
sensorimotor

sensorimotor *(continued)*
   skills, s.
sensorimuscular
sensorineural
sensorium
sensorivascular
sensorivasomotor
sensory
   abnormality, s.
   afferent system, s.
   amusia, s.
   aphasia, s.
   area, s.
   ataxia, s.
   awareness, s.
   changes, s.
   channel, s.
   deficit, s.
   deprivation, s.
   ending, s.
   epilepsy, s.
   evoked potential (SEP), s.
   evoked response (SER), s.
   ganglion, s.
   integration, s.
   level, s.
   loss, s.
   nerve, s.
   nerve action potential (SNAP), s.
   organ, s.
   pathways, s.
   radicular neuropathy, s.
   receptor, s.
   register, s.
   root, s.
   unit, s.
sensual
sensualism
sensuous
sentence completion test
sentience
sentient
sentiment
sentimental
SEP (sensory OR somatosensory evoked
   potential)

separation
  anxiety, s.
separator
septa (pl. of septum)
septic shock
septineuritis
septum (pl. septa)
  pellucidum, s.
  pontis, s.
sequester
sequestered disk
SER (sensory OR somatosensory evoked
  response)
Serentil
serial
  sevens, s.
  threes, s.
serially intact
Sernyl
serotonin
serotoninergic
Serres' angle
serum neuritis
Servo pump
set
Set test
Setchenow's centers
setting-sun sign
seventh cranial nerve
seventh sense
Sewall forceps
sex
  addict, s.
  assignment, s.
  change, s.
  chromosomes, s.
  clinic, s.
  -conditioned, s.
  determination, s.
  differentiation, s.
  education, s.
  incidence, s.
  limitation, s.
  -limited, s.
  -linked recessive trait, s.
  reassignment, s.

sex *(continued)*
  reversal, s.
  role, s.
  steroids, s.
  surrogate, s.
  technique, s.
  therapist, s.
  therapy, s.
sexology
sexopathy
sexual
  abstinence, s.
  abuse, s.
  adaptation, s.
  arousal, s.
  aversion, s.
  behavior, s.
  deviant, s.
  deviation, s.
  dysfunction, s.
  erethism, s.
  exhibitionism, s.
  function, s.
  gratification, s.
  identity, s.
  impotence, s.
  intercourse, s.
  masochism, s.
  orientation, s.
  perversion, s.
  pervert, s.
  promiscuity, s.
  psychopathy, s.
  reassignment, s.
  reflex, s.
  sadism, s.
  torment, s.
sexuality
sexualization
sexually
  active, s.
  dysfunctional, s.
  functional, s.
  inactive, s.
  promiscuous, s.
SF (spinal fluid)

SFEMG (single-fiber electromyography)
SFP (spinal fluid pressure)
SGOT (serum glutamic oxaloacetic trans-
  aminase)
shaggy
Shagreen patch
shaken baby syndrome
shakes
shaking palsy
shallow affect
shallowing of nasolabial fold
sham-movement vertigo
sham rage
shaman
shamanism
shame
shame-based
shameful
shameless
shaping
shared paranoid disorder
sharp waves
Sharpoint microsurgical knife
Shaw scalpel
shawl-like
sheath of Schwann
Sheehan Clinician Rated Anxiety Scale
Sheehan Panic and Anticipatory Anxiety
  Scale
Sheehan Phobia Scale
Sheehy syndrome
sheet sign
Sheldon retractor
Sheldon theory
Sheldon-Pudenz procedure
Sheldon-Pudenz retractor
shell shock
shepherd's crook deformity
Sherrington's law
Sherrington's phenomenon
shifting asymmetry
shingles
shinsplints
Shipley Abstraction Test
Shipley Institute of Living Scale
shiver

shock
  allergic anaphylactic s.
  anaphylactoid s.
  anesthesia s.
  cardiogenic s.
  deferred s.
  electric s.
  endotoxin s.
  epigastric s.
  hemorrhagic s.
  hypoglycemic s.
  hypovolemic s.
  insulin s.
  mental s.
  neurogenic s.
  oligemic s.
  peptone s.
  psychic s.
  secondary s.
  septic s.
  serum s.
  shell s.
  spinal s.
  surgical s.
  toxic s.
  traumatic s.
shock blocks
shock position
shock therapy
shock treatment
shocky
shoemakers' cramp
short wave diathermy (SWD)
shoulder
  girdle, s.
  -hand syndrome, s.
  nerve root, s. of
  shrug, s.
shudder
shuffle gait
shuffling gait
shunt
  Holter s.
  Javid s.
  Pudenz s.
  Ramirez s.

shunt *(continued)*
   Silastic ventriculoperitoneal s.
   subarachnoid s.
   ventriculoatrial s.
   ventriculocisternal s.
   ventriculoperitoneal s.
   ventriculovenous s.
shunted
shunting
shuttlemaker's disease
Shy-Drager syndrome
SI (sacroiliac)
   joint, S.
Sia test
SIADH (syndrome of inappropriate antidiuretic hormone)
sialidosis
sib
sibline
sibling
   rivalry, s.
sibship
Sicard's syndrome
sicca syndrome
sickle cell
   crisis, s.
   disease, s.
   trait, s.
sicklemia
sickling
SIDS (sudden infant death syndrome)
Siegert's sign
sighing respirations
sight
sighted
sigma
   rhythm, s.
   spindle, s.
sigmatism
sign
   Abadie's s.
   Amoss' s.
   Andre-Thomas s.
   Anghelescu's s.
   ankle clonus s.
   anterior tibial s.

sign *(continued)*
   Argyll Robertson pupil s.
   Aschner's s.
   Babinski's s.
   Babinski's platysma s.
   Babinski's pronation s.
   Babinski's toe s.
   Baillarger's s.
   Ballet's s.
   Bamberger's s.
   Barany's s.
   Bard's s.
   Barre's s.
   Barre's pyramidal s.
   Bastian-Bruns s.
   Battle's s.
   Becker's s.
   Beevor's s.
   Bekhterev's s.
   Bell's s.
   Berger's s.
   Biernacki's s.
   Binda's s.
   Bjerrum's s.
   Blumberg's s.
   Bonnet's s.
   Bordier-Frankel s.
   Boston's s.
   Bragard's s.
   Brickner's s.
   Brudzinski's s.
   Cantelli's s.
   Capps' s.
   Carnett's s.
   Chaddock's toe s.
   Chaddock's wrist s.
   Charcot's s.
   chin-retraction s.
   Chvostek's s.
   Chvostek-Weiss s.
   Claude's hyperkinesis s.
   Codman's s.
   cogwheel s.
   complementary opposition s.
   contralateral s.
   Coopernail s.

sign *(continued)*
    coughing s.
    Cowen's s.
    Crichton-Browne's s.
    Dalrymple's s.
    Dejerine's s.
    de la Camp's s.
    Demianoff's s.
    de Musset's s.
    d'Espine's s.
    Dixon Mann's s.
    doll's eye s.
    DTP (distal tingling on percussion) s.
    Duckworth's
    echo s.
    Elliot's s.
    Ely's s.
    Enroth's s.
    Erb's s.
    Erben's s.
    Erichsen's s.
    Escherich's s.
    fabere s.
    Fajersztajn's crossed sciatic s.
    fan s.
    forced grasping s.
    forearm s.
    formication s.
    Frankel's s.
    Froment's paper s.
    Gaenslen's s.
    Galeazzi s.
    Gifford's s.
    Goggia's s.
    Goldstein's s.
    Goldthwait's s.
    Gordon's finger s.
    Gordon's leg s.
    Gottron's s.
    Gowers' s.
    Graefe's s.
    Grasset's s.
    Grasset-Bychowski s.
    Grasset-Gaussel-Hoover s.
    Griffith's s.
    Guilland's s.

sign *(continued)*
    Gunn's s.
    Gunn's pupillary s.
    Hahn's s.
    halo s.
    harlequin s.
    Heilbronner's s.
    Helbing's s.
    Hennebert's s.
    Hirschberg's s.
    Hoffmann's s.
    Holmes' s.
    Homans s.
    Hoover's s.
    Horsley's s.
    Howship-Romberg s.
    Hoyne's s.
    Hueter's s.
    Human's s.
    Huntington's s.
    Hutchinson's s.
    hyperkinesis s.
    impostor s.
    interossei s.
    Itard-Cholewa s.
    Jellinek's s.
    Joffroy's s.
    jugular s.
    Kanavel's s.
    Kashida's s.
    Kerandel's s.
    Kernig's s.
    Kerr's s.
    Kestenbaum's s.
    Kleist's hooking s.
    Klippel-Feil s.
    Knie's s.
    Kocher's s.
    Koranyi's s.
    Lafora's s.
    Lasegue's s.
    leg s.
    Leichtenstern's s.
    Leri's s.
    Leudet's s.
    Lhermitte's s.

sign *(continued)*
    Lichtheim's s.
    Linder's s.
    Livierato's s.
    long tract s.
    Lombardi's s.
    Lust's s.
    Macewen's s.
    Magendie's s.
    Magendie-Hertwig s.
    Magnan's s.
    Mann's s.
    Mannkopf's s.
    Marcus Gunn's pupillary s.
    Marie's s.
    Marie-Foix retraction s.
    Marinesco's s.
    Mayer's s.
    Mayo's s.
    McCarthy's s.
    Means' s.
    Mendel-Bekhterev s.
    Mennell's s.
    Minor's s.
    Mobius' s.
    Moebius' s.
    Morquio's s.
    Munson's s.
    Myerson's s.
    neck s.
    Neri's s.
    Nothnagel's s.
    omega s.
    Oppenheim's s.
    Ortolani's s.
    Parrot's s.
    patellar clonus s.
    Patrick's s.
    Pende's s.
    peroneal s.
    Piltz's s.
    Piotrowski's s.
    Plummer's s.
    pneumatic s.
    Pool-Schlesinger s.
    Pottenger's s.

sign *(continued)*
    Prevost's s.
    pronation s.
    pseudo-Babinski's s.
    pseudo-Graefe's s.
    pyramid s.
    Quant's s.
    Queckenstedt's s.
    Quinquaud's s.
    Radovici's s.
    Raimiste's leg s.
    Rasin's s.
    Raynaud's s.
    Remak's s.
    Revilliod's s.
    Ritter-Rollet s.
    Rivier's s.
    Robertson's s.
    Romana's s.
    Romberg's s.
    Rommelaere's s.
    rope s.
    Rosenbach's s.
    Roser's s.
    Roser-Braun s.
    Rossolimo's s.
    Rumpf's s.
    Saenger's s.
    Sarbo's s.
    Saunders' s.
    Schaefer's s.
    Schepelmann's s.
    Schlesinger's s.
    Schultze's s.
    Schultze-Chvostek s.
    Seeligmuller's s.
    Seguin's s.
    Seidel's s.
    setting-sun s.
    Siegert's s.
    Signorelli's s.
    Simon's s.
    Snellen's s.
    Soto-Hall s.
    Souques' s.
    spinal s.

sign *(continued)*
   spine s.
   Squire's s.
   stairs s.
   Stellwag's s.
   Sterlings's s.
   Stewart-Holmes s.
   Strumpell's s.
   Suker's s.
   swinging flashlight s.
   Theimich's lip s.
   thermic s.
   Thomas' s.
   tibialis s.
   Tinel's s.
   Tournay's s.
   trepidation s.
   Tromner's s.
   Trousseau's s.
   Turyn's s.
   Uhthoff's s.
   Vanzetti's s.
   Vedder's s.
   von Graefe's s.
   Wartenberg's s.
   Weber's s.
   Weiss' s.
   Wernicke's s.
   Westphal's s.
   Widowitz's s.
   Wilder's s.
sign language
signal
   branch, s.
   symptom, s.
significant other
signing
Signorelli's sign
SIJ (sacroiliac joint)
Silastic block
Silastic bur hole cap
Silberer phenomenon
silent myocardial infarction
silent period
Silex's sign
siliqua

siliqua *(continued)*
   olivae, s.
silver clip
Silverskiold's syndrome
Silver's syndrome
simesthesia
simian
   crease, s.
   line, s.
   T-virus (STV), s.
Simmerlin type
Simmerlin's dystrophy
Simmonds' syndrome
Simmons cervical spine fusion
Simon's sign
simple reflex
simultanagnosia
sincipital
sinciput
Sinemet
Sinequan
Singer-Blom valve
single photon emission computed tomography (SPECT)
single-fiber electromyography (SFEMG)
singultation
singultous
singultus
sinister
sinistrad
sinistral
sinistrality
sinistraural
sinistrocerebral
sinistrocular
sinistrogyration
sinistromanual
sinistropedal
sinistrorse
sinistrotorsion
Sinkler's phenomenon
sinsemilla
sinus
   carotid s.
   cavernous s.
   cerebral s.

sinus *(continued)*
  durae matris, s.
  dural s.
  pericranii, s.
  sagital s.
  sagittalis inferior, s.
  sagittalis superior, s.
  subarachnoidal s.
sinusal
sinusitis
Sioux alarm
siriasis
sitieirgia
sitomania
sitophobia
situational
  reaction, s.
  stress, s.
16 Personality Factor Questionnaire
sixth cranial nerve
sixth sense
Sjogren's syndrome
Sjogren-Larsson syndrome
skateboard
skelalgia
skelasthenia
skeletal
  maturity, s.
  metastases, s.
  muscle, s.
  pin, s.
  series, s.
  traction, s.
skew deviation
skewed eye deviation
skills of daily living (SDL)
Skil-Saw
skin
  hook, s.
  turgor, s.
  wheal, s.
Skinner box
skinnerian psychology
skin-popper
Skiodan
Skoog procedure

skull
  cloverleaf s.
  hot cross bun s.
  lacuna s.
  maplike s.
  natiform s.
  steeple s.
  tower s.
  West's lacuna s.
  West-Engstler's s.
skull bur
skull cone bunch
skull films
skull flap
skull fracture
skull plate
skull series
skull survey
skull tongs
skull tractor
skull trephine
skullcap
SLE (systemic lupus erythematosus)
sleep
  active s.
  activated s.
  D s.
  deep s.
  desynchronized s.
  dreaming s.
  electric s.
  electrotherapeutic s.
  fast wave s.
  hypnotic s.
  nonrapid eye movement s.
  NREM s.
  orthodox s.
  paradoxical s.
  paroxysmal s.
  pathological s.
  prolonged s.
  quiet s.
  rapid eye movement s.
  REM s.
  S s.
  slow wave s.

sleep *(continued)*
    spindle s.
    synchronized s.
    temple s.
    twilight s.
sleep activation
sleep activity
sleep apnea
sleep apnea syndrome (SAS)
sleep architecture
sleep cycle
sleep deprivation
sleep disorder
sleep disturbance
sleep drunkenness
sleep efficiency
sleep hallucinations
sleep healing
sleep hygiene
sleep latency
sleep log
sleep onset
sleep onset REM period
sleep paralysis
sleep pattern
sleep periodicity
sleep recording
sleep spindles
sleep start
sleep terror
sleep treatment
sleepiness
sleeping sickness
sleeptalking
sleepwalking
sliding scale insulin
slim disease
slip-angle spondylolisthesis
slipped disk
slipping-clutch gait
slow mentation
slow-wave sleep
slowed speech
slowing of background activity
slows
SLR (straight leg raising)

SLRT (straight leg raising test)
Sluder's neuralgia
Sluder's syndrome
sluggish
    pupils, s.
    reactions, s.
    reflexes, s.
slurred speech
slurring
slurry
Sluyter-Mehta thermocouple electrode
Sly disease
Sly syndrome
SMA (supplementary motor area)
smack (heroin)
smacking of lips
small sharp spikes (SSS)
Smedberg drill
smell-brain
Smellie scissors
Smith clip
Smith-Lemli-Opitz syndrome
Smith-Petersen sacroiliac joint fusion
Smith-Robinson cervical disk approach
Smith-Robinson cervical fusion
Smith-Strang disease
Smithwick forceps
Smithwick nerve hook
Smithwick sympathectomy
SMON (subacute myelo-opticoneuro-
    pathy)
smooth muscle
smooth pursuit
    eye movements (SPEM), s.
smooth retractor
smudging
SNAP (sensory nerve action potential)
Snellen chart
Snellen reflex
Snellen sign
Snellen test
Snitman retractor
snore
snoring
snort (inhale cocaine)
snout reflex

snouting
snowstorm shadows
snuffbox
SOA-MCA (superficial occipital artery to middle cerebral artery)
soapsuds cysts
social
   breakdown syndrome, s.
   effectiveness, s.
   isolation, s.
   phobia, s.
   sex, s.
   situation, s.
   skills, s.
   withdrawal, s.
socialization
socioacusis
sociobiology
sociocultural
socioeconomic
sociology
sociometry
sociopath
sociopathic
sociopathy
sociotherapy
sodium pertechnate
sodomist
sodomize
sodomy
soft finding
soft restraints
soft signs
softening of the brain
Sohval-Soffer syndrome
solace
solar
   sneeze reflex, s.
Solcotrans drainage/reinfusion system
soldier's maneuver
sole reflex
solipsism
solitary lesion
Solu-Medrol
soma
Soma compound

somasthenia
somatalgia
somatesthenia
somatesthesia
somatic
somatist
somatization
   disorder, s.
somatoceptor
somatochrome
somatoform
   disorder, s.
somatogenic
somatomotor
somatopagnosis
somatopathy
somatophrenia
somatopsychic
somatopsychosis
somatosensory
   evoked potential (SEP or SSEP), s.
   evoked response (SER or SSER), s.
somatosexual
somatostatin
somatotherapy
somatotonia
somatotopic
somesthesia
somesthetic
   area, s.
   path, s.
   sensibility, s.
SOMI (skull-occiput-mandibular immobilization)
   brace, S.
   orthosis, S.
somite
somnambulance
somnambule
somnambulism
somnambulist
somnifacient
somniferous
somniloquence
somniloquism
somniloquist

somniloquy
somnipathist
somnipathy
somnocinematograph
somnolence
somnolent
    metabolic rate, s.
somnolentia
somnolism
Somnos
somnus
somopsychosis
sone
sonic curette
sonitus
Sonksen-Silver acuity cards
Sonneberg neurectomy
sonoencephalogram (SEG)
sonogram
sonography
sonolucency
sonolucent
SONOP ultrasonic aspiration system
sophomania
Sophy programmable pressure valve
sopor
soporiferous
soporific
soporose
soporous
sorbinil
Sorbothane heel cushion
sorcerer
sorcery
soroche
Sorsby's syndrome
Soto-Hall sign
Sotos' syndrome of cerebral gigantism
Sottas disease
sound
    intolerance, s.
    level, s.
Souques' phenomenon
Souques' sign
Southwick clip-applying forceps

Southwick-Robinson cervical disk approach
Souttar incision
space
    bregmatic s.
    Broca's s.
    epicerebral s.
    epidural s.
    epispinal s.
    Henke's s.
    His' perivascular s.
    Holzknecht's s.
    Magendie's s.
    Malacarne's s.
    Marie's quadrilateral s.
    Meckel's s,
    medullary s.
    parasinoidal s.
    Parona's s.
    perforated s.
    periaxial s.
    perineuronal s.
    perivascular s.
    personal s.
    quadrilateral s. of Marie
    Schwalbe's s.
    subarachnoid s.
    subdural s.
    subepicranial s.
    thenar s.
    Virchow-Robin s.
space adaptation syndrome
space-occupying lesion
space sickness
Spanish fly
spasm
    athetoid s.
    Bell's s.
    bronchial s,
    canine s.
    carpopedal s.
    cerebral s.
    choreiform s.
    clonic s.
    dancing s.
    facial s.

spasm *(continued)*
 fixed s.
 glottic s.
 habit s.
 histrionic s.
 infantile massive s.
 inspiratory s.
 intention s.
 lock s.
 malleatory s.
 massive s.
 mixed s.
 mobile s.
 muscle s.
 myopathic s.
 nictitating s.
 nodding s.
 paraspinal muscle s.
 paravertebral muscle s.
 phonatory s.
 progressive torsion s.
 respiratory s.
 retrocolic s.
 Romberg's s.
 rotatory s.
 salaam s.
 saltatory s.
 synclonic s.
 tetanic s.
 tonic s.
 tonoclonic s.
 torsion s.
 toxic s.
 winking s.
 writers' s.
spasmatic
 asthma, s.
 croup, s.
 stricture, s.
spasmodic
 synkinesis, s.
 torticollis, s.
spasmogen
spasmogenic
spasmology
spasmolygmus

spasmolysant
spasmolysin
spasmolysis
spasmolytic
spasmophemia
spasmophilia
spasmous
spasmus
 agitans, s.
 bronchialis, s.
 caninus, s.
 coordinatus, s.
 cynicus, s.
 Dubini, s.
 glottidis, s.
 nictitans, s.
 nutans, s.
spastic
 bladder, s.
 bulbar palsy, s.
 diplegia, s.
 gait, s.
 hemiplegia, s.
 paralysis, s.
 paraplegia, s.
 quadriparesis, s.
 quadriplegia, s.
 rigidity, s.
spasticity
spatial
 discrimination, s.
 disorganization, s.
 summation, s.
spatula
Speare dural hook
specific
specificity
SPECT (single photon emission computed tomography)
spectrophotometry
speech
 alaryngeal s.
 aphonic s.
 ataxic s.
 clipped s.
 echo s.

speech *(continued)*
   esophageal s.
   explosive s.
   incoherent s.
   interjectional s.
   jumbled s.
   mirror s.
   plateau s.
   pressured s.
   scamping s.
   scanning s.
   slurring s.
   staccato s.
speech abnormality
speech-aid prosthesis
speech defect
speech discrimination
speech disorder
speech dyspraxia
speech impediment
speech mapping
speech pathologist
speech pathology
speech reading
speech reception threshold (SRT)
speech synthesizer
speech therapist
speech therapy
speed (methamphetamine)
speedballing
SPEM (smooth pursuit eye movements)
Spence forceps
Spence-Adson forceps
spermatophobia
spermoneuralgia
Spetzler lumboperitoneal shunt
sphagiasmus
sphenion
sphenobasilar
sphenocephaly
sphenoethmoid
sphenofrontal
sphenoid
   fissure, s.
   ridge, s.
   wing, s.

sphenoidal
   needle electrode, s.
sphenomalar
sphenomaxillary
spheno-occipital
sphenoparietal
sphenopetrosal
sphenorbital
sphenosquamosal
sphenotemporal
sphenotresia
sphenoturbinal
sphenovomerine
sphenozygomatic
spheresthesia
spherophakia-brachymorphia syndrome
spherules of Fulci
sphincter
   control, s.
   tone, s.
sphincteralgia
sphingoglycolipid
sphingolipid
sphingolipidosis
sphingolipodystrophy
sphingomyelinase
sphingomyelinosis
sphingosine
spicular
spicule
spider cells
spider view
Spielmeyer-Sjogren disease
Spielmeyer-Vogt disease
spigelian line
spike
   activity, s.
   and slow wave rhythm, s.
   and wave complex, s.
   and wave pattern, s.
   complex, s.
   discharges, s.
   pattern, s.
   phenomenon, s.
   potential, s.
   seizure activity, s.

spikeboard
spin echo (SE)
spina (pl. spinae)
spina bifida
    anterior, s.b.
    aperta, s.b.
    cystica, s.b.
    manifesta, s.b.
    occulta, s.b.
    posterior, s.b.
spinae (pl. of spina)
spinal
    accessory nerve, s.
    anesthesia, s.
    arachnoid, s.
    block, s.
    board, s.
    canal, s.
    column, s.
    cord, s.
    cord compression, s.
    cord concussion, s.
    cord decompression, s.
    cord injury, s.
    cordotomy, s.
    curvature, s.
    dura mater, s.
    elevator, s.
    epidural space, s.
    field, s.
    fluid (SF), s.
    fluid culture, s
    fluid pressure (SFP), s.
    fusion, s.
    fusion plate, s.
    ganglion, s.
    headache, s.
    induction, s.
    instability, s.
    manometer, s.
    meningitis, s.
    miosis, s.
    muscle, s.
    muscular atrophy, s.
    needle, s.
    nerve, s.

spinal *(continued)*
    pia mater, s.
    precautions, s.
    puncture, s.
    reflex, s.
    segment, s.
    sensory afferent system, s.
    shock, s.
    sign, s.
    somatosensory evoked potential, s.
    stenosis, s.
    subarachnoid block, s.
    tap, s.
    tract, s.
    trephine, s.
spinalgia
spinalis
spinant
spindle
    Axenfeld-Krukenberg s.
    barbiturate s.
    Krukenberg's s.
    Kuhne's s.
    muscle s.
    neuromuscular s.
    neurotendinal s.
    sleep s.
    tendon s.
    tigroid s.
spindle sleep
spindling
    activity, s.
    pattern, s.
spine
    bamboo s.
    bifid s.
    cervical (C) s.
    cleft s.
    dendritic s.
    dorsal (D) s.
    Erichsen's s.
    hemal s.
    jugular s.
    kissing s.
    iliac s.
    lumbar (L) s.

spine *(continued)*
    lumbosacral (LS) s.
    mental s.
    nasal s.
    neural s.
    occipital s.
    poker s.
    railway s.
    rigid s.
    sacral (S) s.
    sciatic s.
    thoracic (T) s.
    thoracolumbar s.
    typhoid s.
    vertebra, s. of
spine board
spine films
spine immobilization
spine sign
spine precautions
spinifugal
spinipetal
spinning sensation
spinobulbar
spinocerebellar
spinocerebellum
spinocervical
spinocortical
spinogalvanization
spinoglenoid
spinogram
spino-olivary
spinoreticular
spinotectal
spinothalamic
spinous
    point, s.
    process, s.
spintherism
spintheropia
spiral organ
spirit
    possession, s.
spiritual therapy
spiritualism
spirituality

spiritualization
spirituous
spirokinesis
Spitz-Holter valve
Spitzka's nucleus
Spitzka's tract
Spitzka-Lissauer tract
splanchnesthesia
splanchnesthetic sensibility
splanchnic
    block, s.
    nerve, s.
    neurectomy, s.
splanchnicectomy
splanchnicotomy
splanchnocranium
splenium
    corporis callosi, s.
splint
    air s.
    airplane s.
    banjo traction s.
    blow-up s.
    Denis Brown s.
    Gibson walking s.
    inflatable s.
    Kanavel s.
    Thomas' knee s.
splinted
splinter skill
splinting
split-brain syndrome
split personality
splitting
splitting the midline
spodiomyelitis
spondee
spondylalgia
spondylarthritis
    ankylopoietica, s.
spondylarthrocace
spondylexarthrosis
spondylitic
spondylitis
    ankylosing s.
    Bekhterev's s.

spondylitis *(continued)*
  hypertrophic s.
  Kummell's s.
  Marie-Strumpell s.
  muscular s.
  post-traumatic s.
  rheumatoid s.
  rhizomelic s.
  traumatic s.
  tuberculous s.
spondylizema
spondyloarthropathy
spondylocace
spondylodesis
spondylodynia
spondylolisthesis
spondylolisthetic
spondylolysis
spondylomalacia
  traumatica, s.
spondylopathy
spondylophyte impaction set
spondylopyosis
spondyloschisis
spondylosis
  cervical s.
  chronica ankylopoietica, s.
  lumbar s.
  rhizomelic s.
spondylosyndesis
spondylotherapy
spondylotic
  bar, s.
  caudal radiculopathy, s.
spondylotomy
spondylous
spongioblastoma
  multiforme, s.
  unipolare, s.
spongostan
spontaneity
spontaneous
spontaneous fracture
sporadoneure
spoon
spork

spot
  blind s.
  blue s.
  Brushfield's s.
  cafe au lait s.
  cherry-red s.
  cold s.
  cotton-wool s.
  flame s.
  Graefe's s.
  hot s.
  hypnogenetic s.
  Koplik's s.
  Mariotte's s.
  mental s.
  mongolian s.
  pain s.
  sacral s.
  temperature s.
  Trousseau's s.
  vital s.
  warm s.
spotty hypalgesia
spousal rape
sprain
spreader
spreading depression
spring fever
spring finger
spring ligament
springing
  mydriasis, s.
sprue
spur
spurred
spurring
Spurling forceps
Spurling maneuver
Spurling rongeur
Spurling sign
Spurling-Kerrison laminectomy rongeur
Spurway syndrome
squama (pl. squamae)
squamae (pl. of squama)
squamofrontal
squamomastoid

squamo-occipital
squamoparietal
squamopetrosal
squamosoparietal
squamosphenoid
squamotemporal
squamozygomatic
squat
squatting
squeeze dynamometer
SQUID (Superconducting Quantum Interference Device)
Squire's sign
SRT (speech reception threshold)
SSEP (somatosensory evoked potential)
SSER (somatosensory evoked response)
S-sleep (synchronized sleep)
SSPE (subacute sclerosing panencephalitis)
SSS (small sharp spikes)
STA (superficial temporal artery)
stab incision
stability
stable
    vital signs, s.
staccato
    speech, s.
Staderini's nucleus
staff constant
stage
    algid s.
    anal s.
    genital s.
    latency s.
    oral s.
    phallic s.
stage of sleep
staggering gait
staggers
staircase phenomenon
stairs sign
STA-MCA bypass
stammering
    bladder, s. of
stance
    phase, s.

standard deviation of mean
standing balance
standing phase
Stanford-Binet Intelligence Test
staphyloschisis
stare
stared
staring spell
start hesitation
startle reaction
startle reflex
startle syndrome
startled
startle-matching taxon
startling
stasibasiphobia
state
    acute confusional s.
    alpha s.
    anelectrotonic s.
    anxiety s.
    anxiety tension s.
    borderline s.
    catatonic s.
    catelectrotonic s.
    central excitatory s.
    central inhibitory s.
    consciousness, s. of
    correlated s.
    dreamy s.
    drowsy s.
    epileptic s.
    excited s.
    fatigue s.
    hypnogogic s.
    hypnoid s.
    hypnopompic s.
    local excitatory s.
    marble s.
    persistent s.
    vegetative s.
    refractory s.
    resting s.
    steady s.
    twilight s.
State-Trait Anxiety Inventory

static
  activity, s.
  ataxia, s.
  equilibrium, s.
  reflex, s.
  scoliosis, s.
  splint, s.
  tremor, s.
station
station and gait
stationary
statoacoustic
statocyst
statokinetic
  reflexes, s.
statotomic reflex
status
  absence s.
  choreicus, s.
  convulsivis, s.
  cribalis, s.
  cribrosus, s.
  criticus, s.
  dysgraphicus, s.
  dysmyelinatus, s.
  dysmyelinisatus, s.
  dysraphicus., s.
  epilepticus, s.
  hemicranicus, s.
  lacunaris, s.
  lacunosus, s.
  lymphaticus, s.
  marmoratus, s.
  migrainus, s.
  petite mal s.
  praesens, s.
  raptus, s.
  spongiosus, s.
  sternuens, s.
  thymicolymphaticus, s.
  thymicus, s.
  verrucosus, s.
  vertiginosus, s.
statutory rape
statuvolence
staurion

stauroplegia
steadied
steadiness
  apparatus, s.
steady
  membrane potential, s.
  state, s.
Stearns' alcoholic amentia
Stecher arachnoid knife
steel mesh
steel plate
Steele-Richardson-Olszewski syndrome
steely-hair syndrome
steeple skull
Steffe plate
Steffe screw
Stein test
Steinbrocker syndrome
Steiner disease
Steinert disease
Steinmann's extension
stellate
  ganglion, s.
  incision, s.
stellectomy
stellreflexe
Stellwag's sign
Stenger test
stenion
stenobregmatic
stenocephaly
stenopaic
stenopeic
stenosal
stenosed
stenosis
stenotic
step-off
stephanion
steppage gait
stepping reflex
stereoagnosis
stereoanesthesia
stereoarthrolysis
stereocognosy
stereoencephalotome

stereoencephalotomy
stereognosis
stereognostic
stereotactic
stereotaxic
stereotaxis
stereotaxy
stereotropic
stereotropism
stereotype
stereotyped
stereotypic
stereotypy
Sterling's sign
Sternberg's disease
sternocleidomastoid
sternovertebral
sternutament
sternutatio
   convulsiva, s.
sternutation
sternutator
sternutatory
steroid
   dependence, s.
   facies, s.
   myopathy, s.
   psychosis, s.
   withdrawal, s.
stethoparalysis
stethospasm
Stevenson forceps
Stevenson scissors
Stewart-Holmes sign
Stewart-Morel syndrome
St. Guy's dance
sthenia
sthenic
sthenometer
sthenometry
Stierlin theory
stiff
   joint, s.
   -man syndrome, s.
   neck, s.
   -neck fever, s.

stiffness
stigma (pl. stigmata)
   degeneration, s. of
   hysterical s.
   psychic s.
stigmata (pl. of stigma)
stigmatic
stigmatism
stigmatization
Stille drill
Stille osteotome
Stille-Gigli saw
Stille-Gigli saw guide
Stille trephine
Stille-Leksell rongeur
Stille-Leur cutting forceps
Stille-Leur rongeur
Stille-Liston bone-cutting forceps
Stilling syndrome
Stilling-Turk-Duane syndrome
stimulant
stimulate
stimulation
   areal s.
   audio-visual-tactile s.
   carotid sinus s.
   electrical s.
   electrical surface s.
   galvanic s.
   magnetic s.
   nonspecific s.
   paradoxical s.
   paraspecific s.
   photic s.
   punctual s.
   transcutaneous electrical nerve s.
stimulator
stimuli (pl. of stimulus)
stimulus (pl. stimuli)
   adequate s.
   aversive s.
   chemical s.
   conditioned s.
   discriminative s.
   electric s.
   eliciting s.

stimulus (pl. stimuli) *(continued)*
  heterologous s.
  homologous s.
  iatrotropic s.
  liminal s.
  mechanical s.
  minimal s.
  nociceptive s.
  noxious s.
  painful s.
  reinforcing s.
  subliminal s.
  supraliminal s.
  thermal s.
  threshold s.
  unconditioned s.
stimulus-response psychology
stimulus threshold
stimulus wave
Stintzing's tables
stitch
St. John's dance
St. Louis encephalitis
stock words
Stocker's sign
stockinette
stocking distribution
stocking-glove distribution
stocking-glove hypalgesia
stocking-glove hypesthesia
stoic
stoicism
stoker's cramp
Stokes' law
Stokes-Adams syndrome
Stookey reflex
storage disease
stork-leg
STRs (superficial tendon reflexes)
strabismus
Strachan's syndrome
straight back syndrome
straight leg raising (SLR)
strain
  chronic low back s.
  ligamentous s.

strain *(continued)*
  lumbosacral s.
  sacroiliac s.
strain x-ray
straitjacket
strangalesthesia
Stransky reflex
strap muscles
strata (pl. of stratum)
stratum (pl. strata)
streak
  Moore's lightning s.
street drugs
strength
  ego s.
  extrinsic muscle s.
  fatigue s.
  hand grip s.
  intrinsic muscle s.
  motor s.
strephosymbolia
stress
  innoculation, s.
  management, s.
  reaction, s.
  reduction, s.
  ulcer, s.
stressed
stressed-out
stressful
stressor
stretch
  receptor, s.
  reflex, s.
stretching
stria (pl. striae)
  fornicis, s.
  Francke's s.
  habenular s.
  lancisii, s.
  medullares acusticae, s.
  medullares fossae rhomboideae, s.
  medullares ventriculi quarti, s.
  medullaris thalami, s.
  meningitic s.
  olfactory s.

stria (pl. striae) *(continued)*
   pinealis, s.
   terminalis, s.
striae (pl. of stria)
striatal
   hand, s.
   nigral degeneration, s.
striatonigral
striatum
stride length
striding
string sign
striocellular
striocerebellar
striomotor
striomuscular
stripe
stroke
   apoplectic s,
   atherothrombotic s.
   back s.
   cardioembolic s.
   completed s.
   heat s.
   impending s.
   lightning s.
   paralytic s.
   sun s.
stroke syndrome
stroking
stroma (pl. stromata)
stromal
stromata (pl. of stroma)
Stromeyer's cephalhematoma
strontium
structural
   analysis, s.
   lesion, s.
structuralism
structure
structured
Strully scissors
Strumpell's disease
Strumpell's phenomenon
Strumpell's reflex
Strumpell's sign

Strumpell's type
Strumpell-Leichtenstern disease
Strumpell-Marie disease
Strumpell-Westphal pseudosclerosis
strychnine
strychninism
strychninization
strychninomania
strychnize
Stryker frame
Stryker leg exerciser
stump
   hallucination, s.
   neuralgia, s.
   pain, s.
stun
stunned
stupefacient
stupefactive
stupomania
stupor
   anergic s.
   benign s.
   delusion s.
   epileptic s.
   lethargic s.
   postconvulsive s.
   postictal s.
stuporous
   depression, s.
Sturge's disease
Sturge's syndrome
Sturge-Kalischer-Weber syndrome
Sturge-Weber syndrome
Sturge-Weber-Dimitri disease
stutter
stuttering
   labiochoreic s.
STV (simian T-virus)
St. Vitus' dance
St. Vitus' dance of the voice
styloglossus
subacute
   bacterial endocarditis (SBE), s.
   myelo-opticoneuropathy (SMON), s.
   necrotizing encephalopathy, s.

subacute *(continued)*
    sclerosing panencephalitis (SSPE), s.
    spongiform encephalopathy, s.
subarachnoid
    bleed, s.
    cistern, s.
    hemorrhage (SAH), s.
    shunt, s.
    space, s.
subarcuate
subatloidean
subaxial
subbasal projection
subcalcarine
subcallosal gyrus
subcentral
subception
subclavian steal syndrome
subcommissural
subconcussion
subconcussive
subconscious
subconsciousness
subcortex
subcortical
    atherosclerotic encephalopathy
      (SAE), s.
subcranial
subdelirium
subduction
subdural
    abscess, s.
    bleed, s.
    blood patch, s.
    empyema, s.
    hematoma, s.
    hemorrhage, s.
    hygroma, s.
    space, s.
    tap, s.
subendymal
subependymal
    giant-cell astrocytoma, s.
    glioma, s.
subependymoma
subepicranial

subextensibility
subfolium
subfrontal
subgaleal
subgrondation
subgyrus
subhyaloid
subicular
subiculum
subjacent
subjective
    sensation, s.
subjectoscope
subligamentous
sublimate
sublimation
subliminal
    learning, s.
    message, s.
    self, s.
    teaching, s.
    thirst, s.
subluxate
subluxation
subneural
subnormal
subnormality
suboccipital
    triangle, s.
    trigeminal rhizotomy, s.
subparalytic
subparietal
subperiosteal
    elevator, s.
subperiosteum
subpersonalities
subpial
subservient
subspinous
subsplenial
substance
    anterior perforated s.
    black s.
    gray s.
    medullary s.
    molecular s.

substance *(continued)*
  P, s.
  periventricular gray s.
  posterior perforated s.
  prelipid s.
  receptive s.
  Rolando's gelatinous s.
  tigroid s.
  transmitter s.
  white s.
  white s. of Schwann
substance abuse
substance dependence
substantia (pl. substantiae)
  alba, s.
  cinerea, s.
  corticalis cerebelli, s.
  corticalis cerebri, s.
  gelatinosa, s.
  grisea, s.
  innominata, s.
  nigra, s.
  perforata, s.
  reticularis alba gyri fornicati, s.
  reticularis alba medullae oblongatae, s.
  reticularis grisea medullae oblonga-
    tae, s.
  Rolandi, s.
substantiae (pl. of substantia)
substitute
substitution
subsulcus
subsultus
  tendinum, s.
subsylvian
subtemporal
subtentorial
subtetanic
subthalamic
  nucleus, s.
subthalamus
subtile
subtle
subtlety
subtraction films
subvertebral

subvirile
subwaking
successive approximation
suck reflex
suction tube
Sudan stain
sudanophilic leukodystrophy
sudden infant death syndrome (SIDS)
sudden mass assault taxon
sudden unexplained death syndrome
  (SUDS)
Sudeck's atrophy
Sudeck-Leriche syndrome
SUDS (sudden unexplained death syndrome)
suffer
suffered
suffering
Sugar clip
suggestibility
suggestible
suggestive
  medicine, s.
  therapeutics, s.
suggestion
suggestionism
Sugita aneurysm clip
suicidal
  depression, s.
  gestures, s.
  ideation, s.
  intent, s.
  precautions, s.
suicide
  gesture, s.
  precautions, s.
  threat, s.
suicidology
Suker's sign
sulci (pl. of sulcus)
sulcus (pl. sulci)
  anterolateral s.
  basilar s.
  basilaris pontis, s.
  bulbopontine s.
  calcarine s.

sulcus (pl. sulci) *(continued)*
   callosal s.
   central s. of cerebrum
   cerebral s.
   chiasmatic s.
   cingulate s.
   collateralis, s.
   corporis callosi, s.
   corpus callosum, s. of
   dorsolateral s.
   frontal s.
   hippocampal s.
   hippocampi, s.
   hypothalamic s.
   hypothalamicus, s.
   inferior frontomarginal s.
   inferior temporal s.
   intraparietal s.
   lateral occipital s.
   limitans, s.
   lunate s.
   medial frontal s.
   median s.
   middle frontal s.
   middle temporal s.
   occipital s.
   occipitotemporal s.
   oculomotor s.
   olfactory s.
   orbital s.
   paracentral s.
   paramedial s.
   parieto-occipital s.
   petrobasilar s.
   petrosal s.
   pontobulbar s.
   pontopeduncular s.
   postcentral s.
   postclival s.
   postnodular s.
   postpyramidal s.
   precentral s.
   prechiasmatic s.
   preclival s.
   prepyramidal s.
   prerolandic s.

sulcus (pl. sulci) *(continued)*
   rhinal s.
   sagittal s.
   subfrontal s.
   subparietal s.
   superior frontal s.
   superior temporal s.
   temporal s.
   Turner's s.
   ventrolateral s.
Sullivan theory
summation
Sunday morning paralysis
Sunday neurosis
sundowning
Sundt clip
Sundt-Kees clip
sunflower eyes
sunset eyes
sunstroke
superabduction
superactivity
Superconducting Quantum Interference
   Device (SQUID)
superduct
superdural
superego
superexcitation
superextension
superficial
   abdominal reflex, s.
   musculoaponeurotic system
      (SMAS), s.
   reflexes, s.
   tendon reflexes (STRs), s.
superficiality
superflexion
superior
   aperture, s.
   cerebellar artery, s.
   cerebellar peduncle, s.
   cerebral vein, s.
   cervical ganglion, s.
   colliculus, s.
   commissure, s.
   frontal gyrus, s.

superior *(continued)*
    frontal sulcus, s.
    fronto-occipital fasciculus, s.
    occipital gyrus, s.
    olivary nucleus, s.
    orbital fissure syndrome, s.
    parietal lobe, s.
    petrosal sinus, s.
    posterior fissure, s.
    quadrantanopsia, s.
    sagittal sinus, s.
    sensory nucleus, s.
    sulcus tumor syndrome, s.
    temporal gyrus, s.
    temporal sulcus, s.
superiority complex
superjacent
supermoron
supermotility
supernatural
supernormal
supernumerary
superolateral
supersensible
supersensitive
supersensory
superstition
superstitious
supinate
supination
supination and pronation
supinator
    longus reflex, s.
supplementary motor area (SMA)
support
    group, s.
    system, s.
suppressed
suppression
    burst pattern, s.
supracallosal gyrus
suprachiasmatic nucleus
supracranial
supraliminal
supralumbar
supranormal

supranuclear
supranuclear
    palsy, s.
supraoccipital
supraoptic nucleus
supraorbital
suprapontine
suprasegmental
    brain, s.
suprasellar
supraspinal
supraspinatus
supraspinous
suprasylvian
supratemporal
supratentorial
sural nerve
surcingle
surdimute
surdimutism
surdimutitas
surditas
    congenita, s.
surdity
surdomute
surefooted
surexcitation
surface coil technique
surfer's knots
Surgicel
Surgitron
Surgivac
surreptitious
surrogate
    parent, s.
    parenting, s.
    sex partner, s.
    spouse, s.
surveillance
surveilled
survivor guilt
susceptibility
susceptible
suscitate
suscitation
suspended animation

suspenopsia
sustained clonus
susto
sutura (pl. suturae)
suturae (pl. of sutura)
sutural
   ligament, s.
suture
   basilar s.
   bifrontal s.
   biparietal s.
   bregmatomastoid s.
   coronal s.
   cranial s.
   frontal s.
   frontoparietal s.
   frontotemporal s.
   interparietal s.
   jugal s.
   lambdoid s.
   longitudinal s.
   mediofrontal s.
   metopic s.
   occipital s.
   occipitoparietal s.
   parietal s.
   petrobasilar s.
   petrosphenobasilar s.
   petrosphenoccipital s. of Gruber
   petrosquamous s.
   rhabdoid s.
   sagittal s.
   sphenoethmoidal s.
   sphenofrontal s.
   sphenoparietal s.
   sphenopetrosal s.
   sphenosquamous s.
   sphenotemporal s.
   squamosoparietal s.
   squamosophenoid s.
   squamous s.
   temporal s.
   temporo-occipital s.
   temporoparietal s.
   zygomaticofrontal s.
   zygomaticomaxillary s.

suture *(continued)*
   zygomaticotemporal s.
swan-neck deformity
swayback
swaying gait
SWD (short wave diathermy)
Swedish gymnastics
Swedish massage
Sweet clip-applying forceps
swineherd's disease
swing phase
swing-through gait
swing-to gait
swinging flashlight sign
swoon
sycophant
Sydenham's chorea
syllabic utterance
syllable stumbling
sylvian
   aqueduct, s.
   fissure, s.
   fossa, s.
   line, s.
   point, s.
   syndrome, s.
symbiosis
symbiotic
symbol
   phallic s.
Symbol Digit Modalities Test
symbolia
symbolic
symbolism
symbolization
symbolize
symbolophobia
Symmetrel
symmetromania
symmetry
sympathectomize
sympathectomy
   chemical s.
   lumbar s.
   periarterial s.
sympathetic

sympathetic *(continued)*
  activity, s.
  chain, s.
  fiber, s.
  ganglion, s.
  irritation, s.
  nervous system, s.
  plexus, s.
  ramisection, s.
  saliva, s.
  trunk, s.
sympatheticalgia
sympatheticoparalytic
sympatheticotonia
sympathetoblast
sympathicoblastoma
sympathicodiaphtheresis
sympathicogonioma
sympathicomimetic
sympathiconeuritis
sympathicopathy
sympathicotherapy
sympathicotonia
sympathicotripsy
sympathicotropic
sympathicus
sympathin
sympathism
sympathist
sympathoadrenal
sympathoblastoma
sympatholytic
sympathoma
sympathomimetic
sympathy
symphyseal
symphyses(pl. of symphysis)
symphysis (pl. symphyses)
symptom
  behavior, s.
  complex, s.
symptomatic
  pattern, s.
synalgia
synapse
  axoaxonic s.

synapse *(continued)*
  axodendritic s.
  axodendrosomatic s.
  axodomatic s.
  dendrodendritic s.
synapsing
synapsis
synaptic
  blocking agent, s.
  cleft, s.
  field, s.
  transmission, s.
  vesicles, s.
synaptolemma
synaptology
synaptosome
synarthrodial
synarthrophysis
synarthroses (pl. of synarthrosis)
synarthrosis (pl. synarthroses)
synchiria
synchondroses (pl. of synchondrosis)
synchondrosis (pl. synchondroses)
synchronism
synchronization
synchronized sleep (S-sleep)
synchronous
syncinesis
  imitative s.
  spasmodic s.
synciput
synclonic spasm
synclonus
syncopal
  spell, s.
syncope
  anginal s.
  anginosa, s.
  cardiac s.
  carotid sinus s.
  cough s.
  defecation s.
  digital s.
  exertional s.
  hysterical s.
  laryngeal s.

syncope *(continued)*
   local s.
   micturition s.
   postural s.
   stretching s.
   swallow s.
   transient s.
   tussive s.
   vasodepressor s.
   vasovagal s.
syncopic
syncytial
syndesis
syndrome
   Aase s.
   abstinence s.
   Achard s.
   acquired immune deficiency (AIDS) s.
   acute brain s.
   acute organic brain s.
   acute radiation s.
   Adair-Dighton s.
   Adie's s.
   adiposogenital s.
   adrenogenital s.
   Aicardi s.
   Alajouanine's s.
   Albright's s.
   Albright-McCune-Sternberg s.
   Alezzandrini's s.
   Alice in Wonderland s.
   Allemann's s.
   Alport's s.
   Alstrom's s.
   Alzheimer's s.
   amnesic s.
   amnestic s.
   amnestic-confabulatory s.
   Angelucci s.
   anorexia-cachexia s.
   anterior cord s.
   anterior tibial compartment s.
   anticholinergic s.
   anxiety s.
   Apert's s.
   Arnold's nerve reflex cough s.

syndrome *(continued)*
   Arnold-Chiari s.
   Asherson's s.
   ataxia-telangiectasia s.
   auriculotemporal s.
   Avellis' s.
   Baastrup's s.
   Babinski's s.
   Babinski-Frolich s.
   Babinski-Nageotte, s. of
   Babinski-Vaquez s.
   BADS s.
   Balint's s.
   Baller-Gerold s.
   Bannwarth's s.
   Bardet-Biedl s.
   Barre-Gauillain s.
   Barre-Lieou s.
   Bartschi-Rochain s.
   Bartter's s.
   basal cell nevus s.
   battered-child s.
   battered-spouse s.
   battered-wife s.
   Beals' s.
   Beard's s.
   Beck's s.
   Behcet's s.
   Benedikt's s.
   Bernard's s.
   Bernard-Horner s.
   Bernard-Soulier s.
   Bernhardt-Roth s.
   Bertolotti's s.
   Bianchi's s.
   Biemond II s.
   Bjornstad's s.
   Blackfan-Diamond s.
   Bloom s.
   body of Luys s.
   Bonnet's s.
   Bonnier's s.
   Borjeson's s.
   Borjeson-Forssman-Lehmann s.
   Brachmann-de Lange s.
   Briquet's s.

syndrome *(continued)*
    Brissaud-Marie s.
    Brissaud-Sicard s.
    Bristowe's s.
    brittle bone s.
    Brown's vertical retraction s.
    Brown-Sequard s.
    Bruns' s.
    Brushfield-Wyatt s.
    Budd-Chiari s.
    bulbar s.
    burning feet s.
    callosal s.
    camptomelic s.
    Capgras' s.
    capsular thrombosis s.
    capsulothalamic s.
    cardiofacial s.
    carotid sinus s.
    carpal tunnel s.
    Carpenter's s.
    cat's cry s.
    cat's eye s.
    cauda equina s.
    caudal dysplasia s.
    caudal regression s.
    cavernous sinus s.
    central cord s.
    centroposterior s.
    cerebellar s.
    cerebrocardiac s.
    cerebrohepatorenal s.
    cervical s.
    cervical rib s.
    cervicobrachial s.
    Cestan's s.
    Cestan-Chenais s.
    Cestan-Raymond s.
    Charcot's s.
    Charcot-Weiss-Baker s.
    Chiari's s.
    Chiari-Arnold s.
    chiasmatic s.
    Chinese restaurant s.
    Chotzen's s.
    chronic brain s.

syndrome *(continued)*
    chronic organic brain s.
    Churg-Strauss s.
    Citelli's s.
    Claude's s.
    Claude Bernard-Horner s.
    Clerambault's s.
    closed head s.
    Cockayne's s.
    Cogan's s.
    Collet's s.
    Collet-Sicard s.
    combined immunodeficiency s.
    compartmental s.
    compression s.
    concussion s.
    congenital rubella s.
    Conn's s.
    contiguous gene s.
    Cornelia de Lange's s.
    corpus striatum, s. of
    Costen's s.
    costoclavicular s.
    Cotard's s.
    couvade s.
    craniosynostosis-radial aplasia s.
    CREST s.
    Creutzfeldt-Jakob s.
    cricopharyngeal achalasia s.
    cri du chat s.
    Crigler-Najjar s.
    crocodile tears, s. of
    Cross s.
    Cross-McKusick-Breen s.
    CRST s.
    crush s.
    cryptophthalmos s.
    cubital tunnel s.
    culture-specific s.
    Cushing's s.
    Cyriax's s.
    DaCosta's s.
    Dandy-Walker s.
    Danlos' s.
    Debre-Semelaigne s.
    Dejerine's s.

syndrome *(continued)*
    Dejerine-Klumpke s.
    Dejerine-Roussy s.
    Dejerine-Sottas s.
    de Lange's s.
    Dennie-Marfan s.
    depersonalization s.
    depressive s.
    DeSanctis-Cacchione s.
    Devic's s.
    diencephalic s.
    diffuse idiopathic skeletal hyperosto-
        sis (DISH) s.
    DiGeorge s.
    Dighton-Adair s.
    DISH s.
    Donohue's s.
    Down's s.
    Duane's s.
    Duchenne's s.
    Duchenne-Erb s.
    dumping s.
    Dupre's s.
    Dyke-Davidoff s.
    dysmnesic s.
    Eaton-Lambert s.
    ectopic ACTH s.
    Edward's s.
    EEC s.
    effort s.
    Ehlers-Danlos s.
    Ekbom s.
    elfin facies s.
    Ellis-van Creveld s.
    empty-sella s.
    encephalotrigeminal vascular s.
    epiphyseal s.
    Erb's s.
    exomphalos-macroglossia-gigantism s.
    extrapyramidal s.
    faciodigitogenital s.
    Fallot's s.
    Fanconi's s.
    fetal alcohol s.
    fetal face s.
    fetal hydantoin s.

syndrome *(continued)*
    Fevre-Languepin s.
    floppy infant s.
    Foix-Alajouanine s.
    Forsius-Eriksson's s.
    Foster Kennedy s.
    Foville's s.
    fragile X s.
    Francheschetti s.
    Francheschetti-Jadassohn s.
    Francois' s.
    Freeman-Sheldon s.
    Fregoli s.
    Friderichsenn-Waterhouse s.
    Friedmann's vasomotor s.
    Frohlich's s.
    Froin's s.
    G s.
    Ganser s.
    Garcin's s.
    Gardner's s.
    Gardner-Diamond s.
    Gee-Herter-Heubner s.
    Gelineau's s.
    gender dysphoria s.
    general adaptation s.
    Gerhardt's s.
    Gerstmann's s.
    Gilles de la Tourette's s.
    glioma-polyposis s.
    Goldenhar's s.
    Good's s.
    Goodman s.
    Gopalan's s.
    Gorlin's s.
    Gorlin-Goltz s.
    Gougerot-Nulock-Houwer s.
    Gower's s.
    Gradenigo's s.
    gray s.
    gray spinal s.
    Griscelli s.
    Guillain-Barre s.
    Gunn's s.
    gustatory sweating s.
    Hakim's s.

syndrome *(continued)*
 Hallermann-Streiff s.
 Hallermann-Streiff-Francois s.
 Hallervorden-Spatz s.
 hand-shoulder s.
 Hanhart's s.
 Harada's s.
 Hare's s.
 Harris' s.
 Heidenhaim's s.
 Hoffman-Werdnig s.
 Holmes-Adie s.
 Homen's s.
 Horner's s.
 Horner-Bernard s.
 Horton's s.
 Hunt's s.
 Hunt's striatal s.
 Hunter's s.
 Hunter-Hurler s.
 Hurler's s.
 Hurler-Scheie s.
 Hutchinson-Gilford s.
 hyaline membrane s.
 hyperabduction s.
 hyperactive child s.
 hypereosinophilic s.
 hyperkinetic s.
 hypersomnia-bulimia s.
 hyperventilation s.
 hypoglossia-hypodactyly s.
 impostor s.
 inappropriate antidiuretic hormone, s.
  of (SIADH)
 Jackson's s.
 Jahnke's s.
 Jakob-Creutzfeldt s.
 jaw-winking s.
 Jervell and Lange-Nielsen s.
 jugular foramen s.
 Kanner's s.
 Kast's s.
 Kearns-Sayre s.
 Kennedy's s.
 Kiloh-Nevin s.
 kinky-hair s.

syndrome *(continued)*
 Kinsbourne s.
 kleeblattschadel s.
 Kleine-Levin s.
 Klippel-Feil s.
 Klippel-Feldstein s.
 Klumpke-Dejerine s.
 Kluver-Bucy s.
 Kocher-Debre-Semelaigne s.
 Koerber-Salus-Elschnig s.
 Korsakoff's s.
 Kostmann's s.
 Krause's s.
 Lambert-Eaton s.
 Landry's s.
 Larsen's s.
 Launois' s.
 Laurence-Moon s.
 Lawen-Roth s.
 Lawford's s.
 Legg-Calve-Perthes s.
 Leigh s.
 Lennox s.
 Lennox-Gastaut s.
 Lenz's s.
 leopard s.
 Leriche's s.
 Lermoyez's s.
 Lesch-Nyhan s.
 levator s.
 Leyden-Moebius s.
 Lhermitte and McAlpine s.
 Lichtheim's s.
 Lobstein's s.
 locked-in s.
 loculation s.
 Louis-Bar s.
 Loew-Terry-Machiachan s.
 Lowe s.
 lower radicular s.
 McCune-Albright s.
 Mackenzie's s.
 Maffucci's s.
 Marchesani's s.
 Marcus Gunn's s.
 Marfan s.

syndrome *(continued)*
    Marinesco-Sjogren's s.
    Maroteaux-Lamy s.
    Martorell's s.
    mastocytosis s.
    maternal deprivation s.
    Meckel's s.
    Meckel-Gruber s.
    Melkersson's s.
    Melkersson-Rosenthal s.
    Mengert's shock s.
    Meniere's s.
    Menkes' s.
    metameric s.
    methionine malabsorption s.
    Meyer-Schwickerath and Weyers s.
    Millard-Gubler s.
    Mobius' s.
    Mohr s.
    Monakow's s.
    Moore's s.
    Morel s.
    Morgagni's s.
    Morgagni-Stewart-Morel s.
    morning glory s.
    Morquio's s.
    Morquio-Ullrich s.
    Morvan's s.
    Moynahan s.
    Muckle-Wells s.
    mucosal neuroma s.
    multiple lentigines s.
    Munchausen s.
    myasthenia gravis s.
    myasthenic s.
    myelofibrosis-osteosclerosis s.
    myeloproliferative s.
    Naegeli s.
    Naffziger's s.
    Nelson's s.
    neostriatal s.
    Netherton's s.
    neurocutaneous s.
    neuroleptic malignant s.
    Noack's s.
    Nonne's s.

syndrome *(continued)*
    nonsense s.
    Nothnagel's s.
    OAV s.
    oculocerebral-hypopigmentation s.
    oculocerebrorenal s.
    oculomandibulofacial s.
    OFD s.
    Ogilvie's s.
    OMM s.
    Oppenheim's s.
    oral-facial-digital s.
    organic brain s.
    organic delusional s.
    organic mental s.
    organic mood s.
    organic personality s.
    orofaciodigital s.
    Ostrum-Furst s.
    painful bruising s.
    paleostriatal s.
    pallidal s.
    pallidomesencephalic s.
    Pancoast's s.
    pancytopenia-dysmelia s.
    paratrigeminal s.
    Parinaud's s.
    Parkinson's s.
    parkinsonian s.
    Parry-Romberg s.
    Patau's s.
    Pendred's s.
    Pfeiffer's s.
    Pick's s.
    pickwickian s.
    Pierre Robin s.
    Poland's s.
    pontine s.
    postcardiotomy psychosis s.
    postconcussional s.
    posterior cord s.
    posterolateral s.
    postirradiation s.
    postlumbar puncture s.
    postpump s.
    post-traumatic brain s.

syndrome *(continued)*
    Potter's s.
    Prader-Willi s.
    premenstrual s.
    premotor s.
    pseudoclaudication s.
    Putnam-Dana s.
    rabbit s.
    radicular s.
    Raeder's s.
    Ramsay-Hunt s.
    Raymond-Cestan s.
    restless legs s.
    retraction s.
    retroparotid space, s. of
    Rett s.
    Reye's s.
    Richards-Rundle s.
    Rieger's s.
    Riley-Day s.
    Riley-Smith s.
    Rimbaud-Passouant-Vallat s.
    Robin s.
    Robinow's s.
    rolandic vein s.
    Romano-Ward s.
    Rot's s.
    Rot-Bernhardt s.
    Roth's s.
    Roth-Bernhardt s.
    Roussy-Cornil s.
    Roussy-Dejerine s.
    Roussy-Levy s.
    Rubinstein-Taybi s.
    rubrospinal cerebellar peduncle s.
    Rud's s.
    Russell's s.
    Rust's s.
    Sabin-Feldman s.
    Saethre-Chotzen s.
    Sakati-Nyhan s.
    salt-losing s.
    Sanfilippo's s.
    scalenus anticus s.
    Schafer's s.
    Schanz's s.

syndrome *(continued)*
    Scheie's s.
    Schmidt's s.
    Schuller's s.
    Schuller-Christian s.
    Schwartz-Jampel s.
    Seabright bantam s.
    Seckel's s.
    segmentary s.
    Selye s.
    sensory dissociation with brachial
        amyotrophy, s. of
    shoulder-hand s.
    Shy-Drager s.
    Sicard's s.
    sicca s.
    sick sinus s.
    Silver's s.
    Silverskiold's s.
    Simmonds' s.
    Sjogren's s.
    Sjogren-Larsson s.
    skin-eye s.
    sleep apnea s.
    Sluder's s.
    Sly s.
    Smith-Lemli-Opitz s.
    social breakdown s.
    Sohval-Soffer s.
    somnolence s.
    Sorsby's s.
    Sotos' s.
    space adaptation s.
    spherophakia-brachymorphia s.
    Spielmeyer-Sjogren s.
    split-brain s.
    Spurway s.
    Steele-Richardson-Olszewski s.
    steely-hair s.
    Steinbrocker's s.
    Stewart-Morel s.
    stiff-man s.
    Stilling s.
    Stilling-Turk-Duane s.
    straight back s.
    stroke s.

syndrome *(continued)*
    Sturge's s.
    Sturge-Kalischer-Weber s.
    Sturge-Weber s.
    subclavian steal s.
    sudden infant death s.
    sudden unexplained death s.
    superior orbital fissure s.
    superior sulcus tumor s.
    supraspinatus s.
    sylvian aqueduct s.
    syringomelic s.
    Takayasu's s.
    Tapia's s.
    tarsal tunnel s.
    tegmental s.
    temporomandibular joint s.
    tethered cord s.
    thalamic s.
    Thiele s.
    thoracic outlet s.
    tired housewife s.
    Tolosa-Hunt s.
    toxic shock s.
    translocation Down s.
    Treacher-Collins s.
    Treacher-Collins-Franceschetti s.
    trisomy D s.
    trisomy E s.
    trisomy 13-15 s.
    trisomy 16-18 s.
    trisomy 18 s.
    trisomy 21 s.
    Turcot s.
    Turner's s.
    Ullrich-Feichtiger s.
    Ullrich-Turner s.
    ulnar nerve entrapment s.
    Unverricht's s.
    vagoaccessory s.
    van Buchem's s.
    van der Hoeve's s.
    Van der Woude's s.
    Vernet's s.
    Villaret's s.
    Vogt's s.

syndrome *(continued)*
    Vogt-Koyanagi-Harada s.
    Volkmann's s.
    Waardenburg's s.
    Wallenberg's s.
    Ward-Romano s.
    Waterhouse-Friderichsen s.
    Weber, s. of
    Weil's s.
    Weill-Marchesani s.
    Wernicke-Korsakoff s.
    West's s.
    Weyer's oligodactyly s.
    whiplash shake s.
    whistling face s.
    whistling face-windmill vane hand s.
    Williams' s.
    withdrawal s.
    Wolf-Hirschhorn s.
    Wolfram s.
    Wright's s.
    XXY s.
    Zellweger's s.
syndromic
synencephalocele
synergistic
synergy
synesthesia
    algica, s.
synesthesialgia
synkinesia
synkinesis
    imitative s.
    mouth-and-hand s.
    spasmodic s.
synkinetic
synosteotomy
synostosis
    sagittal s.
    tribasilar s.
synostotic
synreflexia
syntactic
syntaxis
syntexis
syntone

syntonic
syntony
syphilis
   meningovascular s.
syphilitic
syphiloma
syphilomania
syphilophobia
syphilopsychosis
syringobulbia
syringocele
syringocephalus
syringocoele
syringoencephalia
syringoencephalomyelia
syringohydromyelia
syringomelia
syringomeningocele
syringomyelia
   atrophica, s.
syringomyelitis
syringomyelocele
syringomyelus
syringopontia
syrinx
system
   association s.
   autonomic nervous s.
   brain cooling s.
   central nervous s.
   cerebrospinal s.
   Conolly's s.
   endocrine s.
   exteroceptive nervous s.
   exterofective s.
   extracorticospinal s.

system *(continued)*
   hypophysioportal s.
   interoceptive nervous s.
   interofective s.
   involuntary nervous s.
   kinesiodic s.
   labyrinthine s.
   limbic s.
   muscular s.
   nervous s.
   parasympathetic nervous s.
   peripheral nervous s.
   periventricular s.
   Pinel's s.
   pituitary portal s.
   proprioceptive nervous s.
   pyramidal s.
   reticular activating s.
   sensory storage s.
   somatic nervous s.
   stomatognathic s.
   sympathetic nervous s.
   vasomotor s.
   vegetative s.
   visceral nervous s.
systema
systematic desensitization
systematization
systematized delusion
systemic
   lupus erythematosus (SLE), s.
   sclerosis, s.
   vasculitis, s.
systremma
Szondi test

Additional entries

Additional entries

T

10-20 placement of electrodes
21-channel EEG
T tubules
TA-55 stapler
Taarnhoj nerve decompression
tabatiere anatomique
tabes
  cerebral t.
  diabetic t.
  dorsalis, t.
  ergotica, t.
  Freidreich's t.
  mesenterica, t.
  spinalis, t.
  vessel t.
tabescent
tabetic
  gait, t.
  mask, t.
  neurosyphilis, t.
tabic
tabid
tabification
tablature
table
taboo
taboparalysis
taboparesis
tabophobia
tabula (pl. tabulae)
tabulae (pl. of tabula)
tabun
Tac gel
TAC (Teller acuity cards)
TACE (tolerance, cut down, eye-opener)
  test for alcoholism
tache
  cerebrale, t.
  meningeale, t.
  motrice, t.
  spinale, t.
tachistoscope
tachyphagia

tachyphasia
tachyphrasia
tachyphrenia
tachypnea
tachypneic
tactile
  agnosia, t.
  anesthesia, t.
  defensiveness, t.
  discrimination, t.
  disk, t.
  elevations, t.
  hypesthesia, t.
  localization, t.
  meniscus, t.
  sensation, t.
  system, t.
tactilogical
taction
tactometer
tactor
tactual
Tactual Performance Test
tactus
  eruditus, t.
taedium
  vitae, t.
taenia (pl. taeniae)
  chorioidea, t.
  cinerea, t.
  fimbriae, t.
  fornicis, t.
  hippocampi, t.
  medullaris thalami optici, t.
  pontis, t.
  semicircularis corporis striati, t.
  tectae, t.
  thalami, t.
  violacea, t.
taeniae (pl. of taenia)
  acusticae, t.
  telarum, t.
taeniola

taeniophobia
tag
tagging
tailor's cramp
Takahashi forceps
Takata-Ara test
Takayasu's arteritis
Takayasu's disease
Takayasu's syndrome
take-down
talalgia
talantropia
talbutal
talipes hobble splint
talipomanus
talking therapy
Talma's disease
tandem gait
tandem walk
tangent screen
tangential
   speech, t.
tangentiality
Tangier disease
tangle
tangoreceptor
Tanner Developmental Scale
Tanner stage (I, II, etc.)
tantalum
   plate, t.
   sheet, t.
   wire, t.
tantrum
tanycyte
tap
   bloody t.
   front t.
   heel t.
   spinal t.
   spinal fluid t.
tapeinocephaly
tapeta (pl. of tapetum)
tapetochoroidal dystrophy
tapetum (pl. tapeta)
   corporis callosi, t.
   ventriculi, t.

taphephobia
taphophilia
Tapia's syndrome
tapir lip
tapotement
Taractan
tarantism
Tarasoff therapy
Tarasoff warning and liability contract
tardive
tardive
   dyskinesia, t.
tardy palsy
Tarlov cyst
tarsal tunnel syndrome
tarsalgia
tarsophalangeal reflex
tasikinesia
tastant
taste
   area, t.
   blindness, t.
   buds, t.
   cells, t.
TAT (Thematic Apperception Test)
tattoo
tattooed
tattooing
tautomer
tautomeral
taxon
Tay Sachs disease
Taylor back brace
Taylor pinwheel
Taylor retractor
Taylor scissors
Taylor splint
T-cell
TCI (transient cerebral ischemia)
TE (echo time)
tease
teasing
tectobulbar
tectocephaly
tectorial
tectospinal

tectum
TED (thromboembolic disease)
 stockings, T.
teenager
Tegaderm dressing
tegmen (pl. tegmina)
tegmenta (pl. of tegmentum)
tegmental
 pons, t.
 sign, t.
tegmentum (pl. tegmenta)
 hypothalamic t.
 mesencephalon, t. of
 pons, t. of
 rhombencephali, t.
 subthalamic t.
tegmina (pl. of tegmen)
Tegretol
teichopsia
teinodynia
tela (pl. telae)
 choroidea, t.
telae
telalgia
telangiectasia
teleceptive
teleceptor
Telectronic electrical stimulation
 apparatus
teledendrite
teledendron
telegraphic phrase
telekinesis
telekinetic
telemnemonic
telencephal
telencephalic
telencephalization
telencephalon
teleneurite
teleneuron
teleopsia
teleotherapeutics
telepathic
telepathist
telepathize

telepathy
telephone scatologia
telesthesia
teletactor
teletherapy
Teletrast
Telfa
Teller acuity cards (TAC)
teloglia
telolemma
telophragma
temazepam
temper
 tantrum, t.
temperament
temperamental
temperantia
temperature senses
temple
tempora
temporal
 arcade, t.
 arteritis, t.
 artery, t.
 epilepsy, t.
 facial nerve, t.
 gyrus, t.
 headache, t.
 hemianopia, t.
 horn, t.
 -limbic dysfunction, t.
 line, t.
 lobe, t.
 lobe seizure, t.
 lobe tumor, t.
 nerve, t.
 operculum, t.
 sulcus, t.
 summation, t.
temporalis
temporoauricular
temporofacial
temporofrontal
temporohyoid
temporomalar
temporomandibular

temporomandibular *(continued)*
   joint (TMJ), t.
   joint syndrome, t.
temporomaxillary
temporo-occipital
temporoparietal
temporopontile
temporopontine
temporospatial
temporosphenoid
temporozygomatic
tenacious
tenacity
tenalgia
   crepitans, t.
tendinitis
tendo Achillis
tendon
   reflex, t.
   spindle, t.
tendril
tenia
   choroidea, t.
   telae, t.
teniola
Tennessee Self-Concept Scale
tenodesis
   splint, t.
tenodynia
tenontomyotomy
tenoreceptor
tenotomy scissors
tenovaginotomy
TENS (transcutaneous electrical nerve
   stimulation)
TENS-Pac
TENS unit
tense
Tensilon test
tension
   headache, t.
tensor
tented
tenth cranial nerve
tenting
   skin, t. of

tenting *(continued)*
   sutures, t.
tentoria (pl. of tentorium)
tentorial
   notch, t.
tentorium (pl. tentoria)
   cerebelli, t.
   hypophysis, t. of
10-20 placement of electrodes
tephromalacia
tephromyelitis
tephrylometer
teratoma
teratophobia
terebinthinism
terebrant
terebration
teres
   major muscle, t.
   minor muscle, t.
tergal
terminal
   buttons, t.
   device, t.
   ganglia, t.
terminationes nervorum liberae
terpenism
terrain treatment
territorial
territoriality
terrified
terror
tertiary lues
tertiary syphilis
test
   letter, t.
   type, t.
tet spell
tetanic
   contraction, t.
   convulsion, t.
   spasm, t.
tetaniform
tetanigenous
tetanilla
tetanism

tetanization
tetanize
tetanode
tetanoid
   paraplegia, t.
tetanolysin
tetanometer
tetanomotor
tetanospasmin
tetanus
   anticus, t.
   artificial t.
   ascending t.
   cephalic t.
   cerebral t.
   chronic t.
   cryptogenic t.
   descending t.
   dorsalis, t.
   extensor t.
   hydrophobic t.
   idiopathic t.
   imitative t.
   infantum, t.
   lateralis, t.
   local t.
   neonatal t.
   neonatorum, t.
   paradoxicus, t.
   physiological t.
   postoperative t.
   puerperal t.
   toxic t.
tetany
   duration t.
   gastric t.
   hyperventilation t.
   latent t.
   neonatal t.
   newborn, t. of
   parathyroid t.
   parathyroprival t.
tetartanopia
tethered cord syndrome
tetraballism
tetrachromic

tetracyclic
tetrad
tetragonum lumbale
tetrahydrocannabinol (THC)
tetralogy
   Eisenmenger, t. of
   Fallot, t. of
tetranopsia
tetraparesis
tetraplegia
tetrapodisis
tetrodotoxin
Texas Scottish Rite Hospital (TSRH)
   Crosslink
TGA (transient global amnesia)
T-griseotomy
THA (transient hemisphere attack)
thalamectomy
thalamencephalic
thalamencephalon
thalami (pl. of thalamus)
thalamic
   syndrome, t.
thalamocele
thalamocoele
thalamocortical
thalamolenticular
thalamomamillary
thalamo-olivary tract
thalamotegmental
thalamotomy
thalamus (pl. thalami)
   dorsal t.
   optic t.
   ventralis, t.
thalassemia
   -sickle cell disease, t.
thalassomania
thalassophobia
thalidomide
   baby, t.
   syndrome, t.
thallium poisoning
thalposis
thalpotic
thanatomania

thanatophobia
Thane's method
THC (tetrahydrocannabinol)
theca (pl. thecae)
    medullare spinalis, t.
    vertebralis, t.
thecae (pl. of theca)
thecal
    puncture, t.
Theimich's lip sign
T-helper cell
Thematic Apperception Test (TAT)
thenar
    cleft, t.
    crease, t.
    eminence, t.
theomania
theophobia
theorize
theory
theque
therapeutic
    exercise, t.
    pessimism, t.
    recreation, t.
therapist
therapy
    aversion t.
    beam t.
    behavior t.
    carbon dioxide t.
    conditioning t.
    confrontation t.
    conjoint t.
    convulsive shock t.
    drug t.
    electric convulsive (ECT) t.
    electric shock (EST) t.
    electroconvulsive (ECT) t.
    electroshock (EST) t.
    family t.
    group t.
    Indoklon convulsive t.
    insulin coma (CCT) t.
    insulin shock (IST) t.
    irritation t.

therapy *(continued)*
    lithium t.
    Metrazol shock t.
    milieu t.
    Morita t.
    myofunctional t.
    narcosis t.
    occupational t.
    pharmacological convulsive t.
    physical t.
    play t.
    primal t.
    reflex t.
    sex t.
    shock t.
    short wave t.
    sleep t.
    speech t.
    spiritual t.
    stimulation t.
    suggestion t.
therapy field
therapy session
thermal
    anesthesia, t.
    hypesthesia, t.
    sense, t.
thermalgesia
thermalgia
thermanalgesia
thermanesthesia
thermesthesia
thermesthesiometer
thermhyperesthesia
thermhypesthesia
thermic
    sense, t.
    sign, t.
thermobiosis
thermogenic anhidrosis
thermohyperalgesia
thermohyperesthesia
thermohypesthesia
thermoinhibitor
thermomassage
thermoneurosis

thermophobia
Thermophore
thermopile
thermoplegia
Thermo-Pulse bed
thermoreceptor
thermoregulatory
thermoregulatory centers
thermostat theory
thermosystaltic
thermosystaltism
thermotonometer
thermotaxis
theta
    activity, t.
    frequency, t.
    rhythm, t.
    wave, t.
thiamine
Thiele syndrome
thigh
    driver's t.
    Heilbronner's t.
thigmesthesia
thigmotactic
thigmotaxis
thigmotropic
thigmotropism
thinking
    autistic t.
    dereistic t.
    disorganized t.
    referential t.
    tangential t.
thiopental sodium
thiothixene
third cranial nerve
third eye
third nerve palsy
third-person hallucinations
thirst
13q-deletion syndrome
thlipsencephalus
Thomas cervical collar
Thomas' sign
Thomas test

Thompson test
Thomsen's disease
thoracalgia
thoracic
    outlet syndrome, t.
    spine (T-spine), t.
    vertebra, t.
    vertebral body, t.
thoracispinal
thoracolumbar
thoracolumbosacral orthosis (TLSO)
thoracomyodynia
Thorazine
thought
    blocking, t.
    broadcasting, t.
    content, t.
    control, t.
    disorder, t.
    insertion, t.
    process, t.
    projection, t.
    transference, t.
    withdrawal, t.
threads of Golgi-Rezzonico
three-beat clonus
three-Hertz spike and slow waves
three-point head fixation device
three-step commands
threshold
    absolute t.
    achromatic t.
    auditory t.
    consciousness, t. of
    convulsant t.
    differential t.
    displacement t.
    double point t.
    flicker fusion t.
    neuron t.
    relational t.
    resolution t.
    sensitivity t.
    stimulus t.
    swallowing t.
    visual sensation, t. of

threshold value
Throckmorton's reflex
throe
thrombi (pl. of thrombus)
thrombin
thrombin-soaked Gelfoam
Thrombinar
thromboangiitis
    obliterans, t.
thrombocytopenic purpura (TP)
thromboembolic
    disease (TED), t.
    phenomenon, t.
thromboembolism
thromboendarterectomy
thrombolysis
thrombolytic
thrombosed
thrombosis
Thrombostat
thrombotic
    occlusion, t.
    thrombocytopenic purpura (TTP), t.
thrombus (pl. thrombi)
thrust
thumb
    pinch, t.
    sign, t.
    sucking, t.
thunderclap headache
Thymatron
thymectomize
thymectomy
thymergastic
thymic
    hyperplasia, t.
thymoleptic
thymoma
thymopathy
thymoprivic
thymus
thymusectomy
thyroactive
thyroid
    crisis, t.
    panel, t.

thyroid *(continued)*
    scan, t.
    -stimulating hormone (TSH), t.
    storm, t.
thyroidectomize
thyrointoxication
thyromegaly
thyroparathyroidectomy
thyroparathyroprivic
thyroprival
thyroprivia
thyrotherapy
thyrotoxic
    myopathy, t.
thyrotoxicosis
thyrotropin
thyroxine
TIA (transient ischemic attack)
tibialis sign
tic
    bowing t.
    convulsif, t.
    convulsive t.
    degenerative t.
    de Guinon, t.
    de pensee, t.
    de sommeil, t.
    diaphragmatic t.
    douloureux, t.
    facial t.
    gesticulatory t.
    laryngeal t.
    local t.
    mimic t.
    motor t.
    nondouloureux, t.
    progressive choreic t.
    respiratory t.
    rotatoire, t.
    rotatory t.
    saltatory t.
    spasmodic t.
tick
    bite, t.
    -borne encephalitis, t.
    -borne rickettsiosis, t.

tick *(continued)*
   paralysis, t.
tickle
tickling
TIE (transient ischemic episode)
Tiedemann's nerve
tigretier
tigroid
   substance, t.
tilmus
tilt vitals
tiltometer
time inventory
Tinel's sign
tingle
tingling
tinnitus
   aurium, t.
   clicking t.
   Leudet's t.
   nervous t.
   nonvibratory t.
   objective t.
   vibratory t.
tinnitus masker
tiqueur
tired housewife syndrome
tires
tissue cyst
tissue plasminogen activator (t-PA)
titanium
   plate, t.
titer
titillate
titillation
Titmus test
titrate
titration
titubant
titubation
   lingual t.
TLSO (thoracolumbosacral orthosis)
TM (transcendental meditation)
TMB (transient monocular blindness)
TMJ (temporomandibular joint)
TNF (tumor necrosis factor)

TNM (tumor, nodes, metastasis)
   staging, T.
to-and-fro tremor
Tobey-Ayer test
tocophobia
Todd's palsy
Todd's paralysis
Todd-Wells guide
toe
   clonus, t.
   drop, t.
   phenomenon, t.
   reflex, t.
   sign, t.
   walking, t.
toes downgoing
toes upgoing
togavirus
toilet seat neuropathy
token economy
Token Test of DeRenzi and Vignolo
Tolosa-Hunt syndrome
tomaculous neuropathy
tomogram
tomography
tomomania
tonaphasia
tone
   feeling t.
   muscle t.
   plastic t.
tone deafness
tone decay test
tongs
tongue
   -biting, t.
   deviation, t.
   protrusion, t.
   test, t.
   thrust, t.
   -tie, t.
tonic
   -clonic seizure, t.
   contraction, t.
   labyrinthine reflex, t.
   neck reflex, t.

tonic *(continued)*
    pupil, t.
    seizure, t.
    spasm, t.
    vibration reflex (TVR), t.
tonicity
tonicize
tonicoclonic
Tonnis clip
tonocionic
    movement, t.
    seizure, t.
    spasm, t.
tonophant
tonoscope
tonotopia
tonus
tooies (secobarbital)
Tooth's atrophy
Tooth's disease
Tooth's type
topagnosia
topagnosis
topalgia
topanesthesia
topectomy
topesthesia
tophophobia
Topinard's angle
Topinard's line
topoalgia
topoanesthesia
topodysesthesia
topognosis
topographagnosia
topography
toponarcosis
toponeurosis
topoparesthesia
topophobia
topothermesthesiometer
torcular Herophili
tori (pl. of torus)
Torkildsen operation
Torkildsen shunt
Torkildsen ventriculocisternostomy

torment
tormented
tormentor
Toronto splint
torpid
torpidity
torpor
torque
torqued
torr
torsed
torsion
    dystonia, t.
    spasm, t.
torsionometer
torsive
Torso-Graph
torticollar
torticollis
    congenital t.
    dermatogenic t.
    fixed t.
    hysteric t.
    intermittent t.
    labyrinthine t.
    mental t.
    myogenic t.
    neurogenic t.
    ocular t.
    reflex t.
    rheumatic t.
    rheumatoid t.
    spasmodic t.
    spurious t.
    symptomatic t.
tortipelvis
tortua facies
torture
tortured
toruli tactiles
torulin
toruloma
torus (pl. tori)
total parental alimentation (TPA)
total parental nutrition (TPN)
total spine precautions

touch
touchdown weightbearing
Tourette's disease
Tourette's syndrome
touretter
Tournay's sign
tourniquet paralysis
Tower fracture table
Tower spinal retractor
Towne projection
toxic
   psychosis, t.
   shock syndrome (TSS), t.
   tremor, t.
toxicity
toxicology screen
toxicomania
toxicophobia
toxiphrenia
toxin
Toxoplasma gondii
toxoplasmosis
TP (thrombocytopenic purpura)
TPA (total parental alimentation)
t-PA (tissue plasminogen activator)
TPI (treponema pallidum immobilization)
   test, T.
T-piece
TPN (total parenteral nutrition)
TR (repetition time)
trabecula (pl. trabeculae)
   cerebri, t.
   cinerea, t.
   cranii, t.
trabeculae (pl. of trabecula)
trabecular
trabs
   cerebri, t.
tracer
   dye, t.
trachelism
trachelismus
trachelocyllosis
trachelokyphosis
trachelomyitis
tracheostomy

tracheotomy
trachoma (pl. trachomata)
trachomata (pl. of trachoma)
trachyphonia
tracing
Tracium
tract
   ascending t.
   Bekhterev's t.
   bulbar t.
   bulboreticulospinal t.
   Burdach's t.
   central t.
   cerebellorubral t.
   cerebellorubrospinal t.
   cerebellospinal t.
   cerebellotegmental t's of bulb
   cerebellothalamic t.
   comma t. of Schultze
   conariohypophyseal t.
   cornucommissural t.
   corticobulbar t.
   corticocerebellar t.
   corticohypothalamic t.
   corticonuclear t.
   corticopontine t.
   corticorubral t.
   corticospinal t.
   Deiters' t.
   descending t.
   dorsolateral t.
   extracorticospinal t.
   extrapyramidal t.
   fastigiobulbar t.
   fiber t's of spinal cord
   Flechsig's t.
   Foville's t.
   Goll's t.
   Gowers' t.
   Helweg's t.
   hypothalamicohypophysial t.
   interomediolateral t.
   internuncial t.
   intersegmental t.
   Lissauer's t.
   Lowenthal's t.

tract *(continued)*
    mamillopeduncular t.
    mamillotegmental t.
    mamillothalamic t.
    Marchi's t.
    mesencephalic t. of trigeminal nerve
    Meynert's t.
    Monakow's t.
    motor t.
    neospinothalamic t.
    occipitopontine t.
    olfactory t.
    olivocerebellar t.
    olivocochlear t.
    olivospinal t.
    optic t.
    parietopontine t.
    peduncular t.
    Phillippe-Gombault, t. of
    pontoreticulospinal t.
    pyramidal t.
    reticulospinal t.
    rubroreticular t.
    rubrospinal t.
    Schultze's t.
    sensory t.
    septomarginal t.
    solitary t. of medulla oblongata
    spinal t. of
    trigeminal nerve t.
    spinocerebellar t.
    spinocervicothalamic t.
    spino-olivary t.
    spinoreticular t.
    spinotectal t.
    spinothalamic t.
    spiral t.
    Spitzka's t.
    Spitzka-Lissauer t.
    strionigral t.
    sulcomarginal t.
    supraopticohypophysial t.
    sympathetic t.
    tectobulbar t.
    tectocerebellar t.
    tectospinal t.

tract *(continued)*
    tegmental t.
    tegmentospinal t.
    temporopontine t.
    thalamo-occipital t.
    thalamo-olivary t.
    triangular t. of Philippe-Gombault
    trigeminothalamic t.
    tuberohypophysial t.
    tuberoinfundibular t.
    vestibulocerebellar t.
    vestibulospinal t.
    Vicq d'Azyr, t. of
tractotomy
tractus
trailing
    phenomenon, t.
Trail Making Test
train
trainable
training
trains
trait
    anxiety, t.
trance
    death t.
    induced t.
trancelike
tranquil
tranquility
tranquilize
tranquilizer
tranquilizing agent
transactional analysis (TA)
transaudient
transaxial
transbasal
transcalvarial
transcendental meditation (TM)
transcortical
transcranial
transcutaneous electrical nerve stimula-
    tion (TENS)
transducer
transdural
transection

transependymal
transfer board
transference
   neurosis, t.
transferring
transforation
transforator
transient
   cerebral ischemia, t.
   global amnesia (TGA), t.
   hemisphere attack (THA), t.
   ischemic attack (TIA), t.
   ischemic episode (TIE), t.
   monocular blindness (TMB), t.
   syncope, t.
   tic, t.
   waves, t.
transients
transisthmian
transitional
   vertebra t.
translabyrinthine labyrinthectomy
translocation
   Down's syndrome, t.
   mongolism, t.
translumbar
   aortogram, t.
   myelogram, t.
transmission
   duplex t.
   ephaptic t.
   neurochemical t.
   neurohumoral t.
   neuromuscular t.
   synaptic t.
transmitter
transorbital
   lobotomy, t.
transoval window exenteration
transpersonal therapy
transphysical science
transround window exenteration
transsexual
   surgery, t.
transsexualism
transsphenoidal

transtemporal
transtentorial
transthalamic
transversalis
transverse
   gyri, t.
   myelitis, t.
   myelopathy, t.
   process, t.
transversectomy
transversocostal
transversospinalis muscle
transversotomy
transversus
transvestic fetishism
transvestism
transvestite
Tranxene
trapeze bar
trapping of aneurysm
trauma
traumasthenia
traumatic
   amaurosis, t.
   amnesia, t.
   neuroma, t.
   psychosis, t.
   shock, t.
traumatism
traumatize
traumatogenic
traumatophilia
traumatosis
Trautmann's triangle
trazadone
Treacher-Collins syndrome
Treacher-Collins-Franceschetti syndrome
tremogram
tremograph
tremor
   action t.
   alcoholic t.
   alternating t.
   anxiety t.
   arsenic t.
   cerebellar t.

tremor *(continued)*
   coarse t.
   continuous t.
   darkness t.
   enhanced physiologic t.
   epileptoid t.
   essential t.
   familial t.
   fibrillary t.
   fine t.
   flapping t.
   forced t.
   hereditary essential t.
   heredofamilial t.
   Hunt's t.
   hysterical t.
   intention t.
   intermittent t.
   kinetic t.
   linguae, t.
   mercurialis, t.
   metallic t.
   motofacient t.
   muscular t.
   opiophagorum, t.
   parkinsonian t.
   passive t.
   persistent t.
   physiologic t.
   pill-rolling t.
   potatorum, t.
   Rendu's t.
   rest t.
   senile t.
   static t.
   striocerebellar t.
   tendinum, t.
   to-and-fro t.
   toxic t.
   trombone t. of tongue
   volitional t.
tremorgram
tremulous
tremulousness
Trendelenburg position
Trendelenburg syndrome

Trendelenburg test
trepan
trepanation
trephination
trephine
trephinement
trepidant
trepidatio
trepidation
   sign, t.
treponema pallidum immobilization (TPI)
treppe
TRH stimulation test
triad
triaditis
triakaidekaphobia
triangle
triangular nucleus of Schwalbe
Triavil
tribadism
tribasilar synostosis
triceps
   surae jerk, t.
Trichinella
trichinophobia
trichinosis
trichion
trichoanesthesia
trichoesthesia
trichoesthesiometer
trichographism
trichokryptomania
trichologia
trichomania
trichomegaly
trichophagia
trichophobia
trichopoliodystrophy
trichorrhexomania
trichotillomania
tricipital
triclofos sodium
Triclos
tricorn
tricyclic antidepressant
Tridione

trifacial
   neuralgia, t.
trigeminal
   cough, t.
   ganglion, t.
   nerve (cranial nerve IV), t.
   neuralgia, t.
   rhizotomy, t.
trigeminus
trigger
   action, t.
   finger, t.
   point, t.
   thumb, t.
   zone, t.
triggered
triggering
trigona (pl. of trigonum)
trigone
trigonocephaly
trigonum (pl. trigona)
   acustici, t.
   cerebrale, t.
   collaterale, t.
   habenulae, t.
   lemnisci, t.
   nervi hypoglossi, t.
   olfactorium, t.
Trilafon
trineural
trineuric
trioclofos sodium
triolism
trip (hallucinations)
tripped out
tripping
triparesis
triphasic waveforms
triple diapers
triple response
triplegia
triploidy
triplopia
tripod
   cane, t.
   position, t.

tripoding
Trippi-Wells tongs
triskaidekaphobia
trismic
trismus
trisomy
   C syndrome, t.
   D syndrome, t.
   E syndrome, t.
   G syndrome, t.
   8 syndrome, t.
   13 syndrome, t.
   13-14 syndrome, t.
   16-18 syndrome, t.
   18 syndrome, t.
   21 syndrome, t.
   22 syndrome, t.
tristimania
tritanomaly
tritanopia
trochlear nerve (cranial nerve IV)
trochocephaly
trombone tremor of tongue
Tromner's sign
tromomania
tromophonia
trophesy
trophic
   changes, t.
trophon
trophoneurosis
   disseminated t.
   facial t.
   muscular t.
trophoneurotic
tropical immersion foot
Trousseau's phenomenon
Trousseau's sign
Trousseau's spot
Trousseau's twitching
true aphasia
true vertigo
truncal
   asynergy, t.
   ataxia, t.
   test, t.

truncal *(continued)*
    vagotomy, t.
trunci (pl. of truncus)
truncus (pl. trunci)
    corporis callosi, t.
    lumbosacralis, t.
    sympathicus, t.
trunk
truth
    serum, t.
truthful
truthfulness
trypanosomiasis
tryptophan test
TSH (thyroid-stimulating hormone)
T-spine (thoracic spine)
TSRH (Texas Scottish Rite Hospital)
    Crosslink
TSS (toxic shock syndrome)
Tsuji laminaplasty
T-suppressor cell
TTP (thrombotic thrombocytopenic pur-
    pura)
tube feeding
tuber (pl. tubera)
    annulare, t.
    anterius hypothalami, t.
    cinereum, t.
    vermis, t.
tubera (pl. of tuber)
tubercle
    Babes t.
    Rolando, t. of
tubercula (pl. of tuberculum)
tubercular
tuberculoma
    en plaque, t.
tuberculosis
tuberculotic
tuberculous
tuberculum (pl. tubercula)
    sella, t.
tuberosity
tuberous sclerosis
tubocurarine chloride
tubular aneurysm

tubulization
tucked lid of Collier
Tuffier retractor
Tuffier-Raney retractor
Tuinal
tularemia
tulip probe
tumescence
tumescent
tumor
    bed, t.
    biopsy, t.
    dose, t.
    headache, t.
    histogenesis, t.
    infiltration, t.
    invasion, t.
    localization, t.
    mass, t.
    metastasis, t.
    necrosis, t.
    necrosis factor (TNF), t.
    registry, t.
    site, t.
    spread, t.
    staging, t.
tumult
tumultuous
tunica (pl. tunicae)
    muscularis, t.
tunicae (pl. of tunica)
tuning fork
tunnel
    disease, t.
    vision, t.
tunnelled
tunneller
tunnelling
Tuohy needle
turban tumor
Turck's bundle
Turck's column
Turck's degeneration
Turck's fasciculus
Turcot syndrome
Turek spreader

turmoil
turmschadel
turned a flap
Turner's sulcus
Turner's syndrome
turricephaly
Turyn's sign
tussive
> syncope, t.

TVR (tonic vibration reflex)
Tweed triangle
tween-brain
twelfth cranial nerve
21-channel EEG
twig
twilight anesthesia
twilight sleep
twilight state
twinge
Twining's line
Twisk forceps
Twisk needleholder
Twisk scissors
twist drill
twitch
twitched
twitching
> fascicular t.
> fibrillar t.
> Trousseau's t.

two-factor learning theory
two-point discrimination
two-point gait
two-poster cervical orthosis
two-step command
type
> amyostatic-kinetic t.
> asthenic t.
> Aztec t.
> bird's head t.
> buffalo t.
> Charcot-Marie t.
> Charcot-Marie-Tooth t.
> Dejerine t.

type *(continued)*
> Dejerine-Landouzy t.
> Duchenne's t.
> Duchenne-Aran t.
> Duchenne-Landouzy t.
> dysplastic t.
> Eichhorst's t.
> Erb-Zimmerlin t.
> Fazio-Londe t.
> Kalmuk t.
> Kretschmer t.
> Landouzy's t.
> Landouzy-Dejerine t.
> leg t.
> Leichtenstern's t.
> Levi-Lorain t.
> Leyden-Mobius t.
> Lorain t.
> Nothnagel's t.
> Putnam's t.
> Raymond's t. of apoplexy
> Remak's t.
> scapulohumeral t.
> Schultze's t.
> Simmerlin t.
> Strumpell's t.
> sympatheticotonic t.
> Tooth's t.
> Werdnig-Hoffman t.
> Wernicke-Hoffmann t.

typhlolexia
typhlology
typhlosis
typhus
tyramine
tyrannism
tyranny
tyrant
tyrosine
> tolerance test, t.

tyrosinemia
tyrosinosis
tyrotoxicosis
tyrotoxism

Additional entries

U

U fibers
UBC (University of British Columbia)
   brace
Uhthoff's sign
ulalgia
ulegyria
Ullman's line
Ullrich retractor
Ullrich-Feichtiger syndrome
Ullrich-Turner syndrome
ulna
ulnad
ulnar
   arch, u.
   drift, u.
   groove, u.
   nerve, u.
   palsy, u.
   reflex, u.
   tunnel syndrome, u.
ulnarward
ultradian
ultrasonics
ultrasonogram
ultrasonography
ultrasound
ultromotivity
ululation
UML-491
UMN (upper motor neuron)
unarousable
unbalanced
uncal
uncarthrosis
uncinate
   bundle of Russell, u.
   convolution, u.
   epilepsy, u.
   fasciculus, u.
   fit, u.
   gyrus, u.
   process, u.
unconditioned reflex

unconscious
unconsciousness
uncoordinated
uncotomy
uncovertebral
uncrossed pyramidal tract
uncus
   corporis, u.
underachiever
underhorn
undersocialized
undertoe
underwater treatment
undifferentiated
   schizophrenia, u.
undinism
undoing
unenhanced
unicornous
unifocal
Unilab Surgibone
unilateral
UNILINK system
unio mystica
unipolar
   depression, u.
   disorder, u.
unirritable
unisex
unisexual
universal cuff
University of British Columbia (UBC)
   brace
unmedullated
unmyelinated
   axon, u.
Unna boot
unorientation
unproductive mania
unrelated paraphasia
unresponsive
unrest
unroof

Unschuld's sign
unsegmented vertebral bar
unstriated
Unverricht's disease
Unverricht's myoclonic epilepsy
Unverricht's syndrome
Unverricht-Lundborg type epilepsy
up and down sheets
upbeat jerk nystagmus
upbiting rongeur
upgoing toes
Upper 7 head halter
upper motor neuron (UMN)
    disease, u.
    paralysis, u.
uptake
uraniscochasma
uraniscolalia
uraniscus

uranoplegia
uranoschisis
uranostaphyloplasty
uranostaphylorrhaphy
uranostaphyloschisis
ur-defense
urecholine supersensitivity test
uremia
uremic
    twitching, u.
urinary director appliance
urolagnia
urophilia
urophobia
using (taking drugs)
Utah arm
uveomeningitis
uvula
uvulopalatopharyngoplasty

Additional entries

V

vaccinia
VACTERL (vertebral, anal, cardiac, tracheal, esophageal, renal, limb) syndrome, V.
vadum
vagabondage
vagal
  attack, v.
  nerve (cranial nerve X), v.
  tone, v.
vagectomy
vagi (pl. of vagus)
vaginismus
vaginoplasty
vagoaccessorius
vagoaccessory syndrome
vagoglossopharyngeal
vagogram
vagolysis
vagolytic
vagomimetic
vagosplanchnic
vagosympathetic
vagotomy
vagotonia
vagotonic
vagotropic
vagotropism
vagovagal
vagrant
vagus (pl. vagi)
  nerve, v.
  pulse, v.
  reflex, v.
  stimulation, v.
vagusstoff
Valentin's corpuscles
valgus
valid
validity
Valium
vallecula
  cerebelli, v.

vallecula *(continued)*
  sylvii, v.
vallecular
Valleix's points
valley of cerebellum
Valli-Ritter law
vallis
valproic acid
Valsalva maneuver
valsalva'd
vampire
vampirism
van Bogaert encephalitis
van Bogaert sclerosing leukoencephalitis
van Buchem's syndrome
van der Hoeve's syndrome
van der Kolk's law
Van der Woude's syndrome
van Gehuchten's cells
van Gieson's stain
Vanzetti's sign
Vaquez's disease
variant
  psychomotor v.
  seizure v.
varicella-zoster virus
varices (pl. of varix)
varix (pl. varices)
varolian
vascular
  compromise, v.
  embarrassment, v.
  headache, v.
vasculomotor
vasculopathy
vasoactive
  amines, v.
vasoconstriction
vasoconstrictive
vasocorona
vasodepression
vasodepressor
  syncope, v.

vasodilation
vasodilator
vasoexcitor
vasogenic edema
vasoinhibitor
vasoinhibitory
vasomotor
    dysfunction, v.
    epilepsy, v.
    hypotonia, v.
    reflex, v.
    response, v.
    rhinitis, v.
    spasm, v.
    tumentia, v.
vasomotorial
vasomotoricity
vasomotorium
vasoneuropathy
vasoneurosis
vasoparesis
vasopressin
vasopressor
vasoreflex
vasosensory
vasospasm
vasospasmolytic
vasospastic
vasostimulant
vasovagal
    attack, v.
    syncope, v.
Vastamaki paralysis
vastus
VATER (vertebral defects, imperforate
    anus, tracheoesophageal fistula, ra-
    dial, ray, or renal defects)
    syndrome, V.
Vater's corpuscles
Vater-Pacini corpuscles
VD (venereal disease)
Vedder's sign
VEE (Venezuelan equine encephalomyeli-
    tis)
vegetate
vegetation

vegetative
    features, v.
    signs, v.
    state, v.
    symptoms, v.
vein of Galen
vela (pl. of velum)
velamenta cerebri
Veley head rest
vellus olivae
velocity
velum (pl. vela)
venereal disease (VD)
venereophobia
Venezuelan equine encephalitis (VEE)
venous
    aneurysm, v.
    hum, v.
    -sinus thrombosis, v.
venter (pl. ventres)
ventilate
ventilation
ventilator
    -dependent, v.
    support, v.
ventrad
ventral
    corticospinal tract, v.
    gray column, v.
    horn, v.
    lumbar nerve, v.
    pontine syndrome, v.
    reticulospinal tract, v.
    root, v.
    sacral nerve, v.
    spinal nerve root, v.
    spinocerebellar tract, v.
    spinothalamic tract, v.
    tegmental decussation, v.
    thalamus, v.
ventralis
ventralward
ventres (pl. of venter)
ventricle
    Arantius, v. of
    brain, v's of

ventricle *(continued)*
  cerebrum, v. of
  cord, v. of
  Duncan's v.
  fifth v.
  first v. of cerebrum
  fourth v. of cerebrum
  lateral v. of cerebrum
  myelon, v. of
  pineal v.
  second v. of cerebrum
  sixth v.
  Sylvius, v. of
  terminal v. of spinal cord
  third v. of cerebrum
  Verga's v.
  Vieussen's v.
ventricornu
ventricornual
ventricose
ventricular
  angiography, v.
  puncture, v.
ventriculi (pl. of ventriculus)
ventriculitis
ventriculoatrial
  shunt, v.
ventriculoatriostomy
ventriculocisternal
  shunt, v.
ventriculocisternostomy
ventriculocordectomy
ventriculogram
ventriculography
ventriculomegaly
ventriculometry
ventriculoperitoneal
  shunt, v.
ventriculopleural shunt
ventriculopuncture
ventriculoscope
ventriculoscopy
ventriculostium
ventriculostomy
ventriculosubarachnoid
ventriculotomy

ventriculovenous
  shunt, v.
ventriculus (pl. ventriculi)
  dexter cerebri, v.
  lateralis cerebri, v.
  quartus cerebri, v.
  sinister cerebri, v.
  terminalis medullae spinalis, v.
  tertius cerebri, v.
ventripyramid
ventroposterolateral (VPL)
  thalamic electrode, v.
VEP (visual evoked potential)
VER (visual evoked response)
Veraguth's folds
veratrin contracture
verbal
  preservation, v.
  tic, v.
verbalization
verbalize
verbigerate
verbigeration
verbomania
Verbrugghen retractor
Verbrugghen-Souttar craniotome
Verga's ventricle
vergence
vergence system
vermiphobia
vermis
  cerebelli, v.
vernal encephalitis
Vernet's rideau phenomenon
Vernet's syndrome
Verneuil's canals
Verneuil's neuroma
Vernier acuity
Vernier caliper
vernoestival encephalitis
Verse's disease
vertebra (pl. vertebrae)
  abdominal v.
  basilar v.
  caudal v.
  caudate v.

vertebra (pl. vertebrae) *(continued)*
   cervical v.
   coccygeal v.
   colli, v.
   cranial v.
   dentata, v.
   dorsal v.
   false v.
   lumbales, v.
   lumbar v.
   magnum, v.
   odontoid v.
   plana, v.
   prominens, v.
   prominent v.
   sacral v.
   sacrales, v.
   sternal v.
   terminal v.
   thoracales, v.
   thoracicae, v.
   transitional v.
   tricuspid v.
   true v.
vertebrae (pl. of vertebra)
   cervical v.
   coccygeal v.
   lumbar v.
   sacral v.
   thoracic v.
vertebral
   arch, v.
   artery, v.
   -basilar artery, v.
   body, v.
   body impactor, v.
   body spreader, v.
   canal, v.
   collapse, v.
   column, v.
   disk, v.
   disk space, v.
   foramen, v.
   groove, v.
   joint, v.
   nerve, v.

vertebral *(continued)*
   notch, v.
   pulp, v.
   ribs, v.
   space, v.
   spine, v.
   spreader, v.
vertebrarium
vertebrarterial
vertebrate
vertebrated
vertebrectomy
vertebroarterial
vertebrobasilar
   artery, v.
   tree, v.
vertebrochondral
vertebrocostal
vertebrofemoral
vertebrogenic
vertebroiliac
vertebromammary
vertebrosacral
vertebrosternal
vertex
   bony cranium, v. of
   cranii, v.
   cranii ossei, v.
vertex sharp waves
vertical gaze
verticality
verticomental
vertiginous
vertigo
   ab stomacho laeso, v.
   alternobaric v.
   angiopathic v.
   apoplectic v.
   arteriosclerotic v.
   auditory v.
   aural v.
   benign paroxysmal positional v.
   benign paroxysmal postural v.
   cardiac v.
   cardiovascular v.
   central v.

vertigo *(continued)*
  cerebral v.
  disabling positional v.
  encephalic v.
  endemic paralytic v.
  epidemic v.
  epileptic v.
  essential v.
  galvanic v.
  gastric v.
  height v.
  horizontal v.
  hysterical v.
  labyrinthine v.
  laryngeal v.
  lateral v.
  lithemic v.
  mechanical v.
  neurasthenic v.
  nocturnal v.
  objective v.
  ocular v.
  organic v.
  paralyzing v.
  peripheral v.
  pilot's v.
  positional v.
  postural v.
  pressure v.
  primary v.
  residual v.
  rider's v.
  rotary v.
  rotatory v.
  sham-movement v.
  special sense v.
  stomachal v.
  subjective v.
  systematic v.
  tenebric v.
  toxemic v.
  toxic v.
  vertical v.
  vestibular v.
  villous v.
  voltaic v.

vesania
vestibular
  nerve, v.
  neuronitis, v.
  nystagmus, v.
vestibule
vestibulocerebellum
vestibulocochlear nerve (cranial nerve
  VIII)
vestibulogenic
vestibulo-ocular
  reflex, v.
vestibulopathy
vestibulospinal
VF (visual field)
Vibram shoe
vibrate
vibratile
vibration
  disease, v.
  sense, v.
  tool syndrome, v.
vibrative
vibrator
  vaginal v.
  whole body v.
vibratory
  sense, v.
vibrometer
vibrotherapeutical
vicarious
  learning, v.
vicious
Vickers microsurgical instruments
Vicq d'Azyr's stripe
Vicq d'Azyr's tract
victim
victimization
vidian canal
vidian nerve
Vi-Drape
Vienna encephalitis
Vieussen's ansa
Vieussen's valve
Vieussen's ventricle
vigil

vigil *(continued)*
    coma v.
vigilambulism
vigilance
vigilant
Villaret's syndrome
villi (pl. of villus)
villus (pl. villi)
    arachnoid v.
vincula (pl. of vinculum)
vinculum (pl. vincula)
Vineland Social Maturity Scale
Vinke tongs
Vira-A
viraginity
Virchow's granulations
Virchow's psammoma
Virchow-Robin space
virile
virilescence
virilism
virility
virilization
visceral
    brain, v.
    skeleton, v.
visceralgia
viscerimotor
viscerocranium
visceromotor
    reflex, v.
visceroreceptor
viscerosensory
    reflex, v.
visceroskeleton
viscerosomatic
    reaction, v.
viscerotome
viscerotonia
viscerovisceral reaction
viscous thinking
visible
    light autokinesis, v.
visile
vision
visna

Vistec x-ray detectable sponge
visual
    acuity, v.
    agnosia, v.
    blurring, v.
    defect, v.
    dimming, v.
    evoked potential (VEP), v.
    evoked response (VER), v.
    field (VF), v.
    field cut, v.
    field defect, v.
    field deficit, v.
    field testing, v.
    function, v.
    graying, v.
    paranomia, v.
    plane, v.
    point, v.
    receptor, v.
visualization
visualize
Visulas Nd-YAG laser
visuoauditory
visuognosis
visuolexic
visuopsychic
visuosensory
visuospatial perception
vital center
Vital Ryder needleholder
Vitallium
vocal
    signs, v.
Vogt's cephalodactyly
Vogt's disease
Vogt's point
Vogt's syndrome
Vogt-Hueter point
Vogt-Koyanagi-Harada syndrome
Vogt-Spielmeyer disease
voiceprint
volar
volardorsal
volarly
volarward

volition
volitional
Volkman curette
Volkmann's contracture
Volkmann's paralysis
Volkmann's syndrome
volley
   antidromic v.
voltage suppression
voltaic vertigo
Voltolini's disease
volubility
voluble
voluntary
   activity, v.
   muscle, v.
volunteer words
voluntomotory
vomer
vomerine
vomerobasilar
von Economo's disease
von Economo's disorder

von Economo's encephalitis
von Graefe's sign
von Hippel disease
von Hippel-Lindau disease
von Lackum surcingle
von Recklinghausen's neurofibromatosis
von Willebrand factor
von Willebrand's knee
voodoo
   death, v.
voodooism
vorbeireden
voyeur
voyeurism
VPL (ventroposterolateral)
   thalamic electrode, V.
Vrolik's disease
vulnerability
vulnerable
Vulpian's atrophy
Vulpian-Heidenhain-Sherrington phenomenon

Additional entries

W

W4D (Worth four-dot test)
Waardenburg syndrome
WACH (wedge, adjustable, cushioned
  heel) shoe
Wada test
Waddell sign
waddling gait
Wagner corpuscles
Wagner skull resection
Wagoner cervical technique
WAIS-R (Wechsler Adult Intelligence
  Scale-Revised Form)
waiter's tip position
wake after sleep onset (WASO)
wakefulness
waking activity
waking state
Waldenstrom's primary macroglobulin-
  emia
walker
walking brace
walking cast
walking system
Wallenberg's syndrome
Waller's law
wallerian
  degeneration, w.
  law, w.
Wallhauser and Whitehead's method
Walter's bromide test
wandering mind
war neurosis
ward milieu
Ward-French needle
Ward-Romano syndrome
warming blanket
Wartenberg disease
Wartenberg pinwheel
Wartenberg sign
washout
WASO (wake after sleep onset)
wasping
wasting

wasting *(continued)*
  disease, w.
  palsy, w.
watch tick test
water on brain
water bed
water intoxication
water rigor
Waterhouse-Friderichsen syndrome
watershed infarct
watsonian psychology
Watson-Schwartz test
wave
  alpha w.
  beta w.
  brain w.
  delta w.
  electroencephalographic w.
  Erb's w.
  excitation w.
  plateau w.
  positive rolandic sharp w.
  random w.
  sharp w.
  slow w.
  sound w.
  spike w.
  stimulus w.
  theta w.
wave complex
wave discharges
waveform
waxy flexibility
Wayne laminectomy seat
Weber's law
Weber's paradox
Weber's paralysis
Weber's sign
Weber's syndrome
Weber test
Weber-Dubler syndrome
Weber-Fechner law
Wechsler Adult Intelligence Scale (WAIS)

Wechsler-Bellevue Intelligence Test
Wechsler Intelligence Scale for Children
   (WISC)
Wechsler Memory Scale
Weck clip
Weck-cel sponge
Wedensky facilitation
Wedensky's phenomenon
wedge
wedge, adjustable, cushioned heel
   (WACH) shoe
wedging of olisthetic vertebra
WEE (western equine encephalomyelitis)
Wegener's granulomatosis
Weichbrodt's reaction
Weichbrodt's test
Weichselbaum's diplococcus
Weigart's myelin sheath stain
Weigart's neuroglia fiber stain
weight-bearing
   axis, w.
weight-lifting syncope
Weil's stain
Weil's syndrome
Weil-Felix reaction
Weill-Marchesani syndrome
Weir Mitchell disease
Weir Mitchell treatment
Weiss' reflex
Weiss' sign
Weitlaner retractor
Welch-Allyn Audioscope
well leg raising
Welland's test
Wellbutrin
Werdnig-Hoffman disease
Werdnig-Hoffman paralysis
Werdnig-Hoffman type
Wernicke's aphasia
Wernicke's area
Wernicke's center
Wernicke's dementia
Wernicke's disease
Wernicke's encephalopathy
Wernicke's hemianopic pupillary phe-
   nomenon

Wernicke's reaction
Wernicke's sign
Wernicke's test
Wernicke-Hoffman type
Wernicke-Korsakoff syndrome
Wernicke-Mann hemiplegia
Wertheim clamp
West-Engstler's skull
West Nile encephalitis
West's lacunar skull
West's syndrome
Western Aphasia Battery
western equine encephalitis (WEE)
Westphal's phenomenon
Westphal's pupillary reflex
Westphal's sign
Westphal's zone
Westphal-Edinger nucleus
Westphal-Piltz phenomenon
Westphal-Piltz reflex
Westphal-Strumpell pseudosclerosis
wet brain
wet field cautery
Weyers' oligodactyly syndrome
wheal
wheelchair
wheelchair-bound
whiplash
   shake syndrome, w.
Whipple's disease
Whipple's triad
whirlpool
whistling face syndrome
whistling face-windmill vane hand syndrome
white
   atrophy, w.
   commissure of spinal cord, w.
   magic, w.
   matter, w.
   matter disease, w.
   noise, w.
white substance
   Schwann, w.s. of
Whitesides-Kelly cervical technique
Whitman frame

Whitman paralysis
whole-body irradiation
whole-brain irradiation
whorl
Whytt's disease
wicca
wide-angle glaucoma
wide-based gait
Widmark's test
Widowitz's sign
Wigraine
Wilbrand's prism test
Wilcoxon rank sum test
Wilde forceps
Wilde's cords
Wilder's law of initial value
Wilder's sign
Willett clamp
Willett forceps
Williams diskectomy
Williams microlumbar diskectomy
   retractor
Williams retractor
Williams syndrome
Williams-Meyerding retractor
Willis' circle
Willis' cords
Willis' paracusis
Wilson laminectomy frame
Wilson's disease
Wiltberger anterior cervical approach
Wiltberger fusion
Wiltberger spreader
Wiltse rods
Winckel's disease
windigo
window
wing
   sphenoid w.
wing-beating
winged scapula
winging of scapula
Winkelman's disease
winking
Winnicott theory
Winter spondylolisthesis

wired
Wirt test
Wisconsin Card-Sorting Test
witchcraft
withdrawal
   syndrome, w.
witigo
Wittenborn Psychiatric Rating Scale
   (WPRS)
witzelsucht
   primary affective w.
Wolf-Hirschhorn syndrome
Wolfram syndrome
Wood's lamp
Wood's sign
Woodcock-Johnson Psychoeducational
   Test Battery
woodcutter's encephalitis
Woodson elevator
Woodson spatula
word blindness
word debris
word retrieval
word salad
work and mental health
work inhibition
workaholic
working through
worried well
worry
Worth four-dot test (W4D)
Wound-Span Bridge II
WPRS (Wittenborn Psychiatric Rating
   Scale)
Wright's stain
Wright's syndrome
Wrisberg's nerve
wrist drop
wrist-flapping
wrist unit
writer's cramp
writhe
writing hand
writhing
wryneck
Wundt-Lamansky law

Additional entries

X

Xanax
xanthochromia
xanthochromic
xanthocyanopia
xanthocyanopsia
xanthogranulomatosis
xanthokyanopy
xanthoma
xanthomatosis
xanthomatous
xanthous albinism
xenon-133
xenophobia

xenophonia
xenorexia
xeroderma
xerodermic idiocy
xerodermoid
Xeroform gauze
xerophagia
X-linked trait
x-ray
    irradiation, s.
X-TEND-O knee flexer
xyrospasm
XXY syndrome

Additional entries

Y

YAG laser
Yasargil bayonet scissors
Yasargil raspatory
Yasargil retractor
Yasargil scoop
Yasargil technique
yellow vision
Yerke-Bridges test

yin-yang
yoga
yogism
yohimbine
yoked muscles
Young-Helmholtz theory
ytterbium DPTA
yttrium

Additional entries

Z

Zaglas' ligament
Zancolli procedure
Zarontin
Zaroxolyn
Zeek necrotizing angiitis
Zeiss operating microscope
zeitgeber
Zellweger's syndrome
zelotypia
Zerssen Adjective Check List
Zervas hypophysectomy kit
Ziehen test
Ziehen-Oppenheim disease
Ziemssen's motor points
zigzagged
Zim jar opener
Zimfoam head halter
Zimmer laminectomy frame
Zimmer Osteo-Stim
Zimmerlin's atrophy
Zimmerlin's type
zincalism
Zinn's corona
zipper pull
zonesthesia
zonula
    occludens, z.
    reticularis, z.
    spongiosa, z.
zonule of Zinn
zooerastia

zooerasty
zoolagnia
zoomania
zoonite
zoophile
zoophilia
zoophilism
zoophobia
zoopsia
zoosadism
zoster
Zostrix
Zuckerkandl's convolution
Zung Self-Rating Depression Scale
Zuntz's theory
Zydone
zygapophyseal
zygapophysis
zygia
zygion
zygoma
zygomatic
    arch, z.
zygomaticofacial
zygomaticofrontal
zygomaticomaxillary
zygomatico-orbital
zygomaticosphenoid
zygomaticotemporal
zygomaxillary
zygostyle

Additional entries